DOCTORS WITHOUT BORDERS

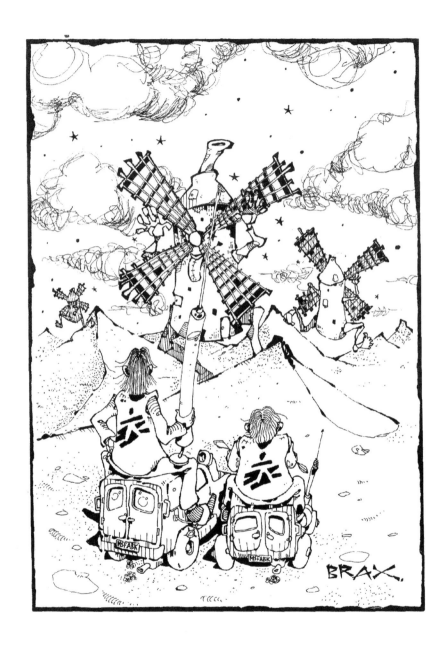

DOCTORS WITHOUT BORDERS

Humanitarian Quests, Impossible Dreams
of Médecins Sans Frontières

RENÉE C. FOX

Johns Hopkins University Press
Baltimore

Johns Hopkins University Press
2715 North Charles Street
Baltimore, Maryland 21218-4363
www.press.jhu.edu

Library of Congress Cataloging-in-Publication Data

Fox, Renée C. (Renée Claire), 1928– author.
  Doctors Without Borders : humanitarian quests, impossible dreams of Médecins
Sans Frontières / Renée C. Fox.
     p. ; cm.
  Includes bibliographical references and index.
  ISBN 978-1-4214-1354-9 (hbk. : alk. paper) — ISBN 1-4214-1354-X (hbk. : alk. paper)
  — ISBN 978-1-4214-1355-6 (electronic) — ISBN 1-4214-1355-8 (electronic)
  I. Title.
  [DNLM: 1. Médecins Sans Frontières (Association) 2. Voluntary Health Agencies.
  3. Epidemics—prevention & control. 4. Medical Missions, Official. 5. Relief Work.
  WA 1]
     RA651
     614.4—dc23   2013032122

A catalog record for this book is available from the British Library.

Frontispiece. Cartoon of Don Quixote and his squire Sancho Panza that appeared on the front of T-shirts worn by members of Doctors Without Borders / Médecins Sans Frontières at their 2005 "La Mancha" conference. Printed on the back of the shirts was the full text of the lyrics of "The Impossible Dream," the theme song of the Broadway musical *Man of La Mancha.* Cartoon reprinted with permission from Samuel Hanryon, a.k.a. "Brax," Rash Brax. Permission for use of lyrics from "The Impossible Dream" has been granted by Alan S. Honig.

Special discounts are available for bulk purchases of this book. For more information, please contact Special Sales at 410-516-6936 or specialsales@press.jhu.edu.

Johns Hopkins University Press uses environmentally friendly book materials, including recycled text paper that is composed of at least 30 percent post-consumer waste, whenever possible.

This book is dedicated to the women and men I have taught over the years, to their dreams, and to the fulfillment of their dreams

Contents

Doctors Without Borders

The Quests

An Introduction

This introduction, and the book to which it is a prelude, encompass two interrelated quests. One is the continuous quest of Doctors Without Borders to provide international medical humanitarian assistance in ways that perpetuate and constantly revitalize its founding principles and ethos. The other is my own quest, through prolonged sociological research, to understand, chronicle, and reflectively analyze its mission, work, and distinctive culture.

Doctors Without Borders/Médecins Sans Frontières (MSF) is an international medical humanitarian organization created by a small group of French doctors and journalists in 1971. Its mission is worldwide. As many as 27,000 MSF personnel, representing dozens of nationalities, provide medical assistance to people in more than sixty countries faced with "violence, neglect, or catastrophe, primarily due to armed conflict, epidemics, malnutrition, exclusion from health care, or natural disaster." The vast majority of these doctors, nurses, logistics experts, laboratory technicians, epidemiologists, mental health professionals, and administrators are members of the communities in crisis; only ten percent of them are drawn from the international staff. In addition to delivering medical care, MSF "reserves the right to speak out to bring attention to neglected crises, challenge inadequacies and abuses of the aid system, and to advocate for improved medical treatments and protocols." Because ninety percent of its funding comes from private, nongovernmental sources, MSF considers itself free to "act independently," without regard to "political, military, or religious agendas."[1]

MSF views itself not just as an international organization but as an "international movement." It is made up of several regional associations and of nineteen "associative" sections—in Australia, Austria, Belgium, Canada, Denmark, France, Germany, Greece, Holland, Hong Kong, Italy, Japan, Luxembourg, Norway, Spain, Sweden, Switzerland, the United Kingdom, and the United States.

In this book, I present a sociological portrait of MSF—of its principles, value commitments, culture, and field missions, and of the medical and moral challenges constantly raised by its humanitarian action. The inquiry from which the book incrementally developed began in 1993.[2] It grew out of my many years of immersion in Belgium, in the Democratic Republic of Congo (Zaïre; the former Belgian Congo), and in France, conducting sociological research centered on phenomena and questions associated with medicine.[3] I first became aware of the existence of MSF during the time that I spent in France and in Belgium, where it established its second section in 1980. There were a number of physicians in the offices of MSF Belgium and MSF France who knew me, or knew of me, chiefly from my extensive research in Belgium. The first MSF headquarters I visited was in Brussels in 1994, where I met with one such physician, Eric Goemaere, then executive director of MSF's Belgian section, who helped to launch me on my research inside MSF. Eight years later, in 2002, we met again, in Cape Town, South Africa. Goemaere had become the director of MSF's mission in South Africa, where he had created its program to provide antiretroviral therapy for persons with HIV/AIDS, which I had traveled to Cape Town to observe.[4]

My experience in the Democratic Republic of Congo played a significant role in my decision to undertake a sociological study of MSF. Africa, and the Congo in particular, which were professionally and personally important to me, were major loci of MSF's work. For a while I entertained the idea of returning to the Congo to conduct firsthand research where MSF had been present since 1981—a quixotic notion in light of the strife and terror, political instability, and social and medical "plagues" wracking that country.

The values that MSF espoused, and that its members pursued and concretized through their medical humanitarian action, drew me to them, and significantly influenced my decision to embark on a long-term study centered on field research. MSF's principles in action coincided with some of my own most basic and strongly felt values. As I have written elsewhere, I hoped that my research would bring me closer to some of "the most crucial social and moral issues associated with health, illness, and medicine: the relationship of disease and sickness to poverty, inequality, . . . and social injustice," and to the human suffering associated with them. "More than occasionally in the past, I had found myself questioning whether the topics to which I had devoted so much of my research and writing [had been] too remotely connected with these issues," and too detached from action to ameliorate them.[5]

I was strongly drawn to MSF as well by the simultaneously realistic and idealistic way in which its members saw "the world as it is"—a world in which there are "suffering and injustice, . . . sickness and premature death" and "natural disasters"—while energetically "refusing to let go of its vision of the world as it ought to be."[6]

The meaning that MSF had for me as a teacher also enhanced my motivation for undertaking research on it. For many of the young nurses and doctors and premedical students I was teaching, MSF exemplified global humanitarian medicine, in which they had a keen interest, and in the case of some, a desire to participate, at least for a while, in the course of their unfolding professional careers.

Clearly, it was impossible for a solo researcher to conduct a firsthand study of all of MSF's sections—its hundreds of projects, located at any one time in as many as seventy countries, and the thousands of people who worked with and for it in numerous different capacities. The decisions that I had to make about crafting and focusing the research so that it would be both feasible and sociologically meaningful were based on pragmatic, opportunistic, empirical, and analytical grounds.[7] In the end, I spent the most concentrated periods with MSF France and MSF Belgium, two of the most important operational sections of the organization. They formed the primary launching pads for the trips that I made to observe MSF in action in the field. During the years of my research I also spent time in the national offices of MSF Australia, Canada, Greece, Holland, Sweden, South Africa, the United Kingdom, and the United States. In addition, the international meetings of MSF that I was invited to attend allowed me to observe the interactions between its multiple sections as they grappled with a range of common questions and problems in a characteristically MSF way.

The three major contexts in which I did intensive field research were in Athens, Greece, Cape Town, South Africa, and Moscow, Russia. These journeys into the field enabled me to make "thickly descriptive"[8] studies of an array of MSF projects in different societal and cultural settings, showing the kinds of issues with which MSF has been confronted in the course of carrying out its humanitarian work. In MSF Greece, I saw firsthand an especially dramatic and crisis-ridden instance of the struggles inside of MSF that striving to live up to the "without borders," and the "independence from all political . . . powers" principles of its Charter have involved.[9]

My research benefited greatly from content analyses of the primary and secondary documents to which I was freely given access. These included communications between MSF staff members within the offices of its various headquarters, from headquarters to the field and from the field to headquarters, and transcripts of internal group discussions and meetings. This messaging was often accompanied by explanatory comments and expressions of opinion from the members of MSF who provided me with the documents. In addition, MSF's many websites were of inestimable value to my research, as chapter 1 demonstrates.

That virtually no restrictions were placed on my participant observation and interviewing or on the documentary material I was permitted to use was testimony to MSF's principles of "transparency" and "accountability." Another MSF principle, "proximity" (its commitment to members "being in the field," physically present with the people whom they assist), was manifest in the receptivity and responsiveness given to my field research. My research was also seen as consistent with MSF's view of itself as "a place of ideas," and with its conviction that "ideas matter for action." In the eyes of the MSFers I met, I was a "semi-outside person." I occupied an "insider-outsider" status, whose observations and interview conversations "fit" their organization's ethos. Some said their oral and written exchanges helped them understand what one long-standing member wittily referred to as "that mystery of nature called MSF," and their "adventures" and experiences within it. Others said my inquiry strengthened their relationship to "the challenges of the world."

However, my research was not free of difficulties. There were many times when it took me a long while to locate the MSF people I was looking for, or to obtain relevant data (which in some instances did not exist in any of MSF's offices).[10] MSF members were invariably willing to assist me. But some of the characteristics of MSF's social organization impeded my task. These included:

- The size to which it has grown over the course of its history
- The global scope of its action
- The complexity of its operations
- The geographical dispersion of its staff, their mobility, and their turnover
- The relative independence of each of its multiple sections
- Its decentralized overall structure and diffuse processes of governance and decision-making
- What some refer to as the latent "informal hierarchy" that exists within MSF, which helps to make it more functionally viable—but whose members and their influence are not always easy to identify
- The hiatuses and lapses in MSF's "institutional memory" that result from these organizational characteristics

Underlying MSF's structural features is its characteristic culture. I had to learn to navigate in it, and it became an important focus of my research. MSF is determined to live up to its collective self-definition as a movement. It seeks to fulfill its commitment to its basic principles and their implementation in action, in ways that replenish the charismatic spirit and the effervescence of its founding days. Yet it is equally determined not to succumb to romantically heroic, evangelical, or ideologically partisan notions of humanitarianism. Integral to MSF's resolute conception of itself is what it calls with some pride, its "culture of debate": the vigorous and often combative self-reflection and self-criticism in which it continually engages as part of its "constant quest to translate [its] principles into [more] effective assistance to people in need," and to "learn from [its] failures as well as successes."[11]

MSF members are mindful that over time, their organization has not only proliferated, but tended to become more formally structured, hierarchically ordered, and bureaucratic. These developments, which have accompanied its growth in personnel, finances, and matériel, as well as the expansion of its activities in range and complexity, are sociologically predictable. To some extent, they contribute to MSF's operational capacity to function efficiently, and are necessary for an organization of this magnitude to do so.[12] However, MSF is inclined to view these trends as problematic: one of the sets of "internal challenges" that it faces at this historical juncture, and as it "looks forward to [its] next decade."[13] Within MSF, such institutional thickening is regarded as antithetic to the value that it places on egalitarianism, participatory democracy, consensual decision-making, the spontaneous exchange of ideas, and effervescence—qualities that MSF associates with its conception of itself as a movement, rather than a formal institution that is "just an organization." Paradoxically, as various case studies in this book demonstrate, some of the steps that MSF has taken over the years to reform its structure have inadvertently added to the elaborateness and complexity of its organization. This has made it less comprehensible to many of its members—and to me as well.

"The efforts of humanitarian . . . workers are remarkable and noble," Craig Calhoun writes. "It takes nothing away from the significance of their labors to say, however, that they are fraught with tensions. Indeed, humanitarian workers are a highly self-critical group, constantly struggling with the contradictions of their work."[14]

As my research progressed, I became increasingly aware that what a member of MSF once called "the numerous dilemmas . . . of the humanitarian act" and "the permanent questioning [that they] engender" permeated the data I was gathering. I saw it in MSF's organization and personnel, its value commitments and culture, its modes of decision-making and operation, its forms of action and field experiences, and the critical events in its history. MSFers were highly aware of these dilemmas, and of the challenges associated with their practical difficulties and ethical complexities. In their office headquarters, in the field, and in most of their prolific meetings, MSF members struggled constantly with these issues—sometimes with angst, sometimes with self-deriding humor, and often with a mixture of both:

- How to be "global" and at the same time "multicultural."[15] This dilemma emanates from MSF's "without borders" vision and founding commitments. It calls for balancing and blending universalism with respect for particularistic differences within and between the many societies and cultures in which MSF works, and also between MSF's national sections and its multinational personnel. It throws into relief the essentially moral question of "whether or not it is feasible, intellectually and practically, to devise a more culturally grounded approach to providing assistance and protection to people in extremis . . . that is based on truly universal values—a sort of 'universal universalism'—rather than on the currently dominant Western universalism."[16]

- How to allocate MSF's commitments, personnel, and material resources in relationship to the world's natural and human-made disasters in a way that is faithful to MSF's principles of globally and impartially responding to "populations in danger." Intricate questions of priorities are involved, including: Where and when should MSF intervene? What actions should it undertake, and which reject? Should projects entailing long-term medical care be pursued, as well as those calling for shorter-term emergency care, and if so, to what extent? How long should MSF maintain particular projects, and when should it withdraw from them, transfer, or terminate them? Issues of triage also arise in this connection. A tension exists between the commitment to care for each patient individually, and to do what is the most beneficial for him or her, and the commitment to safeguarding and furthering the well-being of a community called for in the name of public health—sometimes in disregard of, or at the expense of categories or groups of individuals.
- How to address the sense of many MSF members that "we should, and we can do more and better," which seems to heighten the feelings they bring to such "allocation" questions.[17]
- How to think about and deal with the uncertainties and the paradoxes of humanitarian action—with the unintended negative consequences, and especially the harm that can result even from virtuously motivated, competent, and well-planned interventions.[18]
- How to cope with the finitude of humanitarian action—with its limited ability to change the economic, political, social, and cultural conditions that surround and underlie the forms of human suffering that it addresses. In a Sisyphean way, humanitarian workers must continue to do what they can for those whom they are trying to aid, while recognizing that no matter how hard and ardently they strive, they will never succeed in pushing the huge stone they are trying to budge to the top of the hill, and that in this sense and others their action is "an imperfect offering."[19]

Wrestling with the limits and limitations of humanitarian action also entails confronting its inherent risks. "As volunteers, members understand the risks and dangers of the missions they carry out," MSF's Charter states. While MSF is committed to assuming the risks of providing assistance to people in critical need, it attempts to curtail and manage them through the security rules and regulations that it asks its field workers to observe.[20] MSF personnel have been facing increased dangers of looting, kidnapping, violence, and even death. Such situations raise deeply troubling questions about the "balance between the individual's right to take risks in order to provide assistance" and MSF's right "to limit this risk"—about whether it is "legitimate" for a humanitarian organization like MSF to "refuse to engage in [such] risk," or to withdraw from the field because of it, and if so, under what circumstances with what consequences.[21]

This book begins on the ground—with the women and men of MSF in the field, engaged in the work that is MSF's raison d'être: "assisting people in danger" and in "distress," primarily by providing medical care. On MSF's "blogs from the field" website, they chronicle in moving detail what they experience as they give this care, and also how they feel and see things when they return from the field.

In Part II of the book, key events in MSF's early history and development are recounted and examined. These include its founding by a small group of French physicians and journalists; its connection with the 1967–1970 Nigerian Civil War, and with the International Red Cross in that context; its relationship to the ideological and political climate surrounding the French intelligentsia and student youth in the wake of World War II, and during the 1960s; and, in 1999, its receipt of the Nobel Prize for Peace. One of the most notable characteristics of these first decades of MSF's existence were the inner controversies and schisms with which it was fraught over its "without borders," transnational vision, and its precepts of "neutrality," "impartiality," and "independence." In addition, its conception of itself as a movement was challenged by its growth, its institutionalization, and its success in the world. Throughout this section of the book, MSF's "culture of debate" is pervasive.

Part III illumines the culture of debate and the self-scrutiny integral to it, through a firsthand account and analysis of MSF's 2005 "La Mancha" conference—a pivotal event in an organization-wide reassessment of MSF's operating framework in light of internal and external challenges. MSF's "permanent state of permanent questioning" and its inimitable self-mockery were on full display at this meeting.

Parts IV and V are situated in postapartheid South Africa and postsocialist Russia, two of the countries on two of the continents where MSF has been intensively involved in medical humanitarian action for prolonged periods of time. Based on my field research, we observe national and expatriate staff[22] in the impoverished black township Khayelitsha, Cape Town, and in the penal colonies of Siberia, as they struggle to deal with national epidemics of the infectious diseases that are the most common causes of death globally: HIV/ AIDS, tuberculosis, their synergistic coexistence, and their development into multi-drug-resistant forms. We also join MSFers in Moscow as they create means of medical and social assistance for the thousands of homeless adults and children on that city's streets.

The kinds of witnessing and advocacy in which MSF has engaged in South Africa and Russia are described in these sections of the book. How MSF interacted and dealt with government officials in this connection vividly illustrates the sense in which (in the words of MSF's Nobel Prize acceptance speech) "the humanitarian act is the most apolitical of all acts," with "the most profound of political implications"—implications and consequences that can be beneficial, harmful, or both.

In addition, chapter 9 takes us inside of MSF Africa, with its deeply African spirit and its committed universalistic outlook, as it strives to be granted equal status with the still-predominant western European sections of MSF.

The distinguishing features of MSF's culture and organization, the dilemmas intrinsic to humanitarian action with which it is recurrently and inextricably faced, and MSF's characteristic ways of thinking about and handling them, are saliently present throughout the book. They cross-cut and link its various chapters and sections. They appear prominently again in the final chapter of the book, at the meeting in Paris in 2011 where MSF celebrated its fortieth anniversary, and launched its newly established International General Assembly. That meeting also marked the final episode in my sociological questing, as a participant observer, to understand medical humanitarianism as exemplified by MSF.

I chose the title *Doctors Without Borders: Humanitarian Quests, Impossible Dreams of Médecins Sans Frontières* for this book because I feel that it captures the social and cultural essences of MSF, and the ambience in which it does its humanitarian work. Watching those qualities being dramaturgically played out at MSF's "La Mancha" conference had a lasting impact on me and deeply influenced my choice of this title. At that assemblage, convoked to critically examine MSF's principles, organization, governance, decision-making, and action, its participating members were clad in T-shirts designed to express the

Don Quixote motif of the meeting. On the front of the T-shirts was a cartoon image of Don Quixote and his squire Sancho Panza, who were wearing doublets imprinted with the MSF logo. Sitting astride tiny, dilapidated versions of the Land Rover vehicles that MSF uses on its field missions, they were driving toward eccentric-looking windmills in the near distance that were silhouetted against star-studded skies.[23] Printed on the back of these T-shirts was the full text of the lyrics of "The Impossible Dream," the theme song of the Broadway musical *Man of La Mancha (The Quest)*.[24]

PART I / Overture

CHAPTER ONE

Voices from the Field

A blog (a contraction of the term **web log**) is a discussion or
informational site published on the World Wide Web and consisting
of discrete entries ("posts") . . . Many blogs provide commentary on a
particular subject; others function as more personal online diaries . . .
A majority are interactive, allowing visitors to leave comments . . .
In that sense, blogging can be seen as a form of social networking.

WIKIPEDIA

Darfur is cursed. . . . It's either VERY hot, or VERY windy, or VERY wet or VERY
dry. What is VERY clear is that it's a tough and exacting place. It sings an ancient
song of sadness dusted with weather and socio-political storms alike. Few days
left here for me. I get to return home to [W]oolworth's foods, family and friends.
Here life will go on. A cruel and testing one. The sun will continue to strike and
the guns will continue to run. . . . And [Darfur] will be a periodic headline rearing
its head for the world to remember. We will remember Darfur but not do much
for it. It's hard to say goodbye. It feels like a fracture. You never quite heal back
the way you were. The collage of Darfurians I have encountered on this brief
jaunt will always make me smile. It will always make me know this place exists.
Not just that it exists but that it is. It is—in all its faces, misfortunes, poverty,
richness, complexity, fragility, forgottenness and austere beauty.

   With every goodbye comes the nausea of loss. . . . I feel like a stranger in the
place I have called home for the last 6 months. The petite dispensary, micro-
scopic world I have inhabited feels alien again to me just as it did when I arrived.
. . . I'm struggling to close this chapter. . . . [P]ost mission woe settles in . . . now.
I have to say goodbye to these companions and to the 4 expats I have had to

share every day every meal every thought and every hour with for the last 200 days. What stroke of luck I have to have a Kenyan lass, [and] German and Danish blokes come to be my friends. No trivial acquaintance, but a relationship based on a shared vision, strength, stories of melancholy, luxury, wounds and loads of giggles. So as I spend one of my last nights in the dispensary with a gunshot victim and [a] child with meningitis I know the boomerang is a sad game played in Darfur without game-over potential. I shed a tear for all of it and a smile for the beautiful bambinos.[1]

A South African physician wrote these reflections toward the end of her work with MSF in Serif Umra, a small town along the northwestern border of Darfur, in western Sudan. In this, her final entry in the series of blogs composed during her six-month-long mission there, posted on MSF's international logging platform, she lyrically expressed sentiments and themes found in many blogs written from the field by other MSFers.

We begin our entrance into MSF with voices like hers. As no words of an outside observer can, they take us deeply into the field and the kinds of situations in which the women and men of MSF medically assist the sick and the wounded, know joy, frustration, and sorrow in doing so, and are enlightened and enriched by what they discover about themselves, and by what they receive from those for whom they care.

These blogs not only chronicle in a journal-like way the inner as well as outer trajectories of MSFers' field experiences. They also introduce us to some of the attributes of MSF's ethos that are integral to its culture, and to the motivation, action, and solidarity of its members.

The History of the MSF Blogs and of the Responses to Them

In January 2006, Kenneth M. Tong, the manager of Online/Interactive Media in the Toronto office of MSF Canada, launched what came to be known as MSF's "field blogs." They grew out of the blogs that a member of MSF Canada who was in the field in Darfur, Sudan, at the time, was sending to her family and friends. Reading these messages, some members of MSF France, MSF Holland, and MSF Switzerland became alarmed because the blogger was writing from a politically sensitive area, and describing and relaying possibly controversial and dangerous details about the daily round of the MSF staff in that setting. The perturbed European colleagues asked Tong to stop her blogging.

Tong doubted that this was a good idea. In his view, such prohibitive action "usually pushed things underground, and resulted in less control and higher risk."[2] He proposed instead to set up an MSF platform for blogging, with parameters or guidelines for respecting patient confidentiality, politically sensitive content, and confidential management practices—like those associated with "human resources" (the recruitment, selection, and placement of field staff), or with some financial matters. The bloggers would submit what they wrote to be vetted either by their superiors in the field, such as a head of mission, or by a designated communications advisor overseeing that MSF project. The blogs would only be checked for violations of security and privacy concerns. Their contents would not be modified in any other way; and their language and style would not be altered. The intent was to preserve their personal nature and human feel, and their firsthand observations of MSF fieldwork.

"I saw this as an important way to allow the public to join our field workers on their journeys, in a more-or-less real time way," Tong wrote me.

> MSF previously had static "letters from the field"—Op Ed style entries from field workers, which were invariably singular letters from various contexts and one or two photos, but no continuity, and no interactivity. The Field Blogs were a way to use the new media to continue the journey, use multimedia (photos/videos/ audio) to illustrate stories and add texture, and allow for a dialogue with the field workers via the comments section of the blogging platform.[3]

The field blogs rapidly developed into sites that were more frequently visited than anything else on MSF's web—read by a multitude of persons who avidly followed these narrative field accounts and episodes, and who warmly responded to them. Readers thanked MSF authors for helping to "bring the reality of how people around the world live and die closer to home," and for the way their "beautiful writing captured [these] soulful experiences." They praised the bloggers for their "dedication," for being "out there setting the example of what it means to "live . . . authentically, and give to other people," and told how reading about their "painful, joyful, and ultimately hopeful experiences" had aided them in their lives. Among the responders were college, medical, and nursing students, and also graduate physicians and nurses interested in joining MSF. Primary school students wrote, too—like the sixth grader who asked what he could say in an upcoming presentation to make his classmates understand MSF. Parents said they hoped that they would be "fortunate enough" to raise a child "with as much character and compassion" as the bloggers. And fellow MSFers sent nostalgic greetings to colleagues blogging from a field site where they had worked on a previous mission—wishing them well, and telling them that they would continue to read their posts with great interest, as they came from a place "located in [their] hearts."

A Content Analysis of the MSF Blogs

According to the basic overall, but admittedly "limited and incomplete," data[4] about MSF's archived field blogs and their bloggers made available to me, the countries of origin of the bloggers and the so-called mission countries where they have worked span Africa, Asia, Europe, North America, and Oceania.[5] The largest number of bloggers come from Canada, and the second largest from the United Kingdom. The field sites from which the bloggers write are heavily concentrated in Africa, where MSF has sixty-four percent of its projects in approximately sixty countries. Among the bloggers, physicians and nurses predominate; but they also include a substantial number of logisticians (especially water and sanitation specialists) and non-physician anesthesiologists, some epidemiologists, and several psychologists who were mental health experts. The majority of bloggers appear to have been field or project coordinators. Because a designated person reads the entries before putting them on the web to make sure that nothing recorded in them poses a security threat, a commentary like the following rarely appears among the blogs:

> Two weeks ago in Niger, two French men were kidnapped and killed. One of the men worked for a medical NGO in Niger, and was scheduled to get married this week. The other had recently arrived from France to be the best man at the wedding. The kidnapping happened in a restaurant in the capital city, on the same block as the MSF office. The risks involved in our job have suddenly become more apparent. The kidnappers target the French in Niger, and so MSF has evacuated all of the French staff. The rest of us live with very tight security rules, especially as MSF is perceived as a French organization.
>
> In times like this, you examine the risks. . . . There are risks everywhere in life. The possibility of a Nigerian dying of malnutrition is much higher than the possibility of one of us being kidnapped and killed. So, as the security rules get

tighter for us and it seems like a liberty to go to the bathroom on my own, I wish there were also security rules for children like Bashir and Zara. Security rules to protect them from malnutrition and all of the other risks that come with being a child in a poor, underdeveloped country.[6]

What follows is my content analysis of the seventy-six sets of blogs on the MSF Field Blogs website that I located and accessed. These blogs were written over the course of a five- year period that extended from 2007 through 2011.

Why Blog?

Many of the bloggers begin their narratives with statements about why they decided to chronicle their experiences. They want to share them with their families and friends, they initially say—including the ostensibly "small things in daily life"—in a way that conveys both the "intensity of the moment" and the "longitudinal thread" that runs through these experiences. Blogging is a means of being "contemplative" about them, and about the personal changes veteran MSFers have told them they are likely to undergo. Blogging can also be a form of "witnessing," others state, which fulfills a basic MSF principle, by giving "human identities" and "human voices" to those MSF assists. In addition, "[I]f along the way I create awareness about the issues that inflict our world," a blogger writes, "if I propagate what MSF stands for," and receive logged responses back, "I will be grateful."[7] And some contend that blogging can provide "insurance" in the long term against what in MSF parlance is referred to as "new fridge syndrome":

> There is a joke that goes around MSF: You go off on your mission and you come home. You are sitting at the dinner table with your family and you want to tell them everything about your mission: the poverty, the diseases, the deaths, the happy things, the sadness. Eventually, someone will look at you blankly and say, "Hmmm that's wonderful. Did I tell you we got a new refrigerator?"
>
> Nothing like this happened to me when I got home. There was no "New Fridge Syndrome." I had the feeling that people had a pretty good idea of what it was like. I think it is because they have been reading my blog.[8]

Although they acknowledge these values of blogging, some consider it to be "dangerous" in dimensions other than security. They warn readers of "the traps" that writing them entails—including the stereotyping, "narrow pre-

sumptuousness," "cynical tendencies," and "odd lapse[s] into the superficial"
that might creep into the blogs:

> First of all, there is the danger of reinforcing stereotypes. . . . We immediately
> pull out our cameras when we see what we think is the "real Africa" or the "real"
> country X, Y or Z. . . . When we see the tribal woman on the donkey. The cute
> naked children playing in the dirt. The lone mango tree in the sunset. The kicker
> is that these stereotypes do originate from some grain of truth. . . . But they are
> partial and over-simplified truths. . . .
>
>   Another danger is always being negative, because, well, we are sent to war-
> torn, under-developed, desperately poor places. With, often enough, an epidemic
> of some sort thrown in for good measure. Sure, there are laughing children and
> a perseverance of spirit which serve to inspire. But these things often exist in
> somewhat of a depressing and hopeless context and stand out only because of
> their stark contrast with what is the norm. Even if that is not always the case, it
> is easy to feel that way when you are working long hours, drinking warm water
> all day, and have a multitude of insect bites. . . .
>
>   There is also the danger of superficiality. . . . [I]t is at times too tempting to
> skirt the more complex issues and incessantly lament about how hot it is here
> and how my sweaty forearms stick to my paperwork and smudge the ink.[9]

As the bloggers become immersed in all that their missions ask of them—
physically, emotionally, and morally—their writing and the responses to it
become a way of coping, and a source of support:

> I have written before that when I was at my worst, this helped me through. I am
> particularly grateful to MSF . . . for allowing this forum. . . .
>   I am humbled by the people who have taken the time to read this.[10]

This is likely the last post that I will write; my contract is about done and I am
going home. Thank you, in a gentle way, for reading and taking part in the dialogue, the ranting, the giddiness, the navel-gazing, the aching for clarity, the rage,
the amusing bits. This has become more personal than I expected; it's been an
important part of the mission, this chatter between a traveler and his shadow.[11]

Into the Field: "Why Am I Doing This?" "Why Do We Do It?"

During all these years I have thought of my inclination to do humanitarian work. Am I looking for an adrenaline rush? Travel or adventure? New experiences? Is it so I can test my inner strength? Or is it a quest for social justice that compels me? Do I want to be a witness? Do I want to make a sand-grain contribution towards collective wellbeing? Do I want to rattle my complacency by knowing what it is like to live in a place where your morning doesn't start with a latte and end with a martini?

It was during my interview with MSF, back in April, when the answer to my self-interrogation crystallized.[12]

Often, both at the inception of a mission and at its close, bloggers intently examine their own and their colleagues' reasons for going into the field to do medical humanitarian work. Their motives, they agree, are complex and mixed. Among them are idealism, altruism, moral indignation, a commitment to social justice, a sense of adventure, the desire to "escape an uncomfortable situation back home," or to "put the past behind" one, a search for self-fulfillment, a need to test one's self, and a "because we can" spirit of pragmatism:

Most MSFers I know joined for mostly very noble reasons: a desire to make a positive difference, to help their fellow human beings, and a feeling of outrage regarding the inherent injustice of this World. What is equally true, however, is that most of us are, in one way or another, adrenaline junkies. We like a different kind of adventure though, one that can take the shape of a vaccination campaign, an emergency response to a natural disaster or anything that involve[s] helping a lot of people, in a short period of time, in tricky situations. . . .

My reasons for doing this work are both altruistic and completely selfish. . . . [I believe] that there are things in this world that are simply unacceptable: people suffering and dying, mostly because they were unlucky enough to be born in places where there are no infrastructures, drugs, doctors, clean water, peace or justice. I'm one of the lucky ones who had everything one could wish for and—here's the selfish part—it wasn't enough for me. It didn't feel real, and I wasn't happy.[13]

Many bloggers testify about the transforming meaning their work with MSF has for them:

Why perhaps I have one of the best jobs in the world:

1. I spend most of my days treating countless ill but beautiful children who as they get better smile back at you. Nothing beats the joy of working with children and their families, with medicines that cure.
2. I spend my days with mothers and fathers of beautiful children who smile and laugh at my silly jokes during ward rounds. It is fun to laugh and even more fun to make others laugh.
3. I believe I enjoy the trust of my patients and their families—this is a sacred privilege anywhere in the world.
4. I have a team of MSF volunteers around me, who I would lie down in traffic for, and I believe they would for me. . . .
5. I live in one of the most beautiful places in the world, rural CAR [Central African Republic].
6. I make my own work schedule. . . . As long as the work gets done and done well, I'm free to plan my days.
7. I am mostly surrounded by dedicated national staff who want to learn, get better and work with MSF.
8. I have the privilege to work with a fragile population where . . . our medical interventions can . . . save a life and alleviate suffering. I can do with MSF what I believe most of us MSF'ers signed up to do.
9. I work for MSF who I believe will give me the tools I need to do my job. . . .
10. I work for an organization whose principles and actions inspire (and sometimes challenge) me.[14]

When I worked in Kenya, people would suffer due to the lack of basic things—drugs, equipment, medical items. MSF put a simple solution to this very basic problem in front of me. When you have all the necessary resources to use your skill, it is very gratifying. When you see a child with severe malnutrition, it is very disturbing; it's hard to look at the suffering brought about by lack of good food, where the child's system has actually started to break down its own body tissues. But with the right treatment, the change is incredible—when a child that seemed only a moment away from death smiles for the first time only two or three days after treatment started—when you see them running around a couple of weeks later—that's the motivation. Whether malnutrition or HIV, whether adult or child, the transformation that happens when the right course of treatment is given to someone that [*sic*] was on the verge of death is extremely rewarding, addictive even. I want to see it again and again.[15]

Angst, Anger, and the Limits of Care

Notwithstanding the affirmative ardor of such testimonies, the bloggers are united in their aversion to regarding themselves, or being regarded by others, as "heroic," impregnable, or empowered by their committed work with MSF to "make things better." They write emotionally, in detail, about their body- and soul-draining frustration, anguish, and anger in the face of the "horrifying" suffering and wounds, and all the deaths they witness that are caused, not only by illness and natural disasters, but by poverty, violence, injustice, the forced displacement of populations, and the brokenness of health care systems. The bloggers lament and inveigh against their limited ability to prevent and remedy these conditions:

Twisted swollen hands, the painful legacy of a failing healthcare system. My work here in the Northwest Frontier Province falls into that category. While there always remains the threat of violent conflict in our region, or the possibility of a natural disaster (such as the earthquake which devastated areas of Kashmir in 2005 . . .), the work I am doing here is not addressing any acute emergency. Rather, the team I work with is attempting to prop up or fill the gaps in a national health system that is struggling to meet the needs of the population. . . .

. . . a significant proportion of people suffer the burden of inadequate care.

We hear . . . this in the usually long and complicated stories our patients tell us about their ailments, and it is difficult to suppress the rising frustration and sadness at things being this way.

At the moment under our care is a woman essentially crippled by Rheumatoid Arthritis. Though this is a disease that is difficult to manage even under the best of circumstances, due to delays in her diagnosis and long and tragic gaps in her treatment, she is far more severely affected than she could have been had she received a consistent and appropriate level of care. Though she is only in her 40's, even the most simple movement is an agony. Her hands are twisted and virtually useless, and she requires full-time care from her family.

Talking with her, I am reminded how many others are carrying similar burdens and that we are reaching such a small proportion of those who could use our help.[16]

Since arriving in Farchana, gender roles, writ large in violence, have been one of the largest sources of curiosity, perplexity, frustration, anger, and rage. . . .

The night of Thursday 5 June 2008, seven Sudanese refugee women and girls were tied-up, beaten with whips and sticks, and publicly humiliated by a group of refugee men.

The event was heard and seen by many of the refugees in Farchana camp, some of whom reported the incident to MSF expats the following morning. . . . The beaten women, aged 13–30 years were accused of prostitution. The victims have been "fined"; some money and goods have been seized from them and their families; several have had their or their family's World Food Programme ration cards forcibly removed. The victims have been threatened with further violence if they do not pay the remainder of the fine. . . .

The women were all visibly seriously injured, including several suspected fractured arms. It is alleged that all the victims had their arms damaged or broken in order to prevent them from working for a time. . . .

"Acceptable reasons for beating your wife." This is a mini-list that was told to me by Sudanese women: (1) Refusing sexual relations with your husband, (2) Not doing what you're told, (3) Not doing domestic duties . . . , (4) Leaving home for a non-duty task, such as going to a ceremony without asking permission. . . . "Unacceptable reasons for beating your wife." (1) If you're drunk , (2) If you demand sex in an inappropriate place, . . . (3) If you hit "for no reason", and (4) if you hit her for leaving the house to carry out expected duties.

I am resisting the inclination to trip over superlatives in describing the extent of the suffering that is endured by women at the hands of a patriarchy that leaves them as objects, vessels, chattel, and reproductive systems.[17]

Ntabamhlope is one of my favorite clinics. . . .

Arriving today, though, feels different. I'm greeted by a tense nurse. "We're glad you're here." . . . Suddenly, I'm not glad to be here at all. My heart sinks a little as I'm led into the clinic room.

The patient is a young woman. She's emaciated, exhausted . . . I instinctively reach for her wrist, and find no radial pulse. . . . She's taking a short, shallow breath every second. . . .

The three of us work together. . . . We can't get a drip in and then we do.

Fluids. . . . Whatever intravenous antibiotics we can find. A flurry of activity and then, much, much too quickly, there's nothing else to be done. . . .

We need to transfer her to the provincial hospital, which is nearly ninety kilometers away on terrible, bone-shaking roads. We carry her to the land cruiser and lay her on a sheet in the back. . . . It's a long uncomfortable journey for me, watching my patient's chest rise and fall much too rapidly. Longer for her grandmother. Longer still for her. We take her to the female medical ward and transfer her onto a stained mattress. There's no oxygen. A hospital without oxygen. . . . We hand over to the nurses, and I leave hoping we've offered more to her family than false hope, and the burden of paying to have her body returned ninety bone-shaking kilometers back the way we came. . . .

. . . A couple of days have passed and I'm expecting to hear the worst, hoping to hear better. I go to the nurses' station and enquire after her by name. The nursing sister looks at me. "She just stopped breathing," she says. Just stopped breathing? JUST stopped breathing? Then grab some oxygen, a bag-valve-mask. She's twenty-six years old. Put out a crash call. Do something. But there's nothing to be done, and the nurse in front of me has seen this too many times.

"Does this happen in your country?" she asks. I'm shaking my head. The short answer is no. I could elaborate on this. Of course people die young. Of course people suffer. . . . But I'm talking to a woman who is nursing in a country [Zimbabwe] with one of the lowest life expectancies in the world. The whole world. So, essentially, the answer is no. No. It doesn't happen in my country.

I'm still shaking my head slightly when she turns away. "Does MSF have gloves?" she asks. "Please bring some gloves." How about piped oxygen. A defibrillator? An anesthetist? How about some justice? Gloves. Right. No problem.

Recently, I was talking with a friend at the office who had just returned from yet another family funeral. I'm so sorry. "It happens, Jessica, it happens, it happens. Jessica, it happens." Shaking his head gently with an acceptance that both awes and infuriates me. It happens. But not to everyone, not everywhere. Some people have a greater chance of dying young, or losing someone young, than others. It's the inequality that is the most painful. Life is hard, sure, but it's harder for some than others. Which, I guess, is why we are here. This world is crazy, mixed up. And in the crazy, mixed up world of MSF, the most obvious reason to leave becomes the biggest reason to stay.

We weren't able to save this woman's life. . . . But at least the event won't go unrecorded. At least it will be noted by someone other than the children she has left behind. On Monday, in a small town in southern Africa, a young woman who shouldn't have died, died. Her name was Gunya. This is all we can do. We prevent the suffering we can, and bear witness to the rest.[18]

For the first time since arriving, I felt tired in my bones last week. It's been three months here, and I have since mostly marveled, but. . . . I awoke one morning and felt hesitant about going into the camp and seeing patients. The crush of suffering was daunting, and I just wasn't sure if this would be the day I would lose my grit and have to go back to the compound, or dare the thought enter, just leave altogether. Worse still, the empathy buffer was too thin and I'd show frustration with my patients or colleagues. . . .

. . . Hope is an emotion that operates in accordance with the law of gases: it will expand to fit any container in which it is put. Last week I felt it to be thin, and I wondered selfishly and somewhat ashamedly, how I would survive in this rarefied environment. If hope is some ether of self-preservation mixed with motivation, it is icy clarity and rage that focuses it like a lens. This helps . . . to know in that vital way that things here need to get better.[19]

But as all the bloggers attest, they only gradually and painfully come to see that even their most strenuous efforts to "make things better" may fall short of what they hope to achieve; that their offerings are inevitably "imperfect"; that whatever salutary changes they introduce will come slowly—"one day at a time until [they] can do no more"; and that "some things might even have to be accepted."[20]

We can't do everything and we can't be everywhere. We don't pretend to solve the greater problem or to offer sustainable solutions.

. . . but, wherever we are, we do everything possible for each individual patient. For now that means that Molaw [a ten year-old child suffering from cancer and malnutrition] has a chance for a normal life: fewer headaches, clearer vision, and maybe even school. I had to hold back tears, though, when I realized that "everything possible" is likely not to be enough in the long run.[21]

The Meaning of the Children

Children are central figures in most of the blogs. Working with children is "uniquely hard," everyone says; and seeing a child die is the most devastating experience of all. The children "stay with you in a way that other patients don't." "They imprint themselves in your memory." They "walk [you] down the treacherous road of having [your] heart lacerated and unalterably tattooed."[22] Many of the blogs contain deeply emotional portraits of particular children:

> I've been wanting to write about this little girl since the day I met her. . . . This little girl is very special. She is, indeed, my very first "patient." . . . That she seems to have a very bad and rare form of tuberculosis is not what makes her special, nor that TB treatment is a minefield of adherence strategies, opportunistic diseases (i.e. it could be a consequence of being HIV positive) and fancy drug dosages. Her mother, that African Goddess of strength, begins to explain why she's so special. But really, it's just her: her apparent inherited strength, fighting through the severe malnutrition and swollen abdomen. Yes, but her eyes, how she looks at you, and how through her pain you can still see something incredibly human and dignified; uncanny in an eight-year-old, but especially in this little girl, [who] has everything stacked against her, except for her mother and a team of "crazy humanitarians" who want to give her every possible chance to thrive.
>
> Before I left for my break . . . I went to see her and say good-bye. I don't think she understood the words I was saying, but she did understand that I wanted her to get better and that I could hardly wait to see her progress when I got back. . . . She smiled at me for the first time. I beamed with pride and hope. . . .
>
> I think I haven't written about the little girl because it would make it somehow "final": she wouldn't be "ours" anymore, our little trooper, the embodiment of many things we believe in. . . . She would be "reduced" to this blog entry, and sink into oblivion if she did well, [and] become almost too painful if we lost her.[23]

> 1 kg baby born at our facility to a mom with an illness, which triggered the untimely arrival of simply nothing less than a fighter. She stayed alive for 10 days while I asked repeatedly the mom to hop upon the makeshift ambulance to the bigger health center south of us, and stayed alive while her mom refused to hop due to incalculable contingencies. Encumbrances, hardships, burdens, brutal realities. ALL SORROWFUL WORDS.[24] When premature "her" finally succumbed to the intraventricular hemorrhage she had an appointment with and I was present for her painful farewell, I ponder how I cannot feel responsible for not fighting more, for not plainly forcing her mom to go. How does she walk away bearing the blame and the denouement, and how do I walk away bearing culpability? No sun shining. No moon out to play. Darkness drowns us. I don't have the answer and I especially don't like the question. . . .

I grieve for the little one. I lament for the future [she] lost. . . . I miss her already. I pine to see her again, to see her believe in the future. . . . I guess she will never be sad, never be too late, . . . she'll never have someone see her when no one is there. . . . She is not anymore. They say the blind and seeing are equal but I guess the live and the departed are not.[25]

For the bloggers, these children are imperiled by illness, poverty, and the range of "natural and man-made disasters"[26] to which MSF is humanitarianly committed to respond. And they feel that the children were entrusted to them in a very special and urgent way. As their blogs powerfully indicate, MSFers not only experience the death of a child under their care as a terrible tragedy that fills them with grief, but also as a failure that is hard to forgive—one that confronts them with painful existential questions.

And yet, one of them writes, it is "the children who save you out here."[27] As they recover from a life-threatening illness—if they do—the emerging brightness in the children's faces, their smiles and laughter, help to restore their MSF caretakers' hope, and reassure them that their medical intervention matters:

The therapeutic feeding center is full to capacity this week and the phase 2 or recovery phase has been moved to the tented area near the end of town. . . . My weekly visits to this area are among some of my favorite moments . . . as this is where I see children who came through the ICU, who are now seated on woven mats with their mothers on the sand, some already smiling and playing with sticks or utensils, eagerly awaiting their supplementary food package. This is where I played with little Charifa this week, a 13 month old little girl with Down's syndrome whom I have become attached to, as she for some reason had been smiling already in the ICU while we tried to manage her heart failure. She is always smiling and very little seems threatening to her. Her mother has a very strong bond with her and is entirely oblivious to her special needs, yet fully aware of what a special child she is in every other way. This seems more important at this time in this context and has pushed Charifa to progress rapidly through the phases. She achieved her goal in weight at the end of the week and was discharged home. . . .

A memorable moment for me earlier this week was the discharge of a 4 year old girl in whom we placed a chest tube to drain an infection of her lungs. She came into hospital weighing 6 kilos and after 3 weeks of treatment for TB, she has made a rapid recovery. We were unable to approach her during rounds and she would scream incessantly when we examined her. She made absolutely no eye contact with anyone for weeks. The day of her discharge, she stood giggling, holding her package of therapeutic food and when I finally picked her up, she hugged me and clung to me for several minutes laughing and laughing. After many difficult moments over the last month, Amira's laughter, Charifa's smiles and the privilege of witnessing my patients' first smiles after weeks of illness as they show signs of recovery, has been significant in helping me remain positive in such an urgent environment.[28]

In addition, the bloggers describe the pleasure and amusement they experience in their encounters with the healthy children who crowd around them as they walk to and from work:

The kids are great. There are the ones that we see daily who live on the main route between our office and house—like the group of kids that used to run out to the road and demand to be picked up because one of us did once. That's the same compound where the kids started screaming "you! you! you!" . . .

Mostly kids like to shout "how are you". Today as we were moving by car through our neighborhood, we encountered two groups of kids, acting entirely independently, singing or chanting "how are you" over and over again.[29]

The "Gifts" of a Mission

[T]he project relationship like any other relationship has its "courtship" period. . . . You put on your best smile, look past the mosque waking you up at 4:00, or find some charm in it. Disregard the absence of electricity, find the use of [a] petrol lamp quite romantic and enjoy the absence of Internet as a nice break. In turn, . . . the staff all know your name, smile back, invite you to visit their department, answer all your silly questions. . . . [T]ea in the market; kids smiling and waving at you; women singing joyously in unison in the darkness of the evening.

So the honeymoon phase begins, and everything is perfect and lovely and how could anyone not want to be here now??? The work is fascinating and the team is great. You can now have in-depth conversations, you're getting to the heart of the context and you don't even hear the 4 am call to prayer anymore. Life is beautiful, in its own, twisted, humanitarian way.

If you're really lucky, that's when it happens. Simply, truly, deeply, you fall in love. Whatever hardship, obstacle or problem you will face past this point, you will get through it, you will work hard and as best you can to not only survive, but thrive against all odds.[30]

The MSF bloggers do not confine themselves to the problematic and the painful aspects of their "humanitarian life" in the field. They write with as much detail and emotion about their enjoyable and uplifting experiences— about the support that they receive from both their "expatriate" and "national" colleagues; the occasions of revelry and celebration; the symbolic gifts and the generous hospitality they receive from those they help; their pleasure in participating in cultures other than their own; and their wonder at the physical and human beauty of the landscapes enfolding their work:

> Today it started to snow.... There is a sense of magic in the air—there is no Santa ... but instead old men clustered together to keep themselves warm in their fur hats or turbans or little black caps, and long velvet blue tunics. I walk past the bread shop where a group of them play cards, a daily ritual not disrupted by the cold. Right then, in the morning mist and rising sun, the blue tunics, called "Joma," come alive. The old men, emerging from the mist, with their snowy white beards, look like magicians, as though they will be taken by the wind and turned to snow dust and I love it—a mystical illusion....
>
> So this will be Christmas, away from mum's freshly cooked roti and Indian curry. But our team is a cohesive one ... that resembles the family and loved one that I miss so dearly....
>
> The hospital is having a party on 26th January and there won't be any old man, but an overweight Santa played by our resident logistician, the great Tamas. It is exciting for the kids who I imagine will be happy for any distraction to their institutional lifestyle. The snow is now very thick, and it is beautiful, a sense of peace in this chaotic world. It is hard to hold back my not so dulcet tones singing in true NGO worker [style] John Lennon's "War is Over" as I crumble my snow boots into the dense snow.[31]

> [T]there is an opportunity to learn the ancient language of Tajik so I may eventually get to know this world and speak to the kids in the hospital.... The language sounds like a mix of [U]rdu and [M]andarin to me.... The alphabet is the beautiful Cyrillic alphabet which has shape and music to every letter.... They say the language is poetic and there is a lot of folktale and theatre here but until I have a basic foundation, the nuances of the language are just a dream.

The guards help me a lot here in the office. Our guard is Rasul and he is a tall man worthy of a Tajik medal. He offers me bread, an offering that one must never refuse, and patiently teaches me. I like his style: he smiles and teaches me with lots of repetitions. The basic greetings are to the gods and health, generally followed by a hand to the heart and a bow of the head (I love it).[32]

Something wonderful happened today.

Today was the first day I did Mungele alone. It is the more rural of the two Centres de Santé where I am working. . . . [T]he commute is beautiful.

This part of Maniema province [in the Democratic Republic of Congo] is hilly. The entire way, the road is lined with thick jungle. Every ten minutes or so a small village appears. People wave [and] shout (nicely!) along the way and we often have to slow down for goats or pigs or chickens in the road.

This morning we arrived to the waves and "Bonjour!s" [*sic*] of the staff. As usual, there was a patient waiting for me to see in the small observation room. . . .

I saw patients with the Consultants for the remainder of the morning. . . .

Then the cool thing happened.

The Chief of the largest clan in Mungele came for a call. We shook hands and sat down for a chat. Using an interpreter he thanks MSF and me for coming to his village. He said that the community felt our presence every day. They no longer had to worry about access to good medical care. . . .

And then he gave me the eggs. As a gift to welcome me, he handed me four chicken eggs, wrapped in a piece of cellophane, and tied with a string.

I felt very special today. On the ride back to Lubutu I waved to every person we passed. I arrived at Couvent and I told everyone my story. They agreed this whole Lubutu experience was very "chouette," very cool. Yes, the people here are lucky to have MSF, but we're lucky, too.[33]

On the evenings when meetings don't run over and patients don't arrive too late, I like to walk home from the office. It's a golden walk, with the sun low in the sky behind me and my lengthening shadow ahead.

After leaving the office compound on the main street of Gweru [in central Zimbabwe], the town quickly peters out. My path takes me through the police camp, where I greet the clutch of children who come out to greet me. Then behind the Anglican Church. Sometimes I have the pleasure of hearing the choir practicing and I stop dead to listen. Then my route takes me behind the provincial hospital. I cut through a field of maize and turn and I'm on red earth. Now my path runs alongside the railway track and I'm nearly home. . . .

Today, I'm thinking about a generous gift of avocados from a woman who probably didn't have food to spare. I'm thinking about the color of a stillborn baby's perfect feet and the shadow in the empty crook of her mother's arms. . . . I'm thinking about the pleasure of being chosen by a child. Taking the offered hand, returning the smile. And realizing suddenly that the tuberculosis medication is working and this little boy is miraculously, wonderfully, being restored to health and mischief.[34]

It feels that all that springs forth from this harsh land has been carved from the sky, sitting atop a flat and dusty soil, like miniatures on a piece of softly curving sandpaper: the adobe and straw walls that demarcate the small squares of land allotted to each Sudanese refugee family, the tents constructed by myriad NGOs to house food and supplies; the wood and plastic-sheeting structures that offer sitting areas and consultation rooms for the sick, the malnourished, and those seeking mental health or perinatal care; the concrete slabs that look like a heavy strip mall in the early stages of construction that serves as the school; the water pumps at which women in brightly-colored swaths of fabric move to and fro with pots and buckets balanced on the heads, small children in wobbly tow; the thatch-roofed tukuls in which we sleep; the wandering donkeys and occasional chicken; the thorny brush.

This morning the sky opened up as it has every day since I arrived; it is impossibly large, stark, and embracing. It defies us to enter into it, and we do, out of our camp, through the mango grove, over the dried up wadi . . . , through the small town of several stalls, and into Farchana camp, of about 22,000 Sudanese refugees from the Darfur region.[35]

The first [internally displaced persons] camp I visited was in an old school compound. Small dwellings resembling the forts I would build when I was a small boy. These huts were lined side-by-side; it was difficult to tell where one living space ended and the other began. It seemed impossible to guess how many people lived in each area. It was just a sea of sticks, plastic, grass and other modest building material. Hidden in between some areas were livestock such as cows, horses, donkeys, goats and dogs. Then I got a little lost in the maze. . . . There were a group of about ten children following me, making it more and more difficult for me to fade into the environment. I was embarrassed. One little boy held my hand

and told me an exciting story in Arabic (I had no idea what he said, but he spoke with a lot of expression). The adults would look at my scenario [*sic*] and laugh. With every dead end I encountered, I was greeted with a family who would say: "Fautall" (Sit and be welcome). The community I had originally thought of [as] having nothing was hosting me as a guest—offering me tea, beans and bread. . . . Perhaps stripping away the materialism of life gives people a sense of belonging and "self."[36]

Taking Stock

Preparing their end-of-mission reports for MSF, the bloggers take stock of what they have accomplished and what there is still left to do. They reflect on their relationships with patients and their families, with colleagues, staff, and local employees, and with the community, the culture, and the landscape of the region in which they have worked. They contemplate what it will be like to leave all this. And they examine their own state of being—what they are feeling, what they have learned in the field, and whether they have been significantly changed:

My six month mission with MSF in Pakistan is rapidly drawing to a close. My replacement . . . has arrived and I have the time to look back over what I have done here. Certainly I have not managed to get finished all the things I had (with unrestrained idealism) hoped for at the outset, but some small progress has been made. Some further links with the local community. Some treatment success stories. Perhaps even some lasting influence on the way medicine is practiced here in the Northwest Frontier Province. And if that is all, then it is enough for me. There is much more that still needs to be done, but it will be done by other hands than mine.

As the last few days wind down despite my tiredness and my readiness to move on, I am torn. There are things here with the power to make me want to stay: places, opportunities to use and share my knowledge and experience but most of all, people. I have had a chance to meet and work with—an incredible group of dedicated and talented people from Pakistan and from all around the world. . . .

Moving through town and at work, my brain records snippets of what is going on around me, filing them away. I see a small boy, running alongside the railway track: he is wearing a bright purple woolly hat against the morning chill. He turns

and smiles at me and I wonder: in this place where I have seen the tragic consequences of so much violence, when exactly that innocence will be lost? . . .

The images of patients stays with me: the wizened, gaunt face of a man on his
death bed, dwarfed by the size of his own white beard, his lungs severely scarred
by TB; the history in the eyes and hands of a woman with joint pain, who I am
unable to help in the way I would like. . . .

And other scenes from this other world that I have been a part of for a while
that refuse to be overlooked: heavily armed soldiers on guard duty outside the
fort with the sweeping panorama of the mountain rising above them in the distance; the menagerie of sheep and goats, cows and chickens, donkeys and buf-
falo, walking and grazing and toiling in the narrow streets; the sun setting to the
sound of the evening prayer as I walk on the roof. . . .

All these things will stay with me. For though I will soon leave Pakistan, it will
never leave me as I find myself profoundly changed by having been here.[37]

For every blogger, ending a mission, saying goodbye, and departing from
the field are painful experiences that bring a sense of "loss," and "require some
kind of mourning."[38] The most vivid and wrenching images that they carry
with them are of particular patients—most often of a child:

Remember Molaw? He was the boy with a cancerous growth I wrote about in
one of my first entries after arriving in Dubie [in the Democratic Republic of
Congo]. He came by the office yesterday to say goodbye.

He had made drawings of all the expats and was handing them out, clutching
the coloring book and crayons that [an] expat doctor had given him in the other
hand. . . . We were all holding back tears.

This is the hardest part for me. Of a closure. Of my job. Of the absolute
inequality in which I currently live. I get to go home in a few weeks to hot show-
ers, a big steak and a health care system that will care for me regardless of what
illness I have or how long it takes to treat it.[39]

Molaw will get drugs to manage his pain for a month. But while some of his
treatment is still available at the hospital, the Ministry of Health will install a
user fee putting this largely out of reach for an orphan living with his great aunt.
And that's it. He waves and then climbs into the landcruiser that takes him back
home.

Goodbye Molaw.[40]

so I was in the tb office today thinking about what I will leave behind.[41] as I was balancing the interspace, the one between here and there, then and now, one of the young tb patients walked in. she is about eight years old, and has been on treatment for two months. after the first meeting, I have not seen her parents. she comes every week on her own and always wears the same torn, overlarge black dress. she peeks around the corner, then bashfully slides into the room barefoot, and steps onto the scale. she answers my questions shyly, only with nods. when I finally place the foil packages in her hand,[42] she skips out of the room. I adore her. so brave.

when I saw her this time, for the last time, I had this overwhelming urge to give her everything. I didn't even know what everything was, I just wanted to give it.

and I knew then that I was thinking of things the wrong way. when the plane takes off and the abyei[43] ground falls from beneath my feet for good, the best things I will have left behind are not the ones that can be summarized on my end-of-mission report. they are the bright, beautiful parts of the day that can only be lived here. there are many. I will miss them.[44]

Several of the bloggers' departures from the field coincide with an organizational decision made by MSF that, partly as a consequence of their interventions, conditions had improved sufficiently to warrant turning their work over to local authorities and to the community. A project coordinator and as such, the official representative of MSF in the field, describes the community meeting he convoked to explain this decision to "the local health committees, Ministry of Health nurses from the health center, MSF community outreach workers, the village chief, traditional birth attendants, the local Red Cross, school principals, priests, [and] traditional healers" who were assembled. The "message" to them, he writes, "is a pretty tough one when I know that the level of care will drop":

That the Ministry of Health is present but not nearly as effective as MSF. That even a nominal user fee . . . will exclude a large proportion of the population. . . . That emergency referrals from the health center to the hospital will be by bicycle and will take half a day. That there will be more drug ruptures and the Ministry of Health staff will not be paid well or as often, or at all. . . . [And that] our closure [will have] a huge impact on the 92 national staff currently working in Dubie. . . . [M]ost will be out of work in a country where there really aren't very many jobs.[45]

The angst of bloggers leaving the field during such an MSF "handover" focuses on their patients—particularly on whether a little boy like Molaw or a little girl like the one in "the torn, overlarge black dress" will receive adequate and proper care.

Taking Leave

In the midst of all the busyness of report writing, debriefings, meetings, and farewell festivities that their last days in the field entail, the departing bloggers write thoughtful entries about what they will carry away with them—how their mission has changed them and their "perspective." Some of their reflections are infused with self-mockery; all of them are self-critical; and every one of them affirms that they received more from "the people around [them]"—especially from their patients—than they could have possibly given. In the blunt words of one blogger, "Anyone who thinks that they will give more than they will take from doing work with MSF . . . is off their rocker."[46]

The end of a mission means writing a report of what you did and what's left to do. But it's also a time when I do my own self-assessment, and . . . I find I've gained skills outside my job description. I can catch mice with an old-fashioned mouse trap (use peanuts); I'll use the radio alphabet when spelling my last name on the phone . . . ; the key to lighting a gas heater is to strike the match BEFORE turning on the gas; I can read Russian!

. . . I feel myself changed. I'm even more appreciative of small things (water pressure!), but perhaps I have less tolerance for BS. I've been given loads of opportunities to practice patience, and I'm getting better at it. I still believe in a better world, but I'm becoming more realistic about how to get there, and how long it may take.[47]

[T]hough I will soon leave Pakistan, it will never leave me as I find myself profoundly changed by having been here. Where I go in the world after this, whatever I do, I will carry these images, these snapshots of how life is in this other place. I will be forever grateful for the perspective I have gained, for the things I have learned, and I know that they will help me to be more appreciative of just how fortunate I am in life. Holding onto this, perhaps I can go on to take full advantage of the many opportunities I have with renewed vigor, in the sound knowledge that there are many who cannot even imagine such chances. A worthwhile goal, I think, and a responsibility I now accept with profound gratitude.[48]

As the days go by and my mission in Hebron reaches the end, images are passing through my mind. . . .

One of the most powerful moments that deeply touched me was a teenager girl's wish to conduct [a] session on the ruins of what used to be her house a few days ago. We tried to find a safe "seat" on the cement. [S]he showed me where her room used to be, the living room, the kitchen. She was looking at the ruins as if her room was still standing there. I could almost see the house in her eyes. . . .

Living in Palestine and working with the local people, has urged me [*sic*] to think several times about my relationship with the material aspect of things, with the idea of belongings. How much they mean in my life, how much the idea of happiness and fulfillment are connected with what I have, what I own.

This challenge came to my mind today after visiting a family of seven who suddenly, one morning at 6:00 . . . saw bulldozers coming and demolishing their house within minutes and without allowing them to take anything from inside. Now they live under a tent and on the open roof of a neighbor's house. . . . Their only belongings now are some old mattresses to sleep under the stars, and basic clothes for the kids. . . .

After my visit to this family today I felt that I owe to [*sic*] re-arrange my priorities in life, what really matters and what is just for show off. For some people having a roof above their head or running water is a luxury. For me [it] is a de facto that I need to appreciate more in order to understand better my patients when they are trying to adapt to a tough reality, and also to make my life more meaningful.[49]

This is likely the last post I will write; my contract is almost done and I am going home. . . .

It would be fair to say that before coming to Chad, in the months leading up to this mission, I was expecting something alien. Conditions and life-ways so extreme and dimensionally different from mine that I would struggle to connect with them. In anthropological parlance, I *exoticized the other*. . . .

I thought that *foreign and different* would be more bizarre than *local and different*. . . . And here's what I have come up with: living in Farchana is not so dimensionally different that you can't hit the ground running; I focused on the victimization and unrest and did not project how suffering would become knowledge, strength, and a tighter sense of community than I have ever seen. In what I could only call an honest act of remarkable conceit, I thought that psychiatric training could help me through this. Only insofar as any formal education informs and buttresses one's actionable humanity will it be useful. Pragmatism is primary. The lessons learned have to some extent cleaned off the post-modern/ neurotic shelf . . . sure, the thoughts still spin, but they end with the usual question: now what would be useful?

OK, I have to qualify this. (So much for being less neurotic.) Many things ARE exotic in a way, but so are things back home. Even professionally, the mysterious is ever-present. . . . Some things should have seemed odd for years, but needed to be made contrast with [*sic*] the Farchana sky to become visible. . . .

The light of this computer screen attracts bugs. The rains have come and the air is swarming with insects of all shapes and sizes. Too much![50]

At the end of their last entries, several bloggers feel impelled to speak directly to their readers, exhorting them to savor their lives, and try to fill them with meaning:

And finally, whoever and wherever you may be, take time to appreciate the good things, the special things that you have in your life. If the last six months have taught me anything, it is that to be here (in this life) is an amazing opportunity. [D]on't waste it![51]

I realize that some of the people who are reading this are considering doing a similar thing, either with MSF, or in another way. of course, not everyone needs to practice medical humanitarianism. you simply have to use what you know to effect the change in the world you most want to see. I do not consider [it] a moral overstatement to say that because each of us has a role in making the world, we must take some responsibility for what it is. accept it or change it. . . . live like you have been granted your deathbed wish to do it all over again.[52]

From the Field to "Something Called Home"

I spend my last evening in the field quietly. . . . The next day I am up far too early for my liking. It is cold and all I want to do is stay in bed, but my transport to the capital [Islamabad] is leaving. I say goodbye to my expat team (my family away

from home) and suddenly, after weeks of being ready, I no longer want to leave.
. . .

The distinctive smell of 4am greets my nose as the driver and I shift through the deserted streets on the way to the airport. Silent for most of the way he eventually turns to me and asks: "Is your mission complete?" and despite some reports to finish, despite the never-ending work that I leave behind, I am able to say "Yes." I have done what I came here to do.

We go though one last security check-point on the road: one last slalom between concrete barriers; one last pass in the firing line of the machine-gunner in his sand-bagged bunker; and I am reminded that I have just spent six months in Pakistan and it is the end of what has been a long and difficult year for that country and myself.

The firm fleshy hand of the driver is my final farewell and then, I am gone.[53]

"I am gone." This poignant phrase contains intimations of the writer's feeling that with this departing journey he has entered into a state of limbo, suspended in the "space" between the field, and what another blogger describes as "something that resembles something I used to call home":[54]

I have been home for five weeks. . . . I have spent a lot of time staring at my bedroom ceiling. A good friend told me that it's probably normal and to keep doing it as long as I feel like it, and that eventually I will want to get up and paint the ceiling . . . that hasn't really happened yet.

But I went back to work anyway. I thought it would be better for me to be distracted, to focus on patients and families. I have worked five shifts now in a "developed world" hospital that never runs out of gloves or clean needles or medicine and there is always a doctor there when you need one. There is running water and electricity. Nobody has cholera or measles. It feels very strange. In all honesty I am not really sure what to do with myself.

I keep describing the experience of coming home to people by saying that it feels as if I have been abducted by aliens and dropped on another planet that is vaguely familiar. Vaguely.

People I barely know ask me some pretty personal questions without even realizing it. What was the hardest thing for me? How did it change me as a person? I'm not even sure I can answer any of that for myself. My family is upset because I am not talking about "it," but I don't know what to say. How do you explain an entire year of your life? How do you explain life in another universe?

I miss Kilwa. I miss Congo. I miss my friends, my family in a land far, far away. I am happy to be here now, in Toronto, but I am just not sure I am home yet.[55]

When they return from the field, most people who do medical humanitarian work experience "a rupture"—"an irreconcilable invisible distance between us and others. We talk about how difficult it is to assimilate, to assume routine, to sample familiar pleasures":

> The rift, of course, is not in the world [James Maskalyk writes]: it is within us. And the distance is not only ours. We return from the field, from an Ebola outbreak or violent clashes in Sudan, with no mistake about how the world is. It is a hard place—a beautiful place, but so too an urgent one. And we realize that all of us, through our actions or inactions, make it what it is. . . .
>
> Just as our friends wonder at our distance from their familiar world, we marvel at theirs from the real one. We feel inhabited by it. We plan our return.[56]

Envoi

This book started as a blog that I wrote from my hut in Sudan. It was my attempt to communicate with my family and friends, to help bring them closer to my hot, hot days. It was also a chance to tell the story of Abyei, Sudan, a torn, tiny place straddling a contested border in a difficult country. Mostly, though, it was where I told a story about humans: the people from Abyei who suffered its hardships because it was their home, and those of us who left ours with tools to make it easier for them to endure. It is a story that could be told about many places.

JAMES MASKALYK, *SIX MONTHS IN SUDAN:*
A YOUNG DOCTOR IN A WAR-TORN VILLAGE

In their blogs, MSFers recount many such "stories" about their missions and experiences in the field. Especially notable and sociologically significant is how much these blogs have in common—the recurrent patterns and themes. What makes them so moving is the soul-deep nature of their contents. What makes them "so MSF" is the latent concern present in some of the blogs about the danger of exaggerating how much one's life has been changed by a humanitarian field mission. Why and how doing so violates fundamental MSF values is made eloquently explicit in the following testimony:

Sitting at lunch the other day, a colleague was lamenting the fact that she had yet to participate in an MSF field mission. Based for some years in Brussels, the well-known, if vicious circle of "no prior field experience—no chance of an MSF mission" had crystallized for her into nothing short of an existential crisis. "In my department," she explained, "we need first-hand experience of MSF fieldwork if we are to speak with any legitimacy about the movement." . . .

It was her conviction that an MSF mission would affect her values and perceptions to such a degree that life back in Belgium—relations with friends, lovers, family—might be jeopardized. The prospect of field experience meant embarking on a profound personal transformation at the risk of never seeing things, perhaps even loved ones, the same way again. Her dilemma struck me as typically MSF insofar as it captures the competing sense of solidarity we feel between our commitments at home and the call of conscience triggered by the distant suffering of unfamiliar voices. For those of us who have worked in the field, it is true, the experience infinitely broadens our horizons while it humbles us at the same time. It "changes our life," just as it may shatter us completely—we see peaks and valleys of humanity we never knew existed, and perhaps are not able to bear. What we experience in the field may affect us profoundly, overwhelming our ability to communicate our feelings to those at home. . . . Whatever happens in the field, rare is the individual whose worldview remains unchallenged by an MSF mission.

As common as these feelings and dilemmas are within MSF, this should not legitimate them or exonerate them from critical scrutiny. At bottom, they seem to revolve around a common assumption; namely, that there is a categorical difference between the life I lead "here," and the one I experience in the field. This may seem an innocent and fundamentally accurate way to conceive of the cultural threshold we cross via this strange and wonderful bridge that is international humanitarianism. Certainly the culture shock we experience when moving between field missions and headquarters appears to support this view. Yet the metaphors we employ to explain our experiences are never innocent; they often harbor unquestioned assumptions and deep-rooted prejudices operating underneath the stuff of experience. . . .

If we allow ourselves to see our humanitarian experience as occurring between "two worlds," of seeing crisis situations as involving a difference of essence and not merely of degree vis-à-vis our culture of origin, we fall prey to the romanticization characteristic of colonialism. . . . Each of us is drawn to the challenge of improving the human condition, but the adventure of MSF field experience should not be interpreted as an "initiation" into some higher, more profound form of understanding the human condition. To romanticize it in this way is to mystify the humanitarian experience: to pretend that some fundamental transformation takes place in our way of seeing the world(s) is in effect to exploit the plight of the people we aim to assist as an opportunity for our own personal development. The fantasy of MSF field experience as a "rite of passage" onto some higher plane of human understanding is replete with narcissism—even more repulsive because this so-called initiation is parasitic on the "host" of the suffering we seek to eradicate. . . . In short, there is absolutely nothing "otherworldly" about humanitarian experience in the field: to assume so is to posit an artificial difference in kind between "us" and "them."[57]

PART II / Growing Pains

CHAPTER TWO

Origins, Schisms, Crises

The roots of Médecins Sans Frontières/Doctors Without Borders extend back to the passionate debates of left-wing French intellectuals after World War II, and to the moral anguish and indignation of young physicians from that milieu serving with the International Red Cross during the Nigerian civil war of the late 1960s.

Following the liberation of France in 1944 from its occupation by Nazi Germany, "for a period of about twelve years . . . the issue of communism—its practice, its meaning, its claims upon the future—dominated political and philosophical conversation" among the French intelligentsia, the historian Tony Judt writes:

> The terms of public discussion were shaped by the position one adopted on the behavior of foreign and domestic Communists, and most of the problems of contemporary France were analyzed in terms of a political or ethical position taken with half an eye towards that of Communists and their ideology. . . . The Vichy interlude had served to delegitimize the intellectuals of the Right . . . , while the experience of war and resistance had radicalized the language, if not the practices, of the Left.[1]

"The prestige of the Soviet Union and the French Communist Party was enormous among the French intelligentsia, who were attracted both by the rationalist element in Marxism—the vision of progress and the explanation of history—and by its appeal to faith—the triumph of the oppressed," the polymath social scientist Stanley Hoffmann has commented.[2]

In the mid-1950s, two sets of events precipitated a shift away from this engagement with European Communism and radicalism. On the one hand, there was the death of Joseph Stalin and the disillusioning impact of Nikita Khrushchev's "Secret Speech" denouncing Stalin and the failings and crimes of Stalinism at the Twentieth Congress of the Communist Party of the Soviet Union in 1956. On the other, there was the accelerating wave of anticolonial movements and decolonization engulfing Africa,[3] Asia, and Latin America, which brought in their wake a new preoccupation with the so-called Third World.

In the late 1960s, a post-Stalinist "New Left" movement led by middle-class student youth emerged on the French intellectual scene. Its conception of alienation, liberation, and revolution extended to the Third World, whose political leaders it heroized as true revolutionaries. The movement reached its climax in the May 1968 student uprisings in French universities and the accompanying nationwide general strike of French workers.

Enter Médecins Sans Frontières

The thirteen young Frenchmen (physicians and several medical journalists)[4] who founded Médecins Sans Frontières (MSF) on December 22, 1971, were "inheritors" of this history, as Xavier Emmanuelli, one of its "founding fathers," eloquently testified:

> [W]e were descendants of the ranks of the idealistic Left. Students in medicine, sons of medical families, medicine for us was already idealized; but above all, we had as reference the great antifascist struggles, the heroes of the Resistance, and we grew up in the wake and the mythology of the world war. We had masters, struggles, landmarks.
>
> [Moreover,] the French have always considered an adventure in Africa as educational, and . . . still have a secret emotional esteem for the continent. We had a colonial past.[5]
>
> At the beginning of the 1960s, I was young, and I wanted a destiny.

I was filled with the epic of this century. I ardently wanted to become a son of the adventure, a navigator of the tragic, and to face the blaze of revolution. But I was only a medical student. . . . It seemed to me essential to belong to the race of rebels, of those who had struggled to change the world, and it was completely natural that when my classmates approached me, I joined the Communist Party.[6]

A key element in MSF's historically grounded myth of origin portrays its original members as a small group of young "French doctors," working as volunteers for the French branch of the International Committee of the Red Cross during the Nigerian civil war of 1967–1970, in the seceded southern province of Biafra, whose inhabitants were primarily of Igbo tribal origins. These physicians blamed the famine-stricken plight of the Igbos that they had seen firsthand on the "genocidal" intentions of the Nigerian government in blocking the distribution of food to them.[7] They wanted to denounce the government publicly, but they were constrained from doing so by the contract they had signed, which pledged them to observe a policy of "discretion." The International Committee of the Red Cross (ICRC) explained it this way:

The efficacy of humanitarian action depends largely on the direct and long-term access to victims. In pursuing that objective, the ICRC long ago embraced discretion as a working method. This simply means that it maintains a reserved attitude when it comes to communicating with third parties the observations and findings of its delegates in the course of its activities. It is an approach that allows the authorities concerned to accept on their territory the activities of an institution which they know will not divulge information that could be exploited by their adversaries. It also helps to build up a relationship of trust with the victims in much the same way that medical secrecy does between doctor and patient. . . . The purpose of maintaining discretion with regard to the parties to a conflict is not only to gain access to victims but also to ensure continuing access.[8]

The "French doctors" were morally outraged by this mandatory silence. Out of this experience, when they returned to France, they founded MSF on twin pillars: "acting and speaking" and "treating and witnessing."

The document they drafted in which they formally stated MSF's core principles became its "Charter" (always written with a capital C). The Charter pledged all the members of MSF to "provide assistance to populations in distress, to victims of natural or man-made disasters, and to victims of armed conflict . . . irrespective of race, religion, creed, or political convictions"; to observe "neutrality and impartiality in the name of universal medical ethics and the right to humanitarian assistance"; to "maintain complete independence from all political, economic or religious powers"; and, "as volunteers," to "understand the risks and dangers of the missions they carry out and make no claim for themselves or their assigns for any form of compensation other than that which the association might be able to afford them."

However, the principle of *témoignage*, or witnessing, remained implicit in MSF's ethos until 1995, when the so-called Chantilly Document was drafted, based on agreements reached at an international meeting of MSF held in Chantilly, France. While affirming that the "actions of MSF are first and foremost medical," this document states that "*témoignage*/witnessing [is] an integral complement" to them. "It is expressed through . . . the presence of volunteers with people in danger as they provide medical care, which implies being near and listening; a duty to raise public awareness about these people; [and] the possibility to openly criticize or denounce breaches of international conventions." The latter, the Chantilly document comments, is "a last resort used when MSF volunteers witness mass violations of human rights, including forced displacement of populations, *refoulement* or forced return of refugees, genocide, crimes against humanity and war crimes." The Chantilly document concedes that "[i]n exceptional cases," "it may be in the best interests of the victims for MSF volunteers to provide assistance without speaking out publicly or to denounce without providing assistance."[9] This concession grew out of MSF members' experiences in the field, which confronted them with the fact that however virtuous speaking out might be, it can have unwanted harmful consequences for the provision of medical humanitarian care, for the persons whom that care is intended to assist, and for those delivering the care.

The Boat People

The first of two crises in MSF's early history arose eight years after it was launched, in 1979, when it became entangled, through Bernard Kouchner, its most conspicuous founding member and first president, in a controversy created by the appeal for "Un bateau pour le Vietnam" (A Boat for Vietnam) made by a group of renowned French intellectuals.[10] This project involved chartering a vessel to rescue the so-called boat people—Vietnamese refugees fleeing their embattled country by ship, who were drowning and dying by the thousands in the South China Sea.[11]

Most members of MSF opposed this venture. Its second president, Claude Malhuret, Kouchner's successor,[12] had tasked Rony Brauman—an early member of the second generation of MSF physicians—to investigate its feasibility, and Brauman had deemed it technically impracticable. Brauman's advice was important to Malhuret for several reasons. Between 1975 and 1978, as a physician in the merchant marine, Brauman had been ship's doctor on a vessel laying underwater cables along the west coast of Africa. He had remained in touch with some of the officers with whom he had served, and he solicited their opinion about the Vietnamese boat project. In 1979, moreover, MSF had recruited Brauman as its first permanent physician member, in which capacity he had acquired firsthand knowledge of refugee populations through numerous field missions in refugee camps served by MSF.[13]

In a scathing article, Xavier Emmanuelli, who had become MSF's vice president, attacked Kouchner's "grandstanding" and the "illusory" nature of the venture.[14] Nevertheless, Kouchner and his intellectual companions proceeded to charter a ship called *L'Île de Lumière* (Island of Light). Along with a few other physicians, accompanied by journalists and photographers, Kouchner sailed to the China Sea, where his group provided medical aid to the boat people. The journey received highly theatrical media attention.

Emmanuelli's article helped precipitate a deeper crisis unfolding inside MSF. Concretely, his conflict with Kouchner turned around one of MSF's foundational principles—*témoignage*: its commitment to bear witness to, and to speak out about, the predicament of the individuals and populations to whom MSF provides in-the-field assistance, and where it observes serious abuses, or violations of human rights occurring, to publicly condemn them.

Emmanuelli was no less committed to the principle of witnessing than Kouchner; but what he reacted against passionately was the media "spectacle" made of the plight of the Vietnamese "boat people," of their exodus, and especially of Kouchner's "staging" of the *Île de Lumière* rescue mission. In Emmanuelli's view, the whole episode had been "mediaterized" to a degree that distorted the essence of medically and technically competent humanitarian action.

A schism developed within MSF over the boat people. Kouchner and his *compagnons* (companions), who included most of the founders of MSF—"the elders of Biafra"—espoused politically symbolic action like the rescue of the boat people. Opposing this and supporting Malhuret were the second generation of MSF members—many of whom had worked in refugee camps in Cambodia and Thailand. In contrast to Kouchner, Malhuret focused on practical field action: on the development of a more structured, better administered, more medically competent approach to the emergency and longer-term care that MSF was providing in refugee camps. At the 1979 meeting of MSF's General Assembly, Kouchner's faction was in the minority. In a "solemn speech," Kouchner denounced the "takeover" of MSF by "bureaucrats" and "schemers," predicted that it would destroy MSF, and "left the room," taking with him "the quasi-totality" of MSF's founders, Rony Brauman recalls.[15] Led by Kouchner, this departing group founded another medical humanitarian organization: Médecins du Monde / Doctors of the World.[16]

Médecins Sans Frontières France Versus Médecins Sans Frontières Belgium: The Case of Liberté Sans Frontières

Five years later a second schism shook MSF, pitting MSF France against MSF Belgium. MSF France demanded that the Belgian section of MSF be forbidden to use the name Médecins Sans Frontières and its logo. MSF France alleged that MSF Belgium had "progressively distanced" itself from MSF France, and from its "allegiance" to its *association mère* (mother association) by its "refusal to subscribe to the connection created between MSF France and a foundation named 'Liberté Sans Frontières.'" On July 10, 1985, the case of Médecins Sans Frontières France versus Médecins Sans Frontières Belgium was heard by the Tribunal de Première Instance de Bruxelles (the court of the federal district of Brussels, where the initial trial of a legal action in that district is brought).

The Liberté Sans Frontières Foundation (LSF) had been created by MSF France and approved by its General Assembly in 1984. Its co-originators were two prominent members of MSF France: Rony Brauman and Claude Malhuret. Brauman was named the foundation's director, and Malhuret was elected its president. The board of directors was composed chiefly of members of the editorial committee of the conservatively oriented magazine *Commentaire*.

In presenting their conception of Liberté Sans Frontières to the General Assembly, Brauman and Malhuret had described it, in a calculatedly "euphemistic way," as a "group reflecting on questions of the rights of man and of development in the Third World, free of all ideological prejudice."[17] The documents that MSF France submitted to the court characterized Liberté Sans

Frontières in an equally "euphemistic" manner, as "a center of research on the problems of Human Rights and development":

> The objective of the Liberté Sans Frontières Foundation is to . . . stimulate pragmatic research outside of the assumption that there is only one model possible and that it is necessary to follow it; to analyze the problems of development and Human Rights without making reference to the idea of the *Tiers-monde* [Third World], whose unity does not exist in fact; . . . to draw from this research its consequences for action; . . . [and to] ensure its diffusion among the principal relayers of opinion: the media, the political world, groups and associations.[18]

As Brauman later admitted, deliberate dissembling was involved in the relatively neutral, ideological fashion in which he and Malhuret depicted Liberté Sans Frontières. From the outset, they had conceived of it as "an organ of ideological combat that it was completely legitimate for MSF to establish, because of its action in the field. For us [this] objective was clear."[19] The combat was directed against the valorization of the Third World by much of the French Left.

Another document outlined the "themes" around which Liberté Sans Frontières had organized an inaugural colloquium on *Le Trois-Mondisme en question* [The Third-Worldism in Question], held on January 24–25, 1985, in the chamber of the French Senate in Paris. These themes included: "Neither Third-Worldism nor Cartesianism," "The End of Revolutionary Myths," "The French Colonial Heritage Beyond Legends," "The Third-Worldism of Lenin in Our Time," "How to Reduce Poverty: The Example of Rural Asia," "The New Industrial Asia: History of a Takeoff," "Aid for Development, For or Against?" and "The First Requirement: Political or Socioeconomic Rights?"[20]

MSF Belgium testified that it was not opting for a "rupture" with MSF France, but rather for a "momentary interruption of collaboration" until MSF France "distanced" itself from "being a part of the Liberté Sans Frontières Foundation (LSF)." The core problem, MSF Belgium argued, was that "the support and sponsorship of LSF [was] not compatible with MSF's Charter and the ideological and political independence that is expressed in it."[21] "The difference" between MSF France and MSF Belgium "did not rest on a question of 'allegiance,' but much more fundamentally on the ethical foundation" of MSF, and on the "underlying philosophy as expressed in the common Charter."[22] A basic principle of MSF, the Belgian section affirmed, was its "apoliticism." And in its anti-Third-Worldism, LSF had violated this.

The Belgian court ruled that MSF France's demand was "unfounded" and that it could not prohibit MSF Belgium from using the name Médecins Sans Frontières and its logo. In her decree, the presiding judge stated that "the cornerstone of the litigation is the common Charter of the two parties; that the present litigation must be analyzed in the light of the text of this Charter; that this clear and precise text strongly emphasizes the principles to which the physicians have subscribed." The court then had to determine whether MSF France and MSF Belgium were adhering to Article 2 of the Charter, requiring that Médecins Sans Frontières work "in the strictest neutrality and complete independence, refraining from any involvement in the internal affairs of states, governments, and parties in the territories [in which it is] called to serve." Considering the goals pursued by the Liberté Sans Frontières Foundation that MSF France "has agreed to be part of . . . the judge can say that there is an apparent divergence between the philosophy and goals on the one hand of MSF, and on the other of LSF."[23] In linking itself with LSF, she implied, MSF France was failing to adhere to the principles of the Charter.

Before the trial, Kouchner and two other co-founders of MSF, Dr. Jacques Bérès and Dr. Max Récamier, drafted a public letter defending MSF Belgium. They accused MSF France of having engaged MSF in "ideological and political combat" with the creation of Liberté Sans Frontières:

> That is why [they wrote] in the face of this breach of the ideal, the ethic that animated the founders of MSF, we support our friends of MSF Belgium in their quarrel with the Parisian "apparatchiks." It seems normal to us to support them in the face of the moral and intellectual fraud [*escroquerie*] that the creation of LSF constitutes. It is MSF Belgium that is maintaining the . . . practice and ideal of . . . the Charter and its statutes. It is MSF France that is perverting them.[24]

In a newspaper article, Rony Brauman (who by this time had been president of MSF France for three years) was quoted as calling this "intrusion" of Kouchner in the internal MSF debate "comical." He dismissed this "daughter organization turning against her mother" as a natural psychological phenomenon.

Seen in the sociological perspective of Max Weber, the internal convulsions rocking MSF at this historical juncture were characteristic of organizations that begin as movements under the charismatic inspiration and authority of founder-leaders. As these organizations grow and become more institutionalized, their "charismatic element does not necessarily disappear"; rather, it becomes embodied in a less personal, more rationalized structure and mode of operating. This transition is often accompanied by conflicts erupting around the succession of the movement's leaders, and of the generations of members within it.[25] MSF was undergoing just such a passage from its charismatic origins in the creation of Liberté Sans Frontières and the resulting litigation.

Proliferation of MSF Sections, and Ideological Shifts and Confrontations

MSF was also making another crucial transition. From its inception in 1971 until 1980, it had consisted only of the French group, with its headquarters in Paris. But in 1980, MSF Belgium and MSF Switzerland were founded, followed in 1984 by MSF Holland. MSF Belgium played a proactive role in the creation of these other European sections. It drew up a provisional statute calling for MSF France and MSF Belgium to found an "internationalized" MSF Europe to function within a "common structure," directed by a Comité de Direction Collégiale (Committee of Collegial Direction), made up of different member-sections. Within this framework, each section would have one vote and decisions would have to be unanimous and ratified by all the sections.[26] However, with a few exceptions, the most influential members of MSF France were opposed to the concept of an MSF Europe. Thus, during the period when MSF France launched Liberté Sans Frontières (1984–1986), and of its subsequent lawsuit against MSF Belgium, it was grappling with what it perceived as a threat to its hegemony spearheaded by MSF Belgium. More fundamentally, MSF France was confronting the reality that it was no longer the sole, authoritative embodiment of MSF—of its principles, organization, and decision-making.

In addition, during these years, MSF France was affected by major ideological shifts. The trajectory of French intellectuals' break with Marxism and Communism, their move "towards the non-European world [and] towards *tiers-mondisme*,"[27] and the reaction of *anti-tiers-mondisme* had their parallels inside MSF. These shifts were dramatically played out in the "first public appearance" of Liberté Sans Frontières: the 1985 *Le Trois-Mondisme en question* colloquium. As organized by Brauman and Malhuret, this was designed to be "a frontal attack against *tiers-mondisme*," in Brauman's words. Filling the Senate chamber in Paris and participating vigorously in the discussion were "top tiers-mondistes," as well as "anti-tiers-mondistes"; and newspapers representing the entire Left-to-Right political spectrum of the Paris press gave extensive coverage to the event.

Identifying the content of "tiers-mondisme," the orientation of "tiers-mondistes," and the outlook of "anti-tiers-mondistes" was not easy, French intellectuals having defined these concepts and categories so variously. As Claude Liauzu observed in the historical journal *Vingtième Siècle*:

> Since the colloquium organized by Liberté Sans Frontières in January 1985, a debate as animated as it is confused has periodically recurred. The uninitiated have difficulty in situating its protagonists, in penetrating its meanings, and in defining its ends. . . .
>
> . . . When [French] intellectuals speak of the Third World, they speak about and for themselves. . . .
>
> [T]his debate is fundamental: its stakes concern both representations of the Third World in French opinion, and the ideological relationships between the Right and the Left. . . .
>
> An initial definition of what is called *tiersmondisme* today consisted of taking into consideration that the West was no longer the measure of everything, that the Third World was both a new force and a constituent of what Europe was becoming.[28]

Brauman, the chief architect and spokesman of Liberté Sans Frontières, manifested the ideological vagueness of the Third World debate. He said he was simultaneously "a militant anticommunist" (who earlier had belonged to the "extreme Left"—the "Proletarian Left"), "a tiers-mondiste," and an "anti-tiers-mondiste."[29] What could this mean? He explained: "On the one hand, I was totally centered on countries of the Third World, feeling truly 'good' in many African countries, etc. . . . and, on the other hand, I was ferociously anti-tiers-mondiste, because I found that all that was being recounted about the responsibilities of the North in the economic and social disasters of the South, proposed to us as the new economic order, as perspectives of organized emancipation, were at best derisory sentimentalism, and at worse, a complicity with the bloodiest regimes."[30] Third-Worldism, Brauman asserted, attributed the misfortunes of Third World countries entirely to their exploitation by powerful and prosperous "Northern" and "Western" societies—particularly former colonial powers; it ignored the "primordial" role that Soviet and Communist expansion was playing in the Third World. In "almost all refugee camps in the world," MSF teams reported, "the overwhelming majority" of the displaced persons had "fled from Communist regimes."[31] Brauman strongly condemned Third-Worldism for failing to recognize that in numerous Third World locales, "liberation" movements, often "brandishing . . . Marxist-Leninist emblems," had established "totalitarian regimes" that were despoiling these countries of their wealth and resources and committing acts of brutality that violated human rights.[32] To Brauman, Third-Worldism was "a tropical version" of the most repressive forms of Communism.[33]

The Liberté Sans Frontières Colloquium

The overall tone of the colloquium was accusatory, even combative. Some of the presentations suggested that as used by "tiers-mondistes," the "tiers-monde" concept was a vague, inconsistent, and indefinable "scrap bag." What was more, it was contended that the "Third World" was not a "real-world" entity. It projected a false unity on a wide range of politically, economically, culturally, and ideologically different countries in Africa, Asia, and Latin America, simplifying their complexity and mutual interests, and imputing to them an equally false solidarity. Anti-tiers-mondiste presenters rejected the attribution of the problems of Third World countries, especially those of poverty, to their exploitation by capitalist, imperialist, colonialist, and neocolonialist powers. They claimed that the "disastrous strategies of local governments . . . produced the disasters of the Third World, . . . not the world economic system"; that the "ravages of authoritarian [economic] planning were greater than those of capitalism"; and that liberal, industrial, free enterprise–oriented, democratic societies were the "most efficacious in preventing [economic and political] catastrophe. Third-Worldism was impugned for "almost exclusively" explaining "disparities" in the development of different societies in economic terms, and for slighting political, historical, and anthropological factors.[34]

The colloquium also denounced the "dolorous" and "paternalistic" portrayal of the members of Third World societies as "victims"—in the vivid words of Rony Brauman, as an "infantilized, irresponsible mass, estranged from its history, bent under the weight of the oppression of rich countries." There were elements of "simplifying leftist patterns in this binary conception of a world divided between victims and oppressors," he declared, "expressed in a penitential rather than an insurrectionary version, but mistaken nonetheless." "The persons I saw in hospitals, in refugee camps where I worked were victims of a precise, given situation, of an illness, an aggression, a war that had uprooted them," he recalled. "One can be a victim of something, of a theft, an epidemic, a persecution, but one is not *victim* [Brauman's emphasis] by status, as if that state had become an identity."[35]

The colloquium vehemently upheld human rights as set forth in the Declaration of the Rights of Man and of the Citizen passed by the French National Assembly in 1789, which include the right to liberty, to property, and security; the right to resist oppression; and the right to freedom of thought and expression. The colloquium viewed these "precise and limited" rights, "based on the equality in the law for all individuals," as "categorical imperatives" that pertain to "human nature," and that are universally applicable to, and valid for, all times and places. The claim was made at the colloquium that largely through the influence of Marxism, other concrete economic and social rights had been added to the original Rights of Man and of the Citizen—such as the rights to work, health, material security, housing, development, and education. Although the anti-tiers-monde participants in the colloquium did not dismiss these additional rights, they made it clear that they regarded them as less fundamental, universal, and timelessly important than human rights; and they were critical of what they regarded as a growing tendency to consider material rights more "real." They characterized certain devastating events (most particularly the 1984–1985 famine then ravaging Ethiopia, and the famine, deaths from treatable diseases, and genocide under the Khmer Rouge in Cambodia in 1975–1979) as horrendous outcomes, not only of the failed "social engineering" of Communist insurgencies and regimes, but also of their disregard of basic human rights. They saw a baleful affinity between the priority given to social and economic rights in these countries and the tendency of tiers-mondistes to demand that these rights come first and universal human rights second, as an additional "reward."[36]

The Significance of the 1984–1985 Famine in Ethiopia

The overlap in time between the 1984–1985 famine in Ethiopia, the creation of Médecins Sans Frontières, and its inaugural colloquium had a major influence on how the members of MSF France experienced and participated in this meeting. For them this famine was a catastrophe with which MSF France had been deeply involved in the field, exemplifying the horrific abuses of human rights perpetrated by the "revolutionary" government of a Third World country. This profoundly traumatizing event brought MSF face to face with the realization that "under certain circumstances humanitarian aid can do more harm than good."[37]

The famine that beset northern and southeastern Ethiopia, which resulted in the deaths of hundreds of thousands and the destitution of millions, was as much—perhaps even more—a consequence of the policies of the government of President Mengistu Haile Mariam, and the counterinsurgency campaign of the Ethiopian army and air force against his opponents, as of drought and harvest failure. Mengistu had assumed power as head of state following the overthrow of Emperor Haile Selassie I in 1974 by the Derg, a committee of military officers and enlisted soldiers of which Mengistu was a member. From 1977 to 1978, Mengistu and his Derg regime conducted a reign of terror against the Ethiopian People's Revolutionary Party and constructed what he grandiosely labeled "the first authentically Communist country of Africa." All rural land and foreign- and locally owned companies were nationalized. The Marxist-Leninist Workers' Party of Ethiopia was founded as the country's ruling party, with Mengistu as secretary-general, and members of the Derg were appointed to the Central Committee of its Politburo. The country was renamed the People's Democratic Republic of Ethiopia.

The government's primary response to the drought and famine was a "resettlement" and a "villagization" program, forcibly transferring populations in southern Ethiopia, destroying their villages, and grouping the uprooted into new sites under Party control:

> Ostensibly designed to relocate northerners away from the "famine-prone" region for their benefit, the plan served to deprive . . . opposition movements of a base of local support and to advance the government policy of collectivization. Relief was thoroughly manipulated, denied to areas not held by the government, and used as a weapon to control populations in the north. . . . Food distribution centers became traps, attracting populations to a central location at which many were forcibly recruited into the army or signed up for transfer to the south in accordance with quotas set by Addis Ababa. . . .
>
> The people were deported in deplorable conditions to the south. No effort was made to keep families, villages, or ethnic groups together. Many died en route. Almost all destination villages lacked infrastructure, and the new arrivals were required to clear land and construct their shelter. Due to the lack of health care and sanitation, tropical disease inflicted a high toll on the weakened population.[38]

In 1984, MSF started programs to treat malnutrition in a number of hunger-stricken regions of Ethiopia. Initially reluctant to allow Western aid organizations into the country, the Mengistu government changed its position "as it began to turn the international humanitarian action to its economic, diplomatic, and military advantage. . . . Aid was the bait and the presence of international NGOs gave the [resettlement] program an element of legitimacy and security."[39] In 1985, MSF France confronted the government after some six thousand children "died in a camp where they had adequate materials for assistance but were not allowed to distribute them because, according to government officials, a sufficient number of adults had not agreed to be resettled."[40] Because MSF France spoke out about this tragic incident, and more generally about the government's misuse of aid to relocate millions of its people, the government ordered it to halt its activities, and it was expelled from Ethiopia in December 1985.[41]

Ethiopia was a critical event for MSF France, for Brauman and Malhuret, and for their conception of the Liberté Sans Frontières Foundation and its colloquium. It reinforced their anticommunist and anti-tiers-mondiste outlook, and their inclination to view Communism and tiers-mondisme as antitheses of MSF's democratic, anti-totalitarian, "humanitarian spirit."

The Demise of Liberté Sans Frontières

Notwithstanding the passion surrounding Liberté Sans Frontières, it was short-lived. It became increasingly focused on Third World issues such as health insurance, food, debt, and development. The Foundation produced fifty-five booklets on such topics, which it distributed to a list of some 1,500 national and international "opinion leaders." Brauman found these topics increasingly "boring" and feared that MSF would come to be seen as an agency specializing in Third World issues. To him this was neither appropriate nor desirable.

In 1984, at the time that he had organized the *Trois-Mondisme en question* colloquium, Brauman has said, "if anyone had told [me] that 'tiers-mondisme' was going to collapse like a house of cards, [I] would not have believed it.[42] But already, by 1987–1988, Third-Worldism was foundering. It was a period of transition, Brauman observed. In his view, the core ideas of Liberté Sans Frontières were being increasingly accepted. "Humanitarianism was no longer a subject of contradictory debates but a subject of general consensus . . . of all praise [and] all virtue." Brauman felt that "the work [he] had devoted to the renovation of the philosophical and ethical bases of humanitarianism no longer had a reason for being."[43] It seemed "pointless." So, he "decided to let Liberté Sans Frontières go."[44] In his double capacity of director of Liberté Sans Frontières and president of MSF France, he told the foundation's board of directors that he wished to terminate LSF. Brauman described it as a "very tense meeting," because the board was unwilling to close down LSF, and according to the bylaws of the foundation, a two-thirds vote of approval of its members was required to do so. Brauman, who regarded himself as a "leftist neo-con," had never felt entirely at ease in his discussions with more conservative interlocutors like the LSF board members. "The paradox," he stated, "was that very often, I felt emotionally closer to those whom I criticized than to those who approved of LSF."[45] This contributed to tension in his discussions with the obstinate board. In order to break the impasse, Brauman informed them that MSF France would no longer be able to raise or contribute funds to support LSF, evoking acrimonious responses from the board members. They accused Brauman of manipulating them, of discarding them when he had no further need of them, and of seeking to ingratiate himself politically with his more leftist friends, now that François Mitterand, the leader of the French Socialist Party, had just been elected for a second term as president of France.[46]

Although formally speaking LSF was never voted out of being, by April 1989, its de facto existence had come to an end.[47]

An Event of Enduring Significance

What an MSF member once referred to as the "saga" of Liberté Sans Frontières, with "the ideological adventure"[48] and the associated courtroom confrontation between MSF France and MSF Belgium, could be considered an event of faded significance in MSF's history and collective memory if MSF were not still facing cognate issues. Although under changed and changing circumstances, MSF continues to confront challenges posed by its organizational growth and its increasing geographical and societal scope. It still struggles to realize its "sans frontières" vision more fully, partly through achieving greater "internationalization." It still wrestles with questions about its foundational principles, their interpretation, and their implementation in humanitarian action—including its principles of neutrality, impartiality, and "bearing witness." It still anguishes over humanitarianism's "inherent paradoxes," which "can lead to some negative consequences" that "contradict its fundamental purpose by prolonging the suffering it intends to alleviate."[49] And it is still confronted by the core dilemma that Liberté Sans Frontières threw into relief: how to deal ethically, wisely, and effectively with the fact that (in the words of MSF's Nobel Prize acceptance speech), "the humanitarian act is the most apolitical of acts, but if its actions and its morality are taken seriously, it has the most profound political implications."

CHAPTER THREE

"Nobel or Rebel?"

On October 15, 1999, the Norwegian Nobel Committee announced its decision to award the Nobel Peace Prize for 1999 to Médecins Sans Frontières / Doctors Without Borders "in recognition of the organization's pioneering humanitarian work on several continents." "Since its foundation in the early 1970s," the committee's statement continued, "Doctors Without Borders has adhered to the fundamental principle that all disaster victims, whether the disaster is natural or human in origin, have a right to professional assistance, given as quickly and efficiently as possible":

> National boundaries and political circumstances or sympathies must have no influence on who is to receive humanitarian help. By maintaining a high degree of independence, the organization has succeeded in living up to these ideals.
>
> By intervening so rapidly, Doctors Without Borders calls public attention to humanitarian catastrophes, and by pointing to the causes of such catastrophes, the organization helps to form bodies of public opinion opposed to violations and abuses of power.

In critical situations, marked by violence and brutality, the humanitarian work of Doctor Without Borders enables the organization to create openings for contacts between the opposed parties. At the same time, each fearless and self-sacrificing helper shows each victim a human face, stands for respect for that person's dignity, and is a source of hope for peace and reconciliation.

Although MSF had been nominated for the Nobel Prize many times, and had been considered a runner-up on numerous past occasions, its members reacted to this announcement with collective astonishment, followed by an outburst of celebration. "Staff sang and danced in the hallways" of MSF's Paris office, and others rushed out to buy crates of champagne."[1] In all the other national offices of MSF's nineteen sections, and at its hundreds of field projects in more than eighty countries—with some cultural variation—"the scene was [much] the same."[2] In Tokyo, for example, as in Paris, members of the Japanese section of MSF "expressed surprise at the news saying, 'I can't believe it,' and 'Is that true?' [and] then held a . . . celebration, toasting news of the award with sake and juice"[3]—rather than with French champagne.

However, this wave of excitement and jubilation was soon followed by disquietude and concern:

The day of glory has arrived! It cannot be denied that it caused a warm glow of satisfaction. When the journalists broke the news on TV5, tears almost came to my eyes. A few telephone calls from the embassies, a few letters of congratulation from the UN, and there on the evening of 15 October, we were taking our place, somewhat with gritted teeth, in the Pantheon of Respectability. And then almost immediately I asked myself, why MSF?[4]

I know that this may cast a shadow over the joy of those MSFers who see the prize as a just reward. It is true that the prize warms your heart. But it is also true that the best way to silence a dissident is not to punish him but to reward him."[5]

Today the borders which lie before us are not so much political and national; they are instead those of blind, criminal violence, and of medical exclusion. They radically reduce our capacity to intervene. And in order to face up to them, we must first tackle a third more insidious border, which is eating away at us from the inside, namely institutionalization.[6]

The Nobel Prize triggered a crisis of success inside MSF. The ensuing organization-wide stocktaking was deeply connected with MSF's principles of humanitarian action, its conception of itself as a movement, and its culture. This self-examination brought to the surface tensions among its national sections—particularly between MSF France and the others.

MSF Debates Success

On November 19, 1999, the board of directors of the Belgian section of MSF organized a debate at its Brussels headquarters on the theme "Nobel or Rebel: A Nobel Without a Cause?" The debate focused on why MSF had won the prize, whether MSF deserved it, and on the "dangers" of accepting it. The discussion was premised on MSF's conception of itself as an actively engaged movement of "rebels" dedicated to a mission that was simultaneously medical, humanitarian, and moral. The notion of the "rebel" underlying it drew inspiration from Albert Camus's conception of *l'homme révolté* (the man in revolt):

> What is a rebel? A man who says no, but whose refusal does not imply a renunciation. He is also a man who says yes, from the moment he makes his first gesture of rebellion. . . .
>
> [R]ebellion does not arise only, and necessarily, among the oppressed. . . . [I]t can also be caused by the mere spectacle of oppression of which someone else is a victim. . . . Therefore the individual is not, in himself alone, the embodiment of the values he wishes to defend. . . . When he rebels a man identifies himself with other men and so surpasses himself. . . . Man's solidarity is founded upon rebellion, and rebellion, in turn, can only find its justification in this solidarity. . . .
>
> Rebellion indefatigably confronts evil, from which it can only derive a new impetus. Man should master in himself everything that should be mastered. He should rectify in creation everything that can be rectified. And after he has done so, children will still die unjustly.[7]

Participants in the debate saw a paradox in MSF's being "nobelized": "We are nobelized because we show non-respect for all that creates populations in danger, and we are indignant about the non-respect for human dignity, but the Nobel committee is the most respected committee in the world. All of a sudden we are respectable because we show non-respect."[8]

This "recognition" might cause MSF to develop a "big head" or to "rest on its laurels," or lead to "greater institutionalization." "The Nobel could become a ball and chain, which would prevent us from moving forward, and nothing is more important than that," a member remarked. "The prize should be an opportunity to enlarge our base of action . . . and to avoid arrogance: to continue to work for populations in danger, and not for our own image," another declared.

Other members raised questions about what the image of MSF as a noteworthy recipient of a prize for *peace* would convey to a worldwide public. They were especially concerned about how this could misrepresent their mission, inflate their capacities, and underestimate their limitations:

> The Nobel Prize for Peace. . . . Are we an organization of peace? . . . We cannot change the world, but we can try to infuse a little humanity into situations where human dignity is not respected: relieve their suffering. But we are not actors of peace; we do not try to bring about reconciliations. . . . Also we have been awarded a prize in the name of the "right to intervene." . . . But there is a big difference between the right of states to intervene and "the duty of humanitarians." . . . Humanitarian action is not a panacea. There are circumstances in which we cannot act, and we are not a substitute for political action. It is therefore important that we define our limits.

Some of the themes of the Brussels debate were reiterated in the *Nobel Peace Prize Journal* produced by MSF for circulation among all its members:

> Why were we, the big mouth of humanitarianism, the 28-year-old newcomer to the scene, better known for our arrogance and our impertinence and our stances in defiance of the orthodoxies of international aid, receiving this prize normally conferred on politically correct women, men, and organizations?[9]

> We find it difficult . . . to see ourselves as standard-bearers of the "right to intervention": a right which seems finally to be acknowledged and from now on, considered sacred. Without wishing to appear ungrateful, we cannot allow such a grave misunderstanding to take root. The fact that we are able to contribute on the margins to the development of international laws and practices, and that we are no more inclined than before to venerate national sovereignties, should not be taken to mean that we have become devotees of the cult of that catch-phrase.
> Indeed, this "right of intervention" is a catch-phrase which owes its success to its ambiguity. The expression . . . mixes two approaches, which are not exclusive, but which if confused, bring about the weakening of both:
> —on the one hand, independent humanitarian action;
> —on the other, political and military intervention by the great powers or international coalitions in situations of crime or terror on a massive scale.[10]

The Nobel Prize has sent out a powerful message. It may cause a retreat to the pseudo, "Nobelized" truth, or it may open the door to a new impetus. So, is MSF an institutional temple, or a fledgling rebel movement?[11]

Who Should Give the Speech?

These characteristically impassioned exchanges were partly intended to provoke ideas to include in the Nobel Prize acceptance speech. Deciding on the content of the speech, who should compose it, and who should deliver it, proved to be a controversy-ridden process.

To begin with, MSF aspires to function as a relatively decentralized, non-hierarchical, egalitarian association in which independent thought and participatory democracy prevail and the views of all its members receive equal consideration. But by 1999, MSF had evolved into an international entity, composed of nineteen sections and thousands of physicians, nurses, and allied health professionals, providing medical aid on a global scale.[12] The entire membership of MSF was invited to suggest ideas for the Nobel acceptance speech. But in an organization of this size and scope, attempting to collate all these opinions was problematic—especially within the less than two months between the announcement of the prize in October and the presentation ceremony in Oslo on December 10, 1999. Achieving consensus was made all the more difficult by the quasi-autonomy of MSF's separate sections. Furthermore, notwithstanding the commitment of all the sections to MSF's principles of medical humanitarian action, and their espousal of "without borders" values, significant subcultural differences existed among them. At times in MSF's history, there had been virtually no communication among sections, "amidst periods of profound disagreement on what humanitarian action must mean . . . , and with the risk of breaking up as a movement."[13] As recounted in chapter 2, these conflicts had resulted in the exodus of a whole group of MSF's founders from its ranks. On the threshold of the award ceremony, Alex Parisel, the director of MSF Belgium, was sharply critical of the extent to which the "original impetus" of MSF, "which ignored all borders, ha[d] become a simple sum of each section's *realpolitik*."[14]

By choice and conviction, MSF had no chief executive officer in overall charge of the organization. The International Council, composed of the presidents of all of its sections, loosely coordinated whatever joint decisions were made about important issues and common policies.[15] An elected International

Council president represented MSF as a whole, but he lacked the authority of a CEO. In 1999, James Orbinski, a physician and a founding member of MSF Canada, held this position.[16]

While MSF Belgium was engaged in its "Nobel or Rebel" debate, MSF France's board of directors was engaged in a parallel debate. Philippe Biberson, then president of MSF France, reported to the board on the decision reached about the speech following a month-long series of meetings with various MSF sections, with James Orbinski, with the international office in Brussels,[17] and with the Nobel Prize committee. A consensus had crystallized around "the idea" that someone "from the field representing MSF's volunteers" would be delegated to receive the Nobel medal, and Orbinski would deliver the speech. Because most of the members of MSF France wanted the "special history and role played by Paris in the construction of MSF . . . to be visibly recognized" on this occasion, Biberson had had several conversations with Orbinski about the possibility that the two of them might give talks at the Nobel ceremony. However, Biberson recounted, "certain sections" of MSF, along with the Nobel committee, demurred. And so, in mid-November, he had "voluntarily decided to accept the consensus that had emerged," since he considered that "it was time to concentrate on the content of the speech."[18]

Some members of MSF France's board reacted with outspoken chagrin to Biberson's account:

> *Annemarie*: Personally, I am disappointed because MSF is receiving the Nobel Prize for independence and *témoignage*, and these points are not necessarily captured with the same strength and the same engagement by other sections. That is why I would have strongly wished that MSF France give the speech. I absolutely do not want to disqualify the work of other sections in the field, but it seems to me that it would have been more just to convey the importance of the French section.
>
> *Denis*: The question of the form is not secondary, because what gets organized in the designation of the orator is a transfer of legitimacy. The real legitimacy, located historically in the French section, is sacrificed to the advantage of a bureaucratic, and it seems to me, somewhat demagogic logic. I regret that more of a fight was not put up to occupy the place that we should have, and I fear that the adoption of this form will . . . lead to a speech that is not very provocative.
>
> *Xavier*: I am also very disappointed, but it is we who wanted an International Council, and therefore we no longer have a choice. Nor can we go back on the idea . . . of a volunteer who has been in the field for one or two years, rather than

a person from headquarters in service for many years who, in my view, has much more legitimacy. Well, what we can fight about is the speech, because I don't believe that in gathering ideas from here and there we will be able to construct a muscular speech. It seems to be preferable that the writing of it be done here, and then circulated, amended, and commented upon.

François: I agree with Xavier . . . I am disappointed and I want the board of directors to consider adopting a resolution this evening that asks the other sections to revise this distribution of roles so that it takes into account the history of twenty-eight years of activity to which all the sections did not [contribute equally], and the contribution of *this* section to the Charter and to the big principles of the movement.

At this point Philippe Biberson vehemently declared that he "did not want this board of directors to pose as a giver of lessons to other sections":

I know that is not what François and Denis want to do, but what can't be hidden is that it will be experienced that way by the other sections. It seems to me that there are a thousand other, . . . much more operational ways to transmit our ideas. The Nobel Prize is not the opportunity to do so. I think that your resentment is rooted in a perspective that is entirely turned toward the past, and that it is not possible to obliterate the work of other sections.

"For this reason," he declared, "I will not associate myself with all these deterrents to an international consensus."

Biberson's position was supported by Bruno, another board member, who spoke up in favor of what Biberson had said, and "reminded" his colleagues that it was "not only the French section of MSF that was committed to *témoignage*," and that "at present all the sections [were] making notable contributions to the history of the movement." Nevertheless, Xavier insisted, "the question why it seems to be impossible for the international movement to accept having the speech given by Philippe Biberson and James Orbinski still needs to be asked." "That's because eighteen other sections feel as legitimate as the French section," Bruno retorted. François challenged him:

François: But who has nourished the current of ideas for twenty-eight years? I'm sorry, but the eighteen [other] sections have not played an equal part. What I would like to know is the precise position of each of the sections on this matter. . . . What I fear is that the consensus is a weak one, whose impact on the speech will be disastrous.

> *Bruno*: Let's just say that everyone feels represented by James Orbinski, but as soon as you put a French person alongside of him, the other sections feel that the French section is taking possession.

"MSF Belgium is present in more field situations than MSF France," Bruno added, "so one could also invoke operational legitimacy." "We must find a solution," he exhorted his colleagues.

The verbatim transcript of this meeting ends here. It is followed by a paragraph, headed "Decision," from which it is clear that Biberson's support of MSF's "consensus" in designating Orbinski as the sole speaker at the Nobel ceremony had prevailed over the objections of some of the most vociferous members of the French section's board of directors:

> In conclusion, Philippe [Biberson] refuses to let the question of representation at Oslo be put at stake by legitimacy. The choice of representatives (James Orbinski and a volunteer) constitutes an entirely worthy symbolic solution—both of the primacy of the field and of the non-national character of the movement—and an honorable one for most MSFers, as for MSF itself. Nevertheless, having taken into account the expression of fear of a weak consensus, Philippe proposes to transform it into a strong determination to succeed in producing a text [of the Nobel Prize acceptance speech] that is equal to the cherished ideas of the house.

Writing the Speech

Before the announcement of the Nobel Prize, James Orbinski had planned to travel to Mariinsk, Siberia, to spend several weeks with an MSF team that was working in a group of gulag-like prisons known as Colony 33, where they were treating prisoners afflicted by epidemic-scale tuberculosis, many of whom had developed multi-drug-resistant TB.[19] Although the daunting task of writing the Nobel acceptance speech still lay before him, he decided to go through with his plan, because, he said, after all the hours of being interviewed by the press about the prize, he had begun to "worry that [it] might turn MSF into a 'Nobelized' institution that offered solemn slogans but was divorced from the reality of the people we were trying to help."[20]

Upon his return to his office in Brussels, Orbinski "struggled to complete the speech," meeting with "key people in MSF and canvassing others for ideas and support."[21] In this connection, it was apparent that the MSF sections were not equally influential. Those whom Orbinski considered "key people" were chiefly members of two of MSF's sections, MSF France and MSF Belgium—especially MSF France. MSF France, the founder-section of the organization, and MSF Belgium, the second section to be created, were two of the five designated "operational" sections of MSF. They directly controlled field projects under their aegis, deciding when, where, and what aid was necessary, and when to end a program.[22] (The other, so-called partner sections of MSF did not have such operational authority; their major functions were to recruit volunteers, raise funds, and advocate on behalf of populations in danger.)[23]

On the night before the ceremony, Orbinski worked "into the small hours of the morning" with Philippe Biberson and with Françoise Bouchet-Saulnier, the legal director of MSF France's Paris office and an expert in humanitarian law, to finish writing the speech. "In the course of that long night," Orbinski has written, Biberson helped him to clarify "the relationship between humanitarianism and politics"—an issue with which he had "struggled . . . for years"—and to "find the right words to describe how [he] understood [that] relationship," which he incorporated into the Nobel Prize acceptance speech. "Philippe said that humanitarianism was not about ending or justifying war; it was the struggle to create human spaces in the midst of what is profoundly abnormal. In that moment I understood that to allow that space to exist, we had to be willing to confront political power. It's an imperfect struggle, and it never ends."[24] Both the way that the Nobel speech was composed and how MSF France's board of directors resolved dissent about it provide insight into the making of important decisions in a large organization committed to minimizing formal structure and maximizing egalitarianism. Inside MSF, such decisions are facilitated by what some MSFers refer to as an "informal hierarchy" of influential members.[25]

The Nobel Award Ceremony

The Nobel ceremony protocol authorized MSF to invite sixty of the eight hundred guests in the audience. To avoid giving the impression that it spent large sums of money for travel expenses, MSF chose to invite only thirty guests; and to ensure that governments would not politically exploit the ceremony, it decided that embassy officials would not be among those guests.

On the morning of December 10, the day that the Nobel Prize was awarded,[26] members of the small MSF delegation donned white T-shirts imprinted in Russian with "Stop the Bombing of Civilians in Grozny!" They wore these en masse to the ceremony and immediately afterward joined an Amnesty International protest at the Russian embassy against the siege of Grozny, the capital of Chechnya. This was in protest against Russia's bombing of the capital of Chechnya as part of a military campaign to force Chechnya back under Russian rule.[27]

That afternoon, at precisely 12:59, heralded by the blare of trumpets, and escorted by members of the Nobel Committee, James Orbinski proceeded down the blue-carpeted middle aisle of Oslo City Hall's Central Hall, a grand auditorium decorated with murals depicting scenes from Norwegian legends and history, including many from World War II.[28] Dr. Marie-Eve Raguenaud, an MSF field worker, accompanied him. She had just returned from Burundi, having been chosen to personify the importance that MSF attaches to its members being in the field in a face-to-face, hands-on relationship to those they aid. She felt as though she had been "plucked from a hospital in Burundi," she remarked to Orbinski.[29] They were followed immediately by the king, queen, and crown prince of Norway, and the chairman and secretary of the Nobel Committee.

Dr. Raguenaud was called upon by the chairman of the Nobel Committee, "as MSF's representative doctor," to "come forward and receive the diploma and the gold medal."

Following this ceremonial exchange, Orbinski launched into his speech, beginning with a condemnatory statement about the events that were occurring in Chechnya:

> The people of Chechnya—and the people of Grozny—today, and for more than three months, are enduring indiscriminate bombing by the Russian army. For them, humanitarian assistance is virtually unknown. It is the sick, the old and the infirm who cannot escape Grozny. While the dignity of people in crisis is so central to the honor you give today, what you acknowledge in us is our particular response to it.

In a dramatic gesture, turning to the Russian ambassador seated in the audience, Orbinski said:

> I appeal here today to his excellency the Ambassador of Russia and through him to President Yeltsin, to stop the bombing of defenseless citizens in Chechnya. If conflicts and wars are an affair of the state, violations of humanitarian law, war crimes and crimes against humanity apply to all of us—as civil society, as citizens, and as human beings.

In the body of the speech, Orbinski described MSF as "an imperfect . . . but strong . . . movement," characterized the nature of its humanitarian action, and articulated the moral principles to which it is committed:[30]

Our action is to help people in situations of crisis. And ours is not a contented action. Bringing medical aid to people in distress is an attempt to defend them against what is aggressive to them as human beings. Humanitarian action is more than simple generosity, simple charity. It aims to build spaces of normalcy in the midst of what is abnormal. More than offering material assistance, we aim to enable individuals to regain their rights and dignity as human beings. As an independent volunteer association, we are committed to bringing direct medical aid to people in need. . . . The work that MSF chooses does not occur in a vacuum, but in a social order that both includes and excludes, that both affirms and denies, and that both protects and attacks. Our daily work is a struggle, and it is intensely medical, and it is intensely personal. MSF is not a formal institution, and with any luck at all, it never will be. It is a civil society . . . movement, and today civil society has a new global role, a new informal legitimacy that is rooted in its action and in its support from public opinion. . . . Silence has long been confused with neutrality, and it has been presented as a necessary condition for humanitarian action. From its beginning, MSF was created in opposition to this assumption. We are not sure that words can always save lives, but we know that silence can certainly kill. Over our twenty-eight years we have been—and are today—firmly and irrevocably committed to the ethic of refusal. This is the proud genesis of our identity, and today we struggle as an imperfect movement, but strong in our volunteers and national staff, and with millions of donors who support both financially and morally the project that is MSF.

The speech devoted a great deal of attention to the moral necessity of the humanitarian maintaining its "independence" from the "political." The lines between the humanitarian and the political were being dangerously blurred—through "military humanitarian" action, and the invocation of "the right to intervene," Orbinski averred:

Humanitarian action is by definition universal. Humanitarian responsibility has no frontiers. Wherever in the world there is manifest distress, the humanitarian by vocation, must respond. By contrast, the political knows borders, and where crisis occurs, political response will vary because historical relations, balance of power, and the interests of one or the other must be considered. The time and space of the humanitarian are not those of the political. . . .Humanitarianism occurs where the political has failed or is in crisis. We act not to assume political responsibility, but firstly to relieve the inhuman suffering of that failure. The act must be free of political influence, and the political must recognize its responsibility to ensure that the humanitarian can exist. . . .Today there is confusion and inherent ambiguity in the development of so-called "military-humanitarian operations." We must reaffirm with vigor and clarity the principle of an independent civilian humanitarianism. And we must criticize those interventions called "military-humanitarian." Humanitarian action exists only to preserve life, not to eliminate it. Our weapons are our transparency, the clarity of our intentions, as much as our medicine, and our surgical instruments. Our weapons cannot be fighter jets and tanks, even if we think that sometimes their use may respond to a necessity. The humanitarian is not the military, and the military is not the humanitarian. We are not the same, we cannot be seen to be the same, and we cannot be made to be the same. . . . on the ground, we can work side by side with the presence of armed forces, but certainly not under their authority.

The debate on the "Droit d'Ingérence"—the right of state intervention for so-called humanitarian purpose—is further evidence of this ambiguity. It seems to put at the level of the humanitarian the political question of the abuse of power, and to seek a humanitarian legitimacy for a security action through military means. When one mixes the humanitarian with the need for public security, then one inevitably tars the humanitarian with the security brush.

But one should "not . . . polarize the 'good' NGO against 'bad' governments," Orbinski cautioned, or set the 'virtue' of civil society against the 'vice' of political power." "There are limits to humanitarianism," he said. "No doctor can stop a genocide. No humanitarian can stop ethnic cleansing, just as no humanitarian can make war. And no humanitarian can make peace. These are political responsibilities, not humanitarian imperatives": "Let me say this very clearly: the humanitarian act is the most apolitical of all acts, but if its actions and its morality are taken seriously, it has the most profound of political implications."

Throughout, Orbinski cited instances of suffering, of injustice, and of "moral," "political," or "market failure" that MSF found "unacceptable," and that its "ethic of refusal" dictated it could not, and would not, accept in silence. These included the 1992 crimes against humanity in Bosnia-Herzegovina; the 1994 genocide in Rwanda; the 1997 massacres in Zaïre; "the 1999 . . . attacks on civilians in Chechnya"; and also the fact that "[m]ore than 90% of all death and suffering from infectious disease . . . like AIDS, TB, sleeping sickness and other tropical diseases occurs in the developing world" partly because "life-saving essential medicines are either too expensive, are not available because they are not seen as financially viable, or because there is virtually no new research and development for priority tropical diseases."

Toward the end, Orbinski gave personal testimony to the "inhuman and . . . indescribable suffering," and the "horror," that women, men, and children underwent during the genocide in Rwanda, and to the "sheer courage" with which the Rwandan members of the MSF staff worked during that time. "I was Head of Mission in Kigali then," he said. "And no words can describe the deepest sorrow that I and all in MSF will carry always." At this point, he acknowledged the presence in the audience of Chantal Ndagijimana, who had lost forty members of her family in Rwanda's genocide, and who was now "a part of our team" in Brussels. "She survived the genocide, but like millions of others, her mother and father, brothers and sisters did not." He then paid tribute to a woman he had cared for in Kigali, "who was not just attacked with a machete, but [whose] entire body [was] . . . systematically mutilated":

> There were hundreds of women, children, and men brought to the hospital that day, so many that we had to lay them out on the street. . . . We could do little more for her at that moment than stop the bleeding with a few necessary sutures. We were completely overwhelmed, and she knew that there were so many others. . . . She released me from my own inescapable hell. She said to me in the clearest voice I have ever heard, "Allez, allez . . . ummera, ummera-sha"—"Go, go . . . my friend; find and let live your courage."

"Our volunteers and staff live and work among people whose dignity is violated every day," Orbinski concluded. They "choose freely to use their liberty to make the world a more bearable place":

> Despite grand debates on the world order, the act of humanitarianism comes down to one thing: individual human beings reaching out to their counterparts who find themselves in the most difficult circumstances. One bandage at a time, one suture at a time, one vaccination at a time. And uniquely, for Médecins Sans Frontières, working in around 80 countries, over 20 of which are in conflict, telling the world what they have seen. All this in the hope that the cycles of violence and destruction will not continue endlessly.

What to Do With the Nobel Prize Money?

Orbinski also called attention to what he accusingly called "a growing injustice [that] confronts us . . . in a globalizing market economy": that millions of poor people in developing countries were dying every year from treatable infectious diseases because potentially life-saving medicines were not available, or were unaffordable in those settings. He did not mention that in response to this situation, in the course of 1999, *before* being awarded the Nobel Prize, MSF had launched a "Campaign for Access to Essential Medicines."

There was almost unanimous agreement among MSF members that the prize money, $960,000, be invested in a fund to support pilot projects that would contribute to the clinical development, production, procurement, and distribution of treatments for so-called neglected diseases. The initial target list included sleeping sickness, leishmaniasis, tuberculosis, and malaria. These projects would be implemented within MSF field missions in developing countries, in close collaboration with local initiatives.

Four years later, on July 3, 2003, MSF's International Office in Geneva announced that the Indian Council for Medical Research, the Oswaldo Cruz Foundation in Brazil, the Institut Pasteur in France, and the Ministry of Health of Malaysia would join with MSF to create a new nonprofit entity—the Drugs for Neglected Diseases Initiative (DNDi)—that would work in collaboration with the United Nations' Development Program, the World Bank, and the World Health Organization's Program on Research and Training in Tropical Diseases.

MSF had reached a working consensus about the moral as well as the material use of its Nobel Prize money. But, as we shall see, the organization now faced fresh internal conflicts.

CHAPTER FOUR

MSF Greece Ostracized

To: All The Foreign Media Correspondents
Invitation to Press Conference
MSF Greece: Problematic Concerning
The Humanitarian Movement

Oslo, 6 December 1999. The recent **expulsion of Doctors Without Borders/MSF Greece** from the International Council of the organization because of their decision to provide humanitarian assistance towards the victims of both sides of the Kosovo crisis, did not leave the whole movement untouched [*sic*].

The forthcoming **Nobel Peace Prize** nomination to MSF is a great honor and reward for thousands of volunteers and millions of donors who support the activities of the organization worldwide.

The contribution of MSF Greece—with their **10 years of active involvement**, the commitment and action of more than **200 volunteers** and the support of their **100,000 individual donors**—in the award of the Nobel Prize is already well recognized, although the International Office has decided not to invite MSF Greece to the nomination ceremony. Moreover, MSF Greece seizes the opportunity to raise issues concerning [the] problematic not only within MSF but also in the whole humanitarian movement.

This problematic will be the main point of discussion with you during the Press conference which will be held Friday 10 December 1999, at 9:00 a.m., at the Norwegian International Press Centre ("Saga" room), Vestbannenplassen, near the Town Hall.

With this announcement, the Greek section of MSF invited members of the international press to attend a conference about an internal crisis roiling MSF. The conference—which was presided over by the president of MSF Greece, Odysseas Boudouris, its honorary president, Sotiris Papaspyropoulos, its vice president, Demetrios Pyrros, and the Greek writer Antonis Samarakis, described in the announcement, composed in English, as MSF Greece's "Spiritual [i.e., intellectual] Ambassador"—took place in Oslo, Norway, close to its Town Hall where, only a few hours later, MSF was to be awarded the Nobel Peace Prize. MSF Greece had triggered this crisis on May 7, 1999, when it sent a convoy of MSF vehicles carrying medical supplies, and allegedly flying Greek flags, into Kosovo, in the Federal Republic of Yugoslavia, where they delivered these supplies to the Pristina Hospital. This had occurred in the midst of a war in Kosovo between ethnic Albanians fighting for their autonomy and Serbian forces fighting to hold on to the province. Police, militia, and soldiers of the regime of Slobodan Milošević, president of the Federal Republic of Yugoslavia, were conducting a campaign of forced migration and terror against Albanians. Simultaneously, the North Atlantic Treaty Organization (NATO) was bombing military positions in Kosovo and Serbia to "prevent a humanitarian disaster" and assert "humanitarian values."

This expulsion of the Greek section was a unique event in MSF's history. It took eight years of critical and self-critical analysis, debate, and negotiation before MSF Greece was reintegrated into the MSF movement in mid-January 2007. Its singularity notwithstanding, this MSF Greece episode—its origins, the different ways in which it was perceived and understood by Greek and by non-Greek members of MSF, and MSF's action in response to it—is relevant to recurrent MSF challenges in organization, governance, decision-making, and the implementation of its operational and humanitarian principles. The Greek controversy sheds light on some of the cultural and organizational difficulties of fulfilling international and transnational precepts—even for a movement like MSF, whose foundation is based on a "without borders" vision—and of upholding principles of "neutrality" and "impartiality" in the midst of a conflagration like the Kosovo War.

The History of MSF Greece in MSF

The "unilateral" MSF Greece mission into Kosovo had historical roots in the Greek section's relationship to other MSF sections and to the movement as a whole.

In 1990, a small group of Greek physicians petitioned MSF France to create a Greek section. At a meeting of MSF's International Council on October 11–12, 1990, all agreed to establish it as a "section in the process of construction" (*section en voie de construction*) to function under the sponsorship (*parrainage*) of MSF France. MSF Greece would remain under the supervision of MSF France—its "mother-section"—until it had reached a number of objectives indicating its "maturity."

By 1994, although MSF Greece admitted that it still had some "points of weakness" with regard to the training and technical competence of its members, it not only considered itself to have shown a "satisfactory development," but to have "exceeded all initial forecasts" with regard to the personnel it had recruited, and the funds it had raised from private sources. In its view, it was qualified to become an independent section of MSF. However, the International Council meeting on June 21, 1994, decided otherwise.

Four sections were in favor of making MSF Greece an independent section—MSF Switzerland, Spain, France, and Luxembourg. But the two who were against it, MSF Belgium and Holland, used their veto power to enforce their objection. The final decision of the International Council was "not to create a new section," but to have MSF Belgium "draw up proposals for integrating MSF Greece into the new international framework of [MSF's] delegate offices."[1] MSF Greece was given an "intermediary" status, with MSF Spain as its "mother-section." MSF Greece would not be permitted to participate in the International Council unless invited to do so by MSF Spain; and it would only be allowed to open new projects in countries where a section of MSF was already in the field, under the "coordination" of that section.[2]

On September 7, 1996, the Administrative Council of MSF Greece sent a letter to the International Council asserting that "the weight of the interdiction" on its full membership was becoming "more and more heavy, and less and less justifiable." "We understand that this 'intermediary status' might concern only 'one entity,'" the letter went on to say—particularly that of "a small country—and that it might appear to the International Council to be a 'secondary affair.'" But it is "no less evident that this 'secondary question' is primordial for us."[3]

While MSF Greece was waiting with increasing impatience for a "deadline" on its "intermediary status" to be set, it created a separate organization, Medeco (Medical Development and Cooperation Operations). Medeco had two objectives: "to provide an opening for the volunteers whom MSF [could not] absorb and at the same time keep them in the MSF movement," and "to participate in the investigation of an area of intervention (aid to development) which [was] not an MSF specialty but [was] difficult to ignore because it suit[ed] the structure and the dimension of Greek NGOs." The first Medeco project was to be an aid program for handicapped persons in Gaza, undertaken with the collaboration of local NGOs. In his capacity as president of MSF Greece, Odysseas Boudouris informed MSF Greece's supervisory section, MSF Spain, and MSF's International Council of this undertaking.[4]

Philippe Biberson, president of the International Council, responded to Boudouris with a letter stating that the Council regarded "the creation" and "the structure" of Medeco to be "unacceptable in the framework of MSF." In a more conciliatory tone, Biberson added, "You know that I have always considered that MSF Greece was created with the view to its becoming operational, and that I think that a form of compromise can be found. . . . We understand that the time could seem long to you," Biberson wrote, "but," he then stated forcefully, "the solution that you propose in putting all MSF in front of a fait accompli seems to us badly chosen in its form and in its date":

> Subcontracting its operations to a phantom organization that uses the name of MSF for its resources, its technical support, and its recruitment, is unacceptable. How are you going to account to your public for the actions of Medeco under the cover of MSF?
>
> It is unthinkable that MSF will accept working with Medeco in the field, and MSF Greece, by this fact, will be separated from MSF. Is that what you want?[5]

Answering immediately, Boudouris characterized Biberson's letter as a sort of "closing speech for the prosecution in a trial by custom as unjust in its content as it was in its form." He belligerently asserted that MSF Greece had never "transgressed" any of MSF's "fundamental principles" or any of the recommendations of the International Council, and that MSF Greece had been "transparent" in informing MSF Spain, its "supervisory section" (*section de tutelle*), about the creation of Medeco. While Bourdouris was "entirely in agreement" with Biberson that Medeco was "not acceptable" on a long-term basis, he insisted that any discussion of it had to include the problem from which it stemmed: the "lack of any progress, over the course of two-and-a-half years, regarding the question of MSF Greece's 'intermediary status.' " Boudouris then proposed that a "frank and open discussion" take place at the next meeting of the International Council. "Meanwhile," he offered, "we will freeze all new activity of Medeco."[6]

MSF Greece would have to wait over a year before it finally won a change in its status in March 1998. It was joined with MSF Switzerland to constitute one of MSF's five, newly established operational centers: Operational Center Geneva (OCG). MSF defined this relationship as one of "co-ownership." The boards of MSF Switzerland and MSF Greece would remain autonomous in national matters, but would share responsibility for international operations and the management of field projects. The boards of the two sections would combine to nominate the general director and the operational director of the center and delegate authority on daily operational matters to them. In April 1998, the boards of MSF Switzerland and MSF Greece agreed to appoint MSF Switzerland's director of operations, Thierry Durand, as the operational director of the two sections.

MSF and Greece in the Balkans and Yugoslavia

This was the organizational situation of MSF Greece in 1998–1999 when the Kosovo War erupted. Kosovo was the last tragic act in the disintegration of Yugoslavia, whose constituent republics began breaking away from the Serb-dominated central government in Belgrade in 1991. The Kosovo War was the first full-scale war in Europe since World War II and the first to be formally judged genocidal in character. In the course of it, as many as seven hundred thousand ethnic Albanians, ninety percent of Kosovo's population, were displaced into the neighboring states of Albania and Macedonia by Yugoslav President Slobodan Milošević's forty-thousand-man security forces. The objective was to "ethnically cleanse" all non-Serbs from the province of Kosovo. To prevent this, in March 1999, the North Atlantic Treaty Organization (NATO) launched a six-week bombing campaign against Milošević's troops. NATO's objectives were to end all military action in Kosovo, to prevent atrocities like the massacre the Bosnian Serb army and militias had committed in Srebenica in July 1995,[7] to ensure the safe return of all refugees and displaced persons, and to establish a UN peacekeeping presence in Kosovo.

NATO's bombing of Yugoslavia provoked a great deal of criticism from many quarters. Controversy centered on whether NATO had the right to intervene in a sovereign country, on its choice of targets, and on the five hundred civilians killed by its bombs. However, NATO viewed its campaign as history's first "humanitarian war." It is safe to say that most of the members of MSF regarded the idea of a "humanitarian war" or of a "military-humanitarian coalition" as dangerously incompatible with true humanitarian ideals and action; though some, in their passion to "save Kosovo," were personally and even publicly "pro-NATO."

Three sections of MSF had been operating in the Balkan region at this time: MSF Belgium in Pristina and Belgrade, MSF Holland in Macedonia, and MSF France in Montenegro. However, during the last days of March 1999, MSF Belgium withdrew from Pristina and from Belgrade in reaction against the Serbian forces' systematic campaign of torturing, raping, killing, and expelling Albanian citizens of Kosovo.

Greece is geographically part of the Balkan peninsula, and has for millennia been ethnically, culturally, politically, and economically linked with the region that became Yugoslavia after World War I. In common with the Greek public, the members of MSF Greece felt emotionally identified with a war raging "in their backyard," and they wanted to be centrally and vigorously engaged in responding to it.

Pervasive pro-Serbian sentiment existed in Greece. Some of it had religious roots. In supporting Serbia, the Greeks were exhibiting solidarity with their Eastern Orthodox Christian brethren. (In contrast, the overwhelming majority of the Kosovo population is composed of Muslims, most of them ethnic Albanians.) The Greek government was faced with the challenge of responding to these pro-Serb sentiments, while remaining a member of NATO, which was bombing Serbia. In mid-April, an agreement was reached between the Greek Ministry of Foreign Affairs, NATO, and the Serb government to allow Greek NGOs entry into Kosovo and Belgrade to give humanitarian assistance.

MSF was still highly motivated to resume its humanitarian activities in Yugoslavia but not under the partisan and particularistic conditions negotiated by the Greek government, which MSF viewed as dissonant with its principles of independence and impartiality. On April 11, its Executive Committee held a meeting at which it was decided that an "exploratory mission" under the MSF Switzerland–MSF Greece operational center would "try to go inside Kosovo," in order to ascertain whether "independent humanitarian action" was possible in that setting.

In the meantime, Thierry Durand had resigned as director of the MSF Switzerland–MSF Greece operational center, explicitly citing the difficulties of fulfilling this role from Geneva, the problems of finding a Greek program manager and of "grafting . . . non-Greek transplants" into the organizational structure in Athens, and his growing conviction that "Athens" did not contribute "added value" in running MSF programs abroad. Two unexpressed factors also figured in Durand's resignation: his concern over the nationalistic, pro-Serbian sentiments of the Greek section, and his fear that MSF Greece would go into Yugoslavia on its own.

On May 6, James Orbinski, the president of MSF's International Council, learned via an e-mail copy from Boudouris, that the Greek section was on the point of sending its own exploratory mission into Kosovo. On the same day, Orbinski sent a letter addressed to Boudouris and to Nikos Kemos, MSF Greece's director-general (which he asked them to circulate to all office and field staff, and association and board members of MSF Greece) calling this "unacceptable," inasmuch as it "contravene[d] the spirit and character of the MSF Movement."[8] By unilaterally launching a mission into Kosovo, MSF Greece had contravened the transparent, collaborative, and cooperative system of management among MSF's five operational centers.

"In pursuing these actions, MSF Greece is walking away from the MSF Movement," Orbinski went on to say. "I strongly urge you to come back." But if it were to return to the fold, "MSF Greece must cease immediately all unilateral exploratory missions. . . . Failure to do so will mean that [MSF Greece] is walking further away from the MSF Movement, and that the . . . severest of sanctions by the . . . Movement will have to be considered."

MSF Greece's Mission to Kosovo

On the day that Orbinski dispatched this letter, an all-Greek MSF Greece team of three physicians and a logistician was already en route to Kosovo with eighteen tons of medical supplies destined for the Pristina Hospital. They arrived the next day, May 7, at 11:25 A.M. Eight months later, in a memorandum that he prepared for a January 26, 2000, meeting of MSF's International Council,

Odysseas Boudouris attested that, "In the heart of the tragedy unfolding at the door of, and destroying the Balkans, . . . and given the urgency of the situation," the Greek section had found it "morally unacceptable to wait any longer" to undertake such a mission.[9]

Boudouris contested an "accusation" made by members of MSF's International Office that the MSF Greece convoy had flown the Greek national flag. NATO had required humanitarian convoys to paint identifying insignia—initially a red cross—on the roofs of their vehicles to avoid their being bombed, Boudouris wrote. But when the MSF Greece party arrived at the Yugoslav frontier, NATO representatives had informed them that since the Serbs had been using red cross insignia on conveyances transporting armed troops, they should paint the blue and white stripes of the Greek flag on the tops of their vehicles to protect them from bombing.[10]

Expelling MSF Greece

A "fact-finding" review of the "chronology of events" associated with the Kosovo mission and of MSF Greece's and MSF Switzerland's "version[s] of these events" was presented to a meeting of the International Council in Amsterdam on June 11–12, 1999. MSF Greece was asked to attend, but decided not to. After five-and-a-half hours of discussion and debate, the Council passed the following resolution:

The International Council of MSF resolves that:

Given

1. The unilateral MSF Greece mission into Kosovo lacked the independence necessary to facilitate an objective evaluation of the needs of the population and that unacceptable conditions of access were agreed to by MSF Greece which compromised the mission and undermined future attempts by any MSF section to enter into the FRY [Federal Republic of Yugoslavia];

2. that the actions of MSF Greece were carried out without respecting prior decisions of the IC [International Council] as to how MSF Greece should carry out operations;

3. that the actions of MSF Greece were carried out with a total lack of transparency, were deliberately misleading to members of the IC, and deliberately avoided international debate and coordination, and

4. that the actions of MSF Greece violated the specific decisions taken by the Executive Committee with regard [to] the objectives and conditions necessary for a MSF exploratory mission into Kosovo, the IC considers that the Common Operational Center between Greece and Switzerland has ceased to exist and therefore MSF Greece can no longer carry out operations outside of Greece, effective immediately.

On June 26, MSF Greece's General Assembly voted not only to continue but to *expand* its medical humanitarian missions. In response, on September 16, supported by the votes of seventeen out of eighteen of MSF's sections, the International Council formally expelled the Greek section from MSF. MSF Greece was the only section that voted against the expulsion. This resolution contained a stern statement demanding that the Greek section "immediately cease to use in any way whatsoever . . . the name or logo of MSF / Médecins Sans Frontières and of any related distinctive sign, publicly or privately, in or out of Greece," and that they "refrain from making any misleading representation that they are affiliated, in any way whatsoever, with MSF International or the MSF movement generally."

Subsequently, at a January 26, 2000, meeting of MSF's International Council, the following legally drafted resolution was submitted to a vote:

> The International Council votes to exclude Médecins Sans Frontières–Greek Section, on the basis of a violation of the fundamental principles of the movement and a violation of the International Council's resolution passed at the meeting of 11 and 12 June 1999.

This resolution was adopted by eighteen votes in favor, one vote against (MSF Greece's), and no abstentions.

Its legal expulsion neither altered the Greek section's conviction that it belonged to the MSF movement nor dissuaded it from calling itself "Doctors Without Borders" in Greek and in French. As Boudouris had written in the memorandum he prepared for the January 26 meeting:

> MSF Greece will not change its name, and will continue to call itself Giatroi Choris Synora / Médecins Sans Frontières–Greece, as it has since its creation. On the one hand because it is its legal name, guaranteed by legislation, and on the other, because this name corresponds to a set of principles that constitute its profound identity. The name Doctors Without Borders is not a commercial label, rather it

is an ethical reference to which we have proven our absolute fidelity and have no intention of giving up.[11]

There is a certain irony in this statement. Its defiance of MSF was based on a fervent affirmation of MSF's cardinal principles. And the recalcitrance it expresses is an extreme version of one of those principles—the precept of independence.

A Field Trip to Athens

Dear Renée:
I did not know that you intended to go to Athens to investigate in depth what happened, but I imagine very well your feeling of a mixture of modernity and antiquity, western and eastern worlds. . . . This is exactly what makes the relations with them [MSF Greece] so difficult, but so fascinating as well. And this led to our impossible life together.

PERSONAL COMMUNICATION TO THE AUTHOR FROM A
MEMBER OF MSF'S INTERNATIONAL OFFICE, JANUARY 28, 2001

In February 2001, I made a week-long trip to Athens, Greece. I wanted to see whether the Greek section was functioning since its expulsion from MSF, and, if so, how; and to learn viva voce from its members why they thought their section had been expelled. I was accompanied on this trip by Nicholas Christakis, a physician and sociologist of Greek American origins, then associate professor of medicine and of sociology at the University of Chicago.[12] Out of collegiality and friendship,[13] he had agreed to help me conduct this research in Athens, where he put his fluency in written and spoken modern Greek, his knowledge of Greek society, and his Greek professional and familial relationships at my disposal. In fact, most of the key interviews that we conducted in Athens were arranged by Christakis via his contacts there prior to my departure.

A Visit to the Headquarters of MSF Greece and With Its President

The office of MSF Greece was located in a building near the main campus of the National Technical University of Athens, or Athens Polytechneio (Poly-technic). We were conducted around its offices by the section's general director, Thanassis Papamichos, an occupational therapist by profession.

As we moved from one rather shabby office to another, it was apparent that despite its expulsion, MSF Greece was not only continuing to use the Médecins Sans Frontières name and its logo, but that it was organized into the established MSF departments (Operations, Human Resources, Communications, etc.). In one room, stacks of MSF printed materials were being readied for distribution in public schools. In another, preparations were being made to send a mission to the Indian state of Gujarat, the site of a severe recent earthquake. Because of the Greek section's expulsion, Papamichos lamented, it had been cut off from access to medicines and medical matériel in MSF's logistical supply centers in Europe.

Odysseas Boudouris, a surgeon in part-time practice, was still considered by MSF Greece to be its president. After touring MSF's busy offices, I had a long interview with him, mainly in French, in which he was fluent and felt at ease. He had grown up in Paris and was educated in France, where his parents had migrated from Greece in the early 1950s, in the wake of the Greek civil war. In France, during the 1960s, he first came in contact with MSF, and also with Médecins du Monde/Doctors of the World, the medical humanitarian organization created in 1980 after a split within MSF between members of its first and its second generations.[14] He returned to Greece in 1990, the year MSF Greece was founded.

Initially, he went to work with Médecins du Monde (MDM), but he found its Greek branch insufficiently connected with other sections of the organization—too inclined, he said, to be a "totally Greek organization." So he left MDM and joined MSF Greece, which he admired for its "perseverance" in trying to live up to "the same rules, norms, and principles" of the larger organization. It was almost "obsessed" with doing so, and in that way, it was very different from MDM, which criticized MSF Greece for "not being sufficiently Greek." In fact, even though MSF Greece defined itself as part of an international entity with common principles, Dr. Boudouris remarked, "no section of MSF resembles any other. The French, Belgian, Dutch, and Spanish operational sections have very different cultures."

This launched him into an extensive account of the "tragic" and "tragic-comic drama" that had ended in MSF Greece's expulsion. On the one hand, he began, within the framework of MSF as a whole, MSF Greece was no more than "a grain of sand," which "did not count very much," with only from two to three percent of the organization's volunteers and funds. On the other,

MSF Greece was "symbolically crucial," particularly in connection with the period in MSF's history when it was working through "a crisis of trying to become more international." He was alluding to growing pains MSF endured in the 1980s and early 1990s after its expansion to nearly twenty countries. The period was fraught with conflict among its sections, and with breakdowns in communication among them. In the midst of these tensions, MSF Greece had chafed at the "concentration of power" by MSF's operational sections—France, Belgium, Holland, Switzerland, and Spain. In Bourdouris's view, the Greek controversy should be seen in this context. The tone of voice in which he said this suggested that, like many of his compatriots, he was sensitive and truculent about the domination of Greece by other European powers that considered it to be a "small," "unimportant" country.

Then came "the crisis of Kosovo," Boudouris declared, and "Kosovo is next to us [Greece]." In his version of MSF Greece's mission to Kosovo, as NATO's bombing of Yugoslavia continued, there was an increasing discrepancy between the aid that MSF (along with other NGOs) was giving to both the Albanian population and the Serbs, "victims" of the "crime of the NATO bombardment," as he wrote in a paper circulated among MSF members. According to Boudouris, it was strictly as an intermediary that the Greek Ministry of International Affairs had become involved in NATO's opening up a "humanitarian corridor" free from air strikes that made MSF Greece's mission to Kosovo possible. As for the exploratory mission to Kosovo contemplated by the MSF Switzerland–MSF Greece operational center, it had been stalemated by the refusal of the Federal Republic of Yugoslavia authorities to grant it the necessary visas. Meanwhile, MSF Greece was informed that it would be accorded visas. Although the other MSF sections objected to their undertaking such a mission on their own, because of its questionable "independence" and "impartiality," MSF Greece felt that it was "unethical to tarry" any longer, and on May 7, 1999, "in all transparency," its convoy entered Kosovo. Following NATO's orders, they had painted the alternating blue and white stripes of the Greek flag on the roofs of their vehicles. It was true, he admitted, that even though the mission was defined as exploratory, it had distributed some medical, surgical, and dental supplies. However, he insisted, this was not unprecedented in MSF.

Its "excommunication" notwithstanding, Boudouris declared toward the end of our conversation, MSF Greece was "determined to continue." It had hundreds of volunteers and more than 100,000 donors, and its funds came mainly from private sources. He still hoped, he said, that the misunderstandings that had precipitated MSF's expulsion would be resolved and that it would be reversed.

At the MSF Greece Polyclinic

Thanassis Papamichos picked me up at my hotel to drive me to MSF Greece's polyclinic for a day-long visit. He arrived in a station wagon bearing the logo of MSF. With him was Dr. Demetrios Pyrros, an orthopedic surgeon and "disaster medical consultant," who was a former president of MSF Greece and one of its founding members. Dr. Pyrros was scheduled to attend a planning meeting for the forthcoming Olympic Games in Greece, but before he continued on his way, he invited us to have a cup of coffee with him in the courtyard of the hotel. He wanted to convey to me his enthusiastic support for the continuing existence of MSF Greece and to explain its breakthrough significance. The creation of the Greek section had been inspired by an ideal that "rose above the particularistic attitudes of the Greek reality," he said. The founders of MSF Greece came from different social, political, and religious backgrounds, and they had not originally known one another—atypically of Greek society. They had become meaningfully connected through their mutual commitment to MSF and its "without borders" principles.

The MSF polyclinic, located at the top of a winding staircase on the second floor of a reconditioned old building, was a busy, clean, orderly, and cheerful place. Its walls were decorated with MSF posters, and with a colorful display of children's imaginative drawings of MSF activities. The staff consisted of more women than men: four social workers, three general physicians, a midwife, a lawyer, and two legal counselors. The majority of the patients were immigrants—most of them of illegal status, who came from "different countries all over the world," a staff member said. The number of persons from any one country fluctuated, she observed, but the overall flow of immigrants arriving in Greece by boat had been escalating since the 1980s, owing to the country's location on the border of the European Union, at the crossroads of Africa, Asia, and Europe. This great stream of immigrants, a social worker commented, constituted a "culture shock" for Greeks, who were accustomed to a national population that was not only ethnically homogeneous but also ninety-five percent Greek Orthodox in religion. The staff felt that they were "pioneering" in caring for patients from such diverse backgrounds and helping them to adjust to everyday life in Greece. Their "witnessing" centered on making known, through print and television media, how the rights of their immigrant patients were being violated by the manifestations of intolerance that they were experiencing in Greece.

When a staff member banteringly called their work "a Greek miracle," her colleagues laughed appreciatively. Despite the expulsion of the Greek section, they affirmed, they were "still MSF, in Charter, commitment, and spirit."

At the end of my visit, I received three departing gifts from the staff: a T-shirt imprinted with the MSF Greece logo, several MSF posters, and a CD titled *People and Angels: Something Is Happening Here*, composed and recorded expressly for MSF Greece by Greek musicians.

Upon returning to my hotel, I stopped in the courtyard for a demitasse of Greek coffee. To my surprise, the waitress who took my order asked me (in English) if I was a physician. Looking down at the packet of materials that I had received from the polyclinic, she had recognized the MSF logo on them, and she proceeded to tell me how much she admired their activities.

Some Illuminating Comments

In the course of the summing-up discussions that Nicholas Christakis and I had about our field trip to Athens, he exclaimed that it was "hard to overestimate how novel the . . . MSF movement [was] in Greece." He proceeded to tell me about a relevant incident that had taken place in his youth:

> When my grandmother was dying twenty years ago in Greece, and she needed a blood transfusion, the family had to round up a donor personally. I went to give blood . . . and was told that it would go to my grandmother. . . . I was mystified when a month later I received a very official-looking scroll from the ministry of health, thanking me for what was called my "selfless act." . . . I had been told that my blood would go directly to my grandmother—a member of my own family. . . . Apparently for blood-type incompatibility reasons this did not happen. . . . There was no meaningful anonymous donation of blood in Greece of the sort we are familiar with in the United States . . . or any straightforward way of acknowledging it when it occurred. . . . A semi-deliberate kind of deception had been involved here.

"My point is that Greeks do not have this kind of philanthropic tradition," he continued. "All aid is local, immediate, tied to one's family or village. I cannot stress enough how extraordinary organizations like MSF (and Doctors of the World) are—how much these volunteers are swimming against the tide in Greece." At the same time, he mused, there is a sense in which "they are recreating Greek values in a way that is profoundly Greek, by extending Hellenism."

A Greek doctor I had interviewed earlier made the same point in a letter delivered to my hotel. "Greece is a nation located in the crossroads of the globe where the cultures of the East meet the cultures of the West, [and where] the North intersects the South," wrote Gregory Kyriakos, a general surgeon who had served as an MSF volunteer in Somalia:

> Being in this privileged geographical location, Greece has the chance as well as the responsibility and the obligation to offer humanitarian medicine to near and far incoming populations under distress since many economic refugees are coming from various countries.
>
> [The] Eastern Mediterranean was once called the cradle of human civilization and Greek people have contributed a great deal to this. In the present day, but also in the future, Greek doctors will continue to grant their medical knowledge to suffering people, thanks to the financial help Greeks—rich or poor—donate to the various humanitarian organizations.

CHAPTER FIVE

The Return of MSF Greece

MSF Greece was reintegrated through a prolonged, incremental process, which began at a meeting of the International Council in Barcelona on November 22–24, 2002, where two MSF members appointed to go on a "fact-finding mission" to Greece presented their report. The aim was "to assess whether we feel confident to start negotiations with the former MSF Greece."[1]

The report found that "the former MSF Greece see themselves as MSF [and] followers of the same rules and principles," and wanted to have access again to "the support that comes with being a part of a movement." MSF Greece was active both inside and outside of Greece, and in keeping with MSF's policies, eighty percent of its funds came from private money, rather than governmental sources of any kind. However, it lacked emergency capacity. Moreover, "Mozambique and India [where MSF Greece had sent teams] were quite painful experiences for them in that respect (too small for any impact), they seem to have reached a limit in the number of projects they can manage due to lack of experience and means [of] logistical support."

The report focused on the tension between "humanitarian action and the pressure of [Greek] civil society" on MSF Greece, despite the fact that "they believed they were more independent than any other Greek NGO." "The key is that as part of the conditions for [their] re-integration, a debate needs to be held with them on the political aspects of humanitarianism."

The report attributed Greece's defiant decision to go into Kosovo largely to three "key people" in MSF Greece at the time—especially to Odysseas Boudouris. Since these people were now gone, the present seemed to be "the right time to open up a dialogue with former MSF Greece."

At the end of the discussion, a "resolution on the former MSF Greece section" was drawn up and unanimously accepted:

> The IC decides to open up a dialogue with the former MSF Greece section to look into the possibility of a future reintegration of the former section as a member of MSF–International. The IC states the following clear non-negotiable conditions for a future membership in the movement:
>
> 1. The former MSF–Greece must share with the movement a thorough critical analysis of their actions in Kosovo during spring 1999, and their position on other major crises.
> 2. The operations carried out by the former MSF–Greece section, if to be continued, must be fully incorporated in one of the current five operational directorates of MSF as stated in the International Council resolution on future growth and operationality of MSF.
> 3. The former MSF–Greece must accept that the legal ownership of the name Médecins Sans Frontières, the acronym MSF, its Greek translation and the logo both inside Greece and internationally belongs exclusively to MSF–International, which is a common obligation of the partner sections.
>
> The IC asks the International Office and the executive to appoint two people from MSF to discuss a possible reintegration of the former MSF–Greece section. The commission should report back to the IC no later than November 2003.

It was not until January 13, 2007, that MSF Greece was fully readmitted into MSF International, as an operational cell, with MSF Spain, in the Operational Center Barcelona Athens (OCBA). This occurred at the close of a "Kosovo debate" that took place at an Extraordinary General Assembly meeting of the Greek section, which was also attended by the president and the secretary-general of the International Council and representatives from a number of other MSF sections.[2] The debate was the last of the agreed-upon prerequisites for MSF Greece's reincorporation into the international movement to be fulfilled.

The Kosovo Debate

The tone of the Kosovo meeting was set by Jean-Michel Piedagnel, executive director of MSF UK, in his role as the facilitator of the debate. This was "not a trial," Piedagnel insisted. Rather, it was an opportunity to "move away from black and white positions," to analyze the "big internal and international crisis" that had occurred, with "the maturity to move on" that now existed.[3]

Jean-Hervé Bradol, MSF France's director of operations at the time of the Kosovo crisis, laid out the main points the debate should address. Had the decision to expel MSF Greece been a good one? "Was it a discipline issue?" "MSF's internal discipline is not so strong," he admitted laughingly, and so, "if you exclude someone for discipline matters, then you should exclude a large part of MSF." Looking back on what happened he now felt that the decision about the expulsion of MSF Greece was "maybe not the right one."

Bradol then proceeded to discuss the "dilemmas of action" confronting MSF in dealing with a "humanitarian war in the heart of Europe." MSF had sought to be "present on both sides" by trying to get visas for volunteers from countries outside NATO. Further, it had refused to take money from NATO-involved countries and had sent an exploratory mission to Kosovo to assess the needs of the population, Kosovar and Serb alike. "If we review the facts," he continued, "Kosovar refugees were a very popular issue in Europe at that time. So there were many NGOs functioning in Albania and surrounding areas . . . and I was not convinced that there was space for MSF [in Kosovo]." "The real fight," he declared, "was to establish an independent presence in the area, without military or other help." However, the "pro-NATO" sentiments of many MSF members had affected the public position that MSF took. "It is easy in theory to discuss . . . impartiality," he concluded, "but in practical use, especially during a mission, [impartiality] is not so easy, because trying to be neutral sometimes [means that] you cannot bring relief to the people."

Next, Boudouris took the floor. He continued to believe, he declared, that "if there was violence against Kosovars, then the NATO intervention was a violent one, too." Expelling the Greek section had been an "extreme action," which should have been debated a long time ago. "Movements like MSF first began by pure idealism," he opined, but they then became "huge organizations" that developed "mechanisms of self-defense." This was what had happened to MSF, with the result that it had "a big governance problem." Furthermore, as

Boudouris saw it, each section of MSF had been influenced by its civil society, its own culture, and by the picture of the crisis that its local media were providing. He pointed out that numerous European countries had been involved in the Kosovo war, especially those to which MSF's five operational centers belonged. The "real and difficult dilemma" involved here was "the role of MSF in relation to its civil societies." In his view, Boudouris vehemently stated, the only way to avoid the mistakes that had been made during the Kosovo war in the future was through greater "internationalism of MSF, so that all sections would be able to express their opinions" without risking expulsion.

Other members of the Greek section expressed their pleasure that "the former International Council recognized its mistake" in having expelled MSF Greece—that, in the words of Jean-Hervé Bradol, "We [the International Council] had a range of opinions. We chose the most radical one. It was not the right one." Some members conceded that they "did break the neutrality principles" by painting blue and white bands on the roofs of their vehicles and using the "Greek government's way" to enter Kosovo. "We Greeks should be more self-critical," one averred. "How did MSF Greece believe it had the operational capability to get into a conflict such as the one in Kosovo?" he asked, adding that he thought there had not been "enough transparency" in reaching the decision. A recruiter-member of the Greek section emphasized how "very important" it was for the MSF movement and for each of the sections to "enter the society of MSF bringing with us our culture and opinions." "It is due to the movement's weakness," she said, that "these elements have not been activated efficiently." A panelist commented: "I'm sure that we will be facing dilemmas . . . regarding neutrality . . . from crisis to crisis."

After further reflections from the floor, Christophe Fournier, president of the International Council, declared that MSF Greece was "back in full in the international movement." "Internationalism in the movement may work for impartiality," he noted, "but it doesn't provide a lot of independence for each section's culture and society." Finally, regarding the expulsion, he concluded, "if the same decision was to be made again, it would be made differently and more carefully."

In the summings-up by the panelists that followed, Boudouris had the last word. The Greek section might have "underestimated" the consequences of its expulsion, he said, but, "we were acting by conscience, and not by convenience."

Postlude: MSF Greece in 2012

In 2012, MSF Greece faced a daunting set of conditions, with serious implications for the health of the country's citizens, and of the large number of immigrants who now comprised ten percent of its population. Foremost among these circumstances were the global economic recession and the sovereign-debt crisis that had destabilized the European continent, threatened its common euro currency, and become acutely problematic for several Eurozone countries—among which Greece was especially hard hit.[4] Over the course of 2008 to 2012, the overall rate of unemployment in Greece rose from 6.6 percent to 20 percent, and reached as high as 40 percent for young persons. On May 2, 2010, the European Union countries and the International Monetary Fund agreed to a loan of 110 billion euros for Greece, followed by their agreement on October 27, 2010, to an incremental fifty percent write-off of part of the Greek debt—both conditional on Greece's implementation of harsh austerity measures. In response, in the course of 2010–2011, the Greek government introduced four successive austerity packages, to which, in the wake of the third round of austerity measures, the Greek public reacted with a nationwide general strike and massive protests.

During this period, partly as a consequence of the uprisings in North Africa and the Middle East, there occurred what the executive summary of MSF Greece's 2011 Annual Plan described as a dramatic, "critical surge of asylum seekers / immigrants flooding into South-East Europe and its periphery." Greece was one of the primary destinations of these migrants. They arrived in Greece at a time when, because of the country's economic predicament, its employment opportunities, its social benefits and social programs, and its health services were being challenged and curtailed.[5] MSF Greece expressed concern about how some of these migrants were being "packed in stock-houses as a result of European Union security policies, within societies impacted themselves from the economic and political crisis," and about the dangerous ways in which certain Greek politicians and journalists were contributing to the creation of "a climate of xenophobia" around the country's migrant population.

In formulating its annual plans for 2011 and 2012, MSF Greece sought medical humanitarian ways to respond to the crisis in "access to health care for vulnerable segments of its populations" that would also have "added value" for the Barcelona Athens Operational Center (OCBA), and for the "common good" of the MSF international "movement as a whole," to which, it affirmed, it was "enthusiastically committed."[6] To be "successful in this attempt," its planning documents stated, "we . . . need to continue transforming ourselves." It was recognized that hard choices would have to be made because of the anticipated decrease in the proportion of MSF Greece's income from donations by the Greek public, given the state of the national economy. This did, indeed, happen. Although MSF Greece retained its pool of some forty thousand donors, the average contribution dropped sharply. MSF Greece proactively reduced its expenses by twenty-two percent in all its departments, and the staff in its Athens office from twenty-five to twenty-one persons.

At the end of 2011, MSF Greece drew up plans to tackle some of the communicable diseases that were spreading in the country—tuberculosis, HIV/AIDS, and especially the outbreak of malaria in Laconia, in the southeastern Peloponnese.[7] The intervention against malaria envisioned was to be "limited in scope . . . and in time." It would target the specific geographic area of the outbreak, with its approximately 10,000 inhabitants, of whom 4,850 were Greek residents, and 3,000 were migrant farm workers. It would be focused on "the most vulnerable" persons in the area—the migrant and Roma populations—during "one transmission period," February to November 2012 (when another episode of malaria was expected to occur during the spring). And it would entail bringing to bear on the situation the expertise in malaria screening, diagnosis, treatment, and prevention that the MSF movement had acquired and deployed during the years of its experience in dealing with this communicable disease—particularly in sub-Saharan Africa. Such expertise was virtually absent in Greece, because over the course of the nearly four decades that the country had been malaria-free, it had become an almost "forgotten disease" there.[8]

In addition to migrant workers, MSF Greece also planned to focus on the elderly, pensioners, and the homeless, who were "getting lost in the system" under the present economic and political circumstances.[9]

A Model for the European Union?

These were some of the conditions MSF Greece faced in 2012. What its members described as a "changing new landscape" was being altered by "an unprecedented crisis," which was not only economic, but also societal. Reveka Papadopoulou, MSF Greece's general director, was convinced that for the organization to respond to this optimally would require what she termed "exploratory doing." By this she meant conducting "situational" research and analysis in tandem with medical humanitarian interventions and advocacy that would provide the sort of contextual knowledge and understanding needed to make MSF's action appropriate and effective.

Papadopoulou had initially "joined MSF through MSF Greece" in 1994 and had become its general director in 2008, after the section was reinstated in the movement.[10] Her first MSF mission was a Greek project under the auspices of MSF Belgium in a rural town in Armenia. In 1995, "absolutely convinced that operationality could not/should not be 'monopolized'" by MSF's five operational sections, she helped to launch a project for MSF Greece in the Gaza Strip of the Occupied Palestinian Territories, where MSF Spain and MSF France already had a joint mission. In 1997, after what she termed MSF Greece's "marriage" with MSF Switzerland, she was sent, along with her partner, to the Swiss mission in Liberia. There she found herself in the midst of a heated discussion about the possibility of creating an operational desk in Athens under the direction of Geneva, with the intention of handing the mission over to Athens. She vehemently disagreed with this prospective plan, because she was "not absolutely convinced about the capacity of Athens to manage such an important and complex mission." In 1999, when the war in Kosovo began, Papadopoulou joined the efforts of MSF Greece to explore Greece's northern border in preparation for receiving possible refugees from Kosovo. In the midst of this exploratory mission, MSF Greece was expelled from the movement. She now found herself in the "frustrating" situation of "being between two realities: the one of the colleagues in Athens, and the other of our international colleagues." As a consequence of "being vocal and critical towards Athens"—especially with regard to MSF Greece's failure to "stand up to and speak out against" what was being done to the Albanian Kosovars—she and two other colleagues (one of whom was Greek, the other, Belgian) were "expelled by MSF Greece when MSF Greece was expelled by the MSF movement." The three of them became what they jokingly referred to as "IDPs [International Displaced Persons] from the MSF movement," until the International Office invited her to become a member of MSF Greece's reconstituted board of directors.

Papadopoulou was keenly aware that concentrating its energy on the Greek crisis might confront MSF Greece with a Kosovo-like dilemma: how to be responsive to the Greek situation without compromising MSF's supranational outlook and global commitment. MSF Greece's involvement had to take place "without MSF Greece becoming a Greek NGO." In this connection, she noted a favorable portent. In 2011, when MSF appealed for funds to assist its work in Somalia, the Greek section received the equivalent of 300,000 euros in contributions. To her, this indicated that in spite of all its economic travails, "Greek society understands that our solidarity with people in distress and our assistance to them go beyond frontiers."[11]

In Papadopoulo's view, the Greek crisis should be seen in a larger, "European perspective." What was occurring in Greece was a "worst case" instance of phenomena more generally European. "What is happening in Greece today could happen in Europe tomorrow," she opined. These were events, she felt, that potentially threatened the public-health systems of European nation-states, along with their political and economic stability. The European Union faced the challenge of reconciling diversity, sovereignty, and unity in the relations among its members—the sort of challenge, she noted, with which MSF has long grappled.

Papadopoulou and her colleagues have engaged other European MSF sections to produce a running analysis of the European situation, in collaboration with MSF Greece, on which humanitarian action could be based. In doing this, she said, "we are crossing [some of MSF's] own borders." The initial results have been promising.[12] As Papadopoulou implied, there are striking parallels between the issues raised by the European Union (EU) financial crisis, and the trouble-ridden trajectory through which MSF Greece passed in its relationship to MSF. The EU crisis is rooted in problems that extend well beyond the state of the euro as a common currency, and of economic debt and recession. At stake are the institutional viability of this entity composed of different European societies and their continuing commitment to transnational and transcultural "European-ness," out of which it was forged some sixty years ago. Throughout its four decades of existence, MSF has wrestled time and again with comparable issues over the kind of integration among its multiple sections that best fulfills the "without borders" vision of its movement. The case of MSF Greece constituted the most serious, Europe-based crisis that MSF has faced in this regard.

MSF, in short, is highly conscious of how integration can turn into disintegration. It also knows that it is called upon by the global nature of its "without borders" purview to strive perpetually to extend the scope of its "diversity-in-union" beyond the boundaries of European nation-states and cultures, a task that requires what one of its members calls a "construction and reconstruction that never finishes." This suggests that achieving a "without borders" state of being requires more than the forty years of effort that MSF has devoted to it, and may always be less than perfectly realized. The lesson here for Europe may be that sixty years may not have been long enough for the EU to achieve "union."

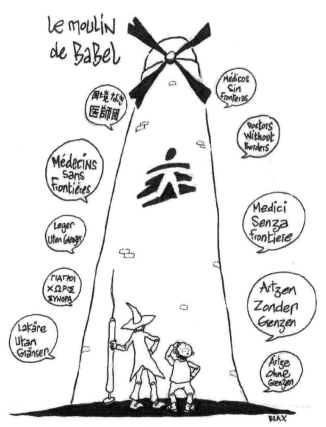

MSF aspires to function as a relatively decentralized, nonhierarchical, egalitarian association in which independent thought and participatory democracy prevail, and the views of all its members receive equal consideration. But by 1999, it had evolved from its genesis in 1971 as a small, charismatic movement of young French doctors into an international entity, composed of nineteen sections and thousands of physicians, nurses, and allied health professionals, providing medical aid on a global scale. In a multilingual organization of this size and scope, collating opinions was problematic. Reproduced by permission of Samuel Hanryon, a.k.a. "Brax," Rash Brax.

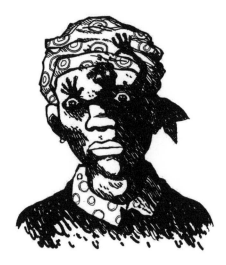

In the field, "gender roles, writ large in violence, have been one of [our] largest sources of curiosity, perplexity, frustration, anger, and rage." Reproduced by permission of Samuel Hanryon, a.k.a. "Brax," Rash Brax.

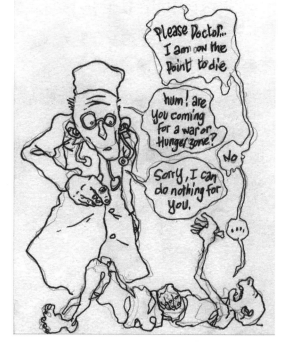

Exchanges took place about the limits of humanitarian action, and about the decisions concerning the allocation of resources that it entails. Reproduced by permission of Samuel Hanryon, a.k.a. "Brax," Rash Brax.

PART III / A Culture of Debate

CHAPTER SIX

La Mancha

To dream the impossible dream,
To fight the unbeatable foe,
To bear with unbearable sorrow,
To run where the brave dare not go.

To right the unrightable wrong,
To love, pure and chaste from afar,
To try when your arms are too weary,
To reach the unreachable star,

This is my quest, to follow that star,
No matter how hopeless, no matter how far,
To fight for the right, without question or pause,
To be willing to march into hell for a heavenly cause.

And I know if I'll only be true to this glorious quest,
That my heart will be peaceful and calm, when I'm laid to my rest,
And the world will be better for this,
That one man, scorned and covered with scars,
Still strove with his last ounce of courage,
To reach the unreachable stars.

"THE IMPOSSIBLE DREAM," FROM *MAN OF LA MANCHA* (1965)

In November 2004, MSF's International Council and its "EXDIR" (general directors of its nineteen sections) launched what was called the La Mancha process. Its aim was to "better define . . . the basic raison d'être" of MSF, its "roles and limitations," and "in what ways [it] should be governed."[1] This was undertaken "in the light of external challenges and internal changes" that, it was felt, were having "a profound impact" on MSF. "The exercise was overdue," International Council President Rowan Gillies commented. "[T]he last such international process took place in Chantilly in 1995—and MSF's good functioning was again being threatened by clashing visions and a governance no longer adapted to an expanded and increasingly interconnected 'multinational' MSF."[2]

As a consequence of the international meeting in Chantilly, France, in 1996, to which Gillies referred, a document called the "Chantilly Agreement" had been drafted and ratified that reaffirmed the foundational principles of MSF's Charter—including impartiality, neutrality, and independence. This document declared that "the actions of MSF are first and foremost medical." It made explicit that *témoignage*" (witnessing) is an "integral complement" of MSF's medical action. It stated that MSF subscribes to the principles of human rights and international humanitarian law. And it emphasized that the "commitment" of each participant in "the MSF movement goes beyond completing a mission." It entails active involvement in "the associative life of the organization and an adherence to the Charter and the Principles of MSF."

From the outset, the La Mancha process was conceived of as a broad effort of consultation and analysis among all members of MSF—particularly those in the field—and also nonmembers knowledgeable about "the humanitarian world." Organization-wide, interviews were conducted around a series of questions:

What attracted you to MSF?
What keeps you involved?
What is the common mission that unites everyone in MSF?
Should the mission evolve?
Which are the most important principles and those no longer relevant
    in the Chantilly documents?
What do you expect from our leaders?
On what issues is it essential for MSF to speak in one voice?
What operating rules must be added to the Chantilly document?
How do you see MSF in 2010?

Members were invited to write short "constructive" papers—which could be "provocative" and "should be fun to write and to read"—on issues of common concern. "More experienced MSF people" were asked to contribute longer papers "related to core questions on identity and mission." In addition, MSF commissioned a group of papers by "outside experts" on "how they read the Chantilly documents" and saw "the challenges faced by humanitarian action in general and MSF in particular."[3] The results were compiled in a four-hundred-page book, consisting of one hundred and fifty articles, entitled *My Sweet La Mancha*, which generated the agenda for the La Mancha conference.

The La Mancha Motif

The name "La Mancha" (a region in central Spain) was bestowed on the project because of its association with Don Quixote, the protagonist of Miguel de Cervantes's literary masterpiece *The Ingenious Gentleman Don Quixote of La Mancha*. Resonant for MSF is the adventure on the La Mancha plain where knight-errant Don Quixote and his squire Sancho Panza come in sight of what Don Quixote imagines are fearful giants whom he heroically intends to charge with his lance until Sancho delicately points out that the giants are in reality windmills.

This allegorical encounter was depicted in a black-and-white cartoon made for MSF by one of its members, who uses "Brax" as his nom de plume.[4] It was reproduced as the frontispiece of *My Sweet La Mancha*, facing a page with a quotation from the philosopher George Santayana: "The mass of mankind is divided into two classes, the Sancho Panzas who have a sense for reality, but no ideals, and the Don Quixotes with a sense of ideals, but mad." It was also printed on the front of the T-shirts that were worn by everyone attending the La Mancha conference. Printed on the back were the lyrics of "The Impossible Dream," the principal song in the musical *Man of La Mancha*.

In Brax's cartoon (which is also the frontispiece to the present book), Don Quixote and Sancho Panza are portrayed as riding on top of two miniature, dilapidated-looking vehicles with MSF license plates. Their feet are in stirrups, and they have spurs on their shoes, as if they were astride horses. The two men are wearing sleeveless vests over their long-sleeved shirts, with the logo of MSF printed on the backs. Don Quixote is holding a large instrument in his right hand that looks more like a huge hypodermic needle than a lance. Looming up directly in front of them is a large windmill, surrounded by two smaller ones—all three of which are strange in appearance because they look as though there are human hands, arms, feet, and legs protruding from them. The small windmills seem to be prancing about on their bare feet, with their arms akimbo. On the horizon, the sky overhead is filled with stars that have emerged from a few gentle clouds.

This cartoon expressed MSF's self-critical perspective on the loftiness of its ideals, its supposed heroism in pursuing them, the "tilting at windmills" nature of some of its missions, and the misperceptions and imperfections that can arise from pursuing its ideals.

The Don Quixote–Sancho Panza cartoon was only one of the more than forty that Brax drew in connection with the La Mancha events. Throughout the conference, he made on-the-spot sketches ironically and satirically commenting on the speakers' presentations and the discussion following them. Projected onto a large public screen, these caricatures were instantly visible to all the participants in the conference.

The La Mancha Conference

The conference took place on March 8–10, 2006, in Luxembourg, in the Neumünster Abbey, which was founded as a Benedictine abbey in the sixteenth century and opened to the public as a cultural center in 2004.[5] This locale was the context for one of the first cartoons drawn by Brax. Under a caption that read "From a Luxembourg Church to a New Bible," it depicted two faceless figures attired in the hooded robes of monks, with stethoscopes around their necks, who, with their hands folded prayerfully, were genuflecting before a voluminous book, with the title CHANTILLY in capital letters, and a large image of the MSF logo printed on its cover. This graphically reflected the humor-accompanied admonitions repeatedly voiced during the conference about the danger, in questing for "moral purity," of "enshrining" MSF's Chantilly Principles—of treating them, and MSF's Charter from which they derive, "too religiously" and dogmatically, as if they were immutable "sacred documents."

More than two hundred members of MSF attended the meeting. Simultaneous translations into English, French, and Spanish were available. However, most of the participants spoke in English, which has superseded French as MSF's lingua franca.[6] Some members of MSF France stayed with French—but only when making extended remarks.

The participants' vocabulary was strikingly apolitical, although many of the issues discussed had political implications.[7] A longtime member of MSF explained that this was a deliberate policy, reflecting MSF's "nonideological, apolitical ideology":[8]

> Ideological/political terms are almost banned from most speeches or analysis. Where this comes from . . . is a proactive censure, and not just ignorance or lack

of political culture. . . . [It] is linked to political neutrality in the movement, which is very cautious not to be associated with any political party or tendency, either in headquarter[s] country or in mission country. . . . [It is] a sort of de-politicization of MSF . . . as humanitarian beliefs are supposed to transcend political ideology.[9]

Rowan Gillies began the conference with a surgical image. "The belly of MSF is open," he declared. He was followed by Secretary-General Marine Buissonière, who gave an overview of MSF's activities, operations, and resources, and the challenging internal and external changes that the organization was facing—about which "everyone . . . in our movement . . . has an opinion." She invoked the ancient tale of a group of blind men in a village who each touch a different part of an elephant, cannot agree on what it is, and not only end up fighting amongst themselves but draw the entire village into the melée.[10] "In the field, encounters between patients and care-givers weave the fabric of our reality," Buissonnère said. "In headquarters, national perspectives and sometimes group dynamics prevail. Like the blind villagers and their elephant, it is sometimes difficult to grasp what MSF has become."[11]

"Surprising" and "Shocking" Revelations

The picture of MSF that Buissonnière presented seemed to surprise many in the audience. MSF had grown rapidly and its activities had expanded greatly since 1999. It had become a very large organization, with an annual revenue of 450 million euros,[12] an average of 300 million euros in cash reserves, nineteen sections, five operational centers, twenty presidents, twenty directors, and more than two hundred board members. Operating three hundred and sixty-five projects in seventy-seven countries, it was heavily present in Africa, where more than sixty-four percent of its activities were currently taking place (predominantly in Sudan, the Democratic Republic of Congo, Angola, Liberia, Ivory Coast, Chad, Burundi, Ethiopia, Kenya, Uganda, and Sierra Leone).[13] Deployed in stable, unstable, armed conflict, and post-conflict contexts, MSF was carrying out ten million consultations annually—vaccinating hundreds of thousands against meningitis or measles, performing 43,000 surgical operations, delivering 73,000 babies a year, and caring for patients suffering from malnutrition, mental health problems, the aftermath of rape and sexual violence, and increasingly, from HIV/AIDS, tuberculosis, and their co-infection. The number of staff in the field had more than doubled, from 11,253 to 24,666. So-called national staff—those working with MSF projects located in

the countries where they resided—filled ninety-two percent of all field positions, whereas expatriate staff—the 2,026 persons who were associated with
projects situated outside their countries—occupied only about eight percent
of such positions.

Hearing that "nationals" made up the overwhelming majority of MSF personnel in the field not only surprised the attendees. It also triggered a *prise de
conscience*. It became a focus of collective dismay, self-criticism and self-blame,
and a subject to which the conference returned again and again. "Our national
colleagues . . . provide the corner stone of MSF's activities," Marine Buissonnière commented. "But . . . [we] have never tried to understand who they are
and the nature of their relationship with MSF." In addition, [a]ccess to posts
of responsibility [and] associative life" in MSF has "remained marginal" to
them.[14] "All too often," another speaker self-accusingly declared, "our attitude
towards our national colleagues" is not only "characterized by . . . arrogance,
and an extraordinary degree of ignorance," but also by a "form of discrimination" that is "racist," "colonialist," and "neo-colonialist":

> Why is it that, still today, a Liberian doctor at the conference speaks about dis-
> crimination, lack of respect, lack of recognition within MSF? And feels compelled
> to say several times, "We too are humans beings. We too have an education. We
> too have experience and can take responsibility." Shocking![15]

These exchanges provoked a series of fierce Brax cartoons. One of them,
with the title "90% of All Staff Are National Staff," depicts a white man with
a horrified expression on his face, exclaiming, "You are telling me that almost
all MSF people are black??" Another shows a white, male "expat-staff" member
being carried in a sedan chair by two barefooted African men, clad in tattered
leopard skins, who are being commanded by their "passenger" to transport
him quickly to the scene of an "emergency" to which he is pointing. A third
cartoon, headed by the question "Why Promote National Staff?" features the
head and torso of a grinning white man with huge teeth, who responds that
"all Heads of Mission agree" that the answer is "Not to bother with expats." He
points to three caricatured white "expats" standing behind him: a male tourist
in a Panama hat and large sunglasses, with a camera slung around his neck;
an unshaven, balding man, holding a liquor bottle; and a saucily smiling nun,
without a veil, wearing a cross, with piously folded hands.

Organization Versus Movement

The La Mancha conferees agreed that the growth of MSF, the mix of health and medical problems that it was now addressing, along with its being "Nobel-prized," had both enhanced and worsened its governance problems:

> Our organization is expanding, more sections are taking on
>   operationality, we improve the quality of our performances, others
>   take over our guidelines and tools.
> If we were a company, we would be very happy.
> As we are a humanitarian NGO, we get worried.
> Worried about our capacity to respond adequately to all these needs,
>   worried about our organization losing its original humanitarian fiber,
>   its reactivity, its flexibility and creativity.[16]

Underlying MSF's persistent worrying about its structure and governance is its conception of itself as a pathmaking "Movement"—not "just an organiza-tion."[17] MSF sees itself as an "association" of individuals, assembled as a com-pany of equals, gathered in the spirit of "voluntarism" around medical and humanitarian ideas and actions, with a social, as well as medical, "mission." While recognizing that "if a movement is to be operationally . . . effective, it needs at least a minimum of organizational structure," MSF is cautiously aware of the danger that "in designing structures" it could "kill the very thing that [it] seeks to be—a movement . . . [and] become ossified, sclerosed, institu-tionalized."[18] Throughout the conference, adjectives like "institutionalized," "bureaucratized," "routinized," "standardized," "hierarchical," "pyramidical," and "centralized" were used to characterize organizational developments in-imical to "the movement's . . . culture of debate," "capacity for medical inno-vation," and "sense of humanity."

MSF's convictions about participatory democracy energized discussion about decision-making. There was palpable uneasiness about voting as a basis for making binding collective decisions. One person suggested that there was "an embarrassment about voting" in MSF—even "a strange taboo." Some said they preferred to reach agreement by consensus. Others argued that "in an organization expanding the way that MSF is, diversity will increase, and vot-ing is the only way to ascertain the majority and the minority." "Our very, very consensual way of proceeding," someone exclaimed, "is the worst we can have in terms of size!" Particular concern was expressed over the difficulty of forming a common "international MSF position," while maintaining the "diversity of opinion in MSF [that] is critical to the vitality of the movement."[19]

Two Brax cartoons satirized these aspects of the discussion. In one of them the torso of a hydralike figure, with grotesque, multiple male heads, wearing a stethoscope, is seated in front of a microphone labeled "MSF." From the mouth of one of his heads comes the utterance: "One day we will find a consensus." In the other cartoon, a group of MSF members, clearly identified by the logo on their shirts, are engaged in a mass fistfight. "Do we agree to disagree publicly?" the overhead caption reads. "Yes, we agree!" is the captioned response that comes from someone, somewhere in the brawling group.

MSF's moral association of maintaining a decentralized structure with its perpetuation as a movement precipitated discussion at the conference about what mechanisms existed within the organization, if any, that facilitated the making of "coherent," binding decisions representing all its sections and its entire membership. The limited, equivocal governing authority of the International Council and president, despite their supposed responsibility for overseeing MSF's mission, became a focus of intense discussion:

> We need to reinforce the President of the International Council, who should be elected by all members. . . .
> We are not an organization with a central office and a CEO. . . .
> I'm not convinced that the International Council should be given more power before we see whether we can function well among ourselves.

This debate became fodder for another Brax cartoon, depicting the International Council as a group of unidentifiable, inscrutable hooded figures, sitting around a conference table, gazing down on a tiny, bewildered man, dressed in shorts, who stands before them, leaning on a crutch.

"Nationalism," "Sectionalism," and "Internationalism"

"Are we French, European, international, global?" a speaker asked, broaching the fraught issue of identity that had riven MSF over the years: "Some of our internal tussles seem to come from a reluctance . . . to accept that MSF is international. . . . And ongoing discussions reveal that we are torn between the myth that we are a truly international organization, and the reality that almost all our decision-makers (and resources) come from the Western world."[20]

On the one hand, MSF had to deal more equitably with its internal national and cultural differences. On the other, it had to strengthen its common identity and solidarity through movement-wide commitment to its "without borders" principles. Questions were raised over whether MSF's supposedly "universal" principles could be applied to the many cultural traditions in the countries where it had projects: "How do we negotiate the notion of humanitarian action, which has roots so firmly in the European Judaeo-Christian tradition, with value systems from the Muslim, Hindu or Buddhist world, from Africa or Asia?"[21]

However, Rowan Gillies contended, now that MSF's nineteen sections were organized into five operational centers (France, Belgium, Holland, Spain, and Switzerland), and shared operations within these centers, there was a sense in which they had become more international, or at least, "more 'sectionalist' than nationalist."[22] Nonetheless, unresolved tensions still existed around how domineering the "Big Five" operational centers were, and over the claims to "individuality," "independence," or "sovereignty" that the sections continued to make.

In response to the exchanges about MSF's "sectionalism," Brax produced several cartoons. One depicts a wounded man with a bandaged head being carried on a stretcher by two men with stethoscopes around their necks. He is asking them—in French—"By the way, what section of MSF are you from?" Another portrays a giant windmill emblazoned with the MSF logo as "The Tower of Babel" (in French). The windmill is encircled by cartoon balloons, each of which contains the name "Doctors Without Borders" in the national language of a particular MSF section. Ballooned question marks hang over the heads of the two small figures standing in front of the tower/windmill (one of whom has a gigantic hypodermic needle by his side, and is wearing a peaked wizard's hat).

HIV/AIDS

It was uncontroversially assumed at the conference that the development of a global pandemic of HIV/AIDS and MSF's involvement in its prevention and treatment were the sources of the movement's greatest medical changes. HIV/AIDS had catalyzed MSF's "remedicalization." Ten years earlier, long, intensive debate had begun to take place "between those who thought that [MSF] could and should conduct AIDS-related activities, and those who thought that it was not within the organization's scope" or competence,[23] because MSF was primarily experienced in dealing with emergency medicine, and caring for AIDS patients required a lifetime commitment. But by 2005, MSF was treating more than forty thousand persons for HIV/AIDS in fifty-five projects in twenty-seven different countries. The global magnitude of the pandemic, its prevalence in eastern, southern, and central Africa, where MSF had so many programs, and the development of a first-line, three-drug regimen of antiretroviral drugs (ARVs) to treat the disease were among the factors that thrust MSF into the fight against HIV/AIDS. MSF had not confined itself to conventional forms of prevention and treatment. To make AIDS prevention and treatment available in resource-poor, high-prevalence areas, it engaged in advocacy, especially through the initiative of its international Campaign for Access to Essential Medicines.[24] It promoted reduction in the cost of antiretroviral drugs by expanding the use of generics. It pressured pharmaceutical firms and worked for the establishment of more flexible world trade rules about patents and patent pools. It lobbied for funding—continuing, long-term, national, and international—to "scale up" HIV treatment and prevention. And it instituted community-based approaches to HIV care.

However, in keeping with the ethos of MSF and its distinctive cultural atmosphere, affirmations about its success in preventing and treating HIV/AIDS were overshadowed by self-examination and self-criticism. HIV/AIDS programs were growing more rapidly than any other MSF projects, utilizing as much as thirty-five percent of the financial resources of some operational centers. All signs pointed to the likelihood that the number of persons being cared for in these programs—indefinitely long-term care since treatment with antiretroviral drugs had become possible—would continually escalate. " If "today 35%, why not 75% tomorrow?"[25] Was that a justifiable allocation of MSF's material and human resources? Should MSF limit its involvement in this sphere of its action? If so, on what medical, practical, and ethical grounds?

MSF's advocacy for the prevention and treatment of HIV/AIDS sparked more controversy at the conference. Advocacy was acknowledged to be a vigorous form of *témoignage*, or witnessing, and viewed as an essential component of MSF's commitment to human rights. Nevertheless, what worried some La Mancha conferees was whether MSF's collaboration with local organizations, national governments, and international agencies in the fight against HIV/AIDS was jeopardizing its independence by politicizing its action. In the opinion of longtime member of MSF Eric Goemaere (its medical coordinator in South Africa, who had launched MSF's second HIV/AIDS program),[26] the creation of such programs had "basically reconciled MSF with politics":

> [W]e feel a much stronger legitimacy for "social and political changes" in the field of communicable diseases, where access to drugs and access to treatment are directly linked to political choices, than we ever felt in any war or refugee situation.
>
> With these programs we initiated, starting from the patient's bed up to the Campaign for Access to Essential Drugs, a subtle synergy, a well synchronized momentum, acting at very different political levels, which induced a dramatic change like never before in MSF's history.
>
> Looking back in time where we started from, AIDS treatment is five years later [*sic*] on everybody's agenda. . . . Rarely in our history have medical action and témoignage been coupled in such a synergistic way, legitimizing each other in a virtuous circle: hardly anyone thought 5 years go we would reach such results. . . .
>
> [O]ne should acknowledge that one of the key success factors has been a clear, legitimate, assumed MSF involvement in addressing the political roots of the problem, involvement which allowed us to identify and denounce them one by one . . . [as] barrier[s] . . . to treatment.[27]

Goemaere conceded that "the political responsibility" taken by MSF in this field raised the question of "how far" this might carry the organization into the sphere of political advocacy—since the "root causes" of HIV/AIDS "are linked to other, deeper root causes [that] like Russian dolls are contained within each other."[28]

Sexual Violence and the Limits of Humanitarian Action

Comparable questions were asked about MSF's response to other forms of suffering. One such situation to which repeated reference was made was the escalating occurrence of sexual violence in places where MSF was in the field—most notably in Darfur, Sudan, and in the Kivu region of the Democratic Republic of Congo, where the massive raping of women had become a weapon of war. Was it enough that MSF offered medical assistance and psychological counseling to rape victims? No, it is not doing enough, the audience agreed. "Humanitarian action never does enough," a seasoned MSFer declared. "We alleviate problems without solving them." We should not only be aware of these "limits of assistance," he went on to say. "We should "rage against [the] ongoing tragedy that these limits imply."[29]

More Cartoons

The exchanges that took place about the limits of humanitarian action, and about the decisions concerning the allocation of resources that it entails, called forth two more cartoons. In one, a man in agony, reduced to skin and bones by his suffering, is lying on the ground, pleading for help from a physician wearing a stethoscope and a surgical cap, who is looking down on him. "Please," the man entreats the doctor, "I am on the point to die [sic]." "Hum! are you coming [from] a war or hunger zone?" the physician asks him. "No," the prostrate man answers. "Sorry, I can do nothing for you," the physician responds.

In the other cartoon, headed "Limits of Advocacy," a diminutive man mounted on a little soapbox is holding a small megaphone to his mouth, through which he appears to be speaking, though he has no visible audience. He is standing within a bounded area, where he is miniaturized by the vast sky with its faraway sun that stretches beyond him.

The Risks of Humanitarian Action

Bearing witness, providing medical assistance, bringing public attention to the predicament of "people in precarious situations": these MSF missions could jeopardize the security of its patients and its staff. The report that MSF Holland had written on sexual violence in Darfur was cited as an example: the Sudanese government had arrested two MSF staff members for crimes against the state, namely, publishing false information.

Furthermore, it was agreed that in the wake of the increase in rebel movements, internecine tribal warfare, terrorism, and failed governments, the risks of humanitarian action had grown in recent years. Carrying personal identification as a member of a humanitarian organization or driving a vehicle marked with its insignia had once afforded protection. But no more.

Participants spoke grimly of five MSF colleagues murdered in Afghanistan in June 2004, of the kidnapping of two MSF staff members in the Democratic Republic of Congo, and of two kidnapped in Russia. Special attention was paid to what Kenny Gluck had to say about these happenings. In January 2001, Gluck was abducted by unidentified armed men while he was traveling in a humanitarian convoy in Chechnya, working as head of MSF Holland's North Caucasus project in Russia.[30]

In Gluck's spoken comments, and more fully in the article he contributed to *My Sweet La Mancha* volume, he articulated the risks and choices of humanitarian work, and where he stood in relation to them.

> The choices that MSF has made in assisting victims of violence, abuse and deliberate neglect have to be accompanied with the recognition that humanitarian action inherently involves risk not only because we respond to needs in dangerous places, but because the attempt to stand by and assist the victims of violence brings us in confrontation with those who control violence.
>
> The recognition that aid is inherently risky doesn't mean that everywhere it is dangerous, but it does mean that there is no means by which MSF can manage risk out of our programs.

Gluck's emphasis on safeguarding "the individual right to take risks" was sharply challenged by the general director of MSF France, Pierre Salignon: "Can our willingness to aid populations in the most extreme situations— sometimes when we no longer know how, as in Afghanistan and Iraq—justify *all* the risks we take and lead us to putting *our very lives* at risk? This question is intended to be provocative."[31]

As suggested by some contributions to the La Mancha debate, risk-taking was a collective matter, "particularly when it concerns the security of the teams. Without it, we risk maintaining the demagogic and deceptive myth of the *heroic* humanitarian; of seeing the development, as in other organizations, of *missionary* tendencies accepting *sacrificial* mindsets far removed from our humanitarian responsibilities, and finally, of cultivating a feeling of being *all powerful*."[32]

Humanitarianism "Militarized"

Salignon's reference to Afghanistan and Iraq, the kind of "war against terror" being waged there, and MSF's presence on the ground touched on another security risk much discussed at the conference. In Iraq and Afghanistan, U.S. and other armed forces were providing assistance to civilian populations— distributing food, water, and medicine—which the coalition explicitly called "humanitarian acts." In a 2001 speech to the leaders of American humanitarian NGOs, General Colin Powell had referred to NGOs like MSF as "an important part of our combat team . . . committed to the same, singular purpose to help humankind."[33]

As the spirited discussion at La Mancha made plain, most MSF members regarded any attempt to identify humanitarian action with military operations as exceedingly dangerous. Conflating the two seriously threatened one of MSF's basic principles: its commitment to "strict independence from all structures or powers, whether political, religious, economic, or other," and its "refusal to serve or be used as an instrument of foreign policy by any government."[34] Linking NGO humanitarian workers with troops blurred the distinction between them in ways that confused their respective auspices and roles, increasing the possibility that MSF staff might be kidnapped, wounded, or murdered.

The menacing Brax cartoon that emerged from this discussion of the dangers of "militarizing" humanitarian action portrayed a squat, fierce-looking soldier clad in a military uniform, a helmet, and combat boots, carrying a machine gun in his right hand and a first-aid kit, with what looks like a red cross insignia on it, in his left. He is identified in French, in a cartooned balloon, as a "salaried military." The French-language caption over his head reads: "The State Imposes a New Status of Humanitarian Worker."[35]

A Serenade

The La Mancha conference concluded on a high note. It was serenaded bilingually—in French and in English—by a chorus of nine MSF France members who dubbed themselves "the Parisian party committee." The two songs performed were based on the interwoven melodies of the Beatles' "Yellow Submarine," the French singer-songwriter Michel Polnareff's "On Ira Tous Au Paradis" ("We Will All Go to Paradise"), and "La Carmagnole" (a song dating from 1790 that was the hymn of the sans culottes, the radical militants of the revolutionary army during the early years of the French Revolution). Taking great poetic liberty with the lyrics, the choristers conveyed a musical message to the La Mancha assemblage that parodied MSF's idealism, revolutionary spirit, and optimism, its foibles and conflicts, and its failures to live up to its principles. As they sang, they returned self-mockingly to the refrain, "Ah ça ira! ça ira! ça ira!" ("Oh, things will be all right" / "It will be fine").

Rowan Gillies closed the conference with a positive statement about what the meeting had accomplished, and about the work of drafting a "La Mancha Agreement" based upon it that now lay ahead. "At least we ended up with a song," was his final remark.

The "La Mancha Agreement"

Immediately following the conference, MSF's International Council prepared a draft of a "La Mancha Agreement" text, which was then sent to the nineteen MSF sections for consideration at the annual meetings of their general assemblies.[36]

There was one overarching concern about the La Mancha document: the possibility that it would be construed to have as "high" a status as MSF's Charter and its Chantilly Principles, and considered as fundamental and morally binding. Lest the La Mancha Agreement be interpreted in this way, its drafters stated in its initial paragraphs:[37]

> **Our basic principles remain those expressed in the Charter and Chantilly documents.** These principles should be referred to when taking and reviewing decisions, with the acknowledgment that every decision is a singular act and not made by the mechanical application of principles.
>
> **Complementary to the Charter and the Chantilly Principles, the La Mancha Agreement is not a comprehensive description of MSF action.** It outlines aspects of our action on which we agree and feel are indispensable, taking into account our past experiences, and identifying current and future challenges to this action.

The La Mancha Agreement affirmed the strength of MSF's culture—its openness to diversity of opinion, its reliance on persons who "live and work in the countries of intervention"—while calling for MSF to strike a better balance between its commitments to "decentralization" and "coherence."

Threaded through the Agreement are references to situations in which MSF had to confront its limitations, mistakes, and failures. For example:

- The "massive diversion of humanitarian aid"—including MSF's— "for the benefit of war criminals" in 1994–1996 in Rwandan refugee camps, and in 1991–2003 in Liberia.
- The "multiplication of military interventions that included the deployment of a "humanitarian" component among their strategic goals (Kosovo 1999, Afghanistan 2001, Iraq 2003), and the challenge this posed for MSF's "understanding of risk," and its "independence from political influence."

- In Burundi, with the support of the Ministry of Health, MSF's backing of a medical cost-recovery program that involved payment by patients of a lump sum for all their care, which unintentionally "led to the exclusion of a great number of people from treatment both within and outside [MSF's] programs."
- And notwithstanding whatever "success" MSF's introduction of antiretroviral drugs in its HIV/AIDS programs and its "comprehensive approach to treatment, care and prevention" might constitute," the fact that its "medical action has not provided a solution to the global pandemic" of this "life-long disease."

Stocktaking

Unsurprisingly, the post hoc evaluation of La Mancha's content and achievements varied greatly, as personal communications I received from some of the conferees indicated. Here are extracts from two of them:

> At the moment, due to this meeting and the overall atmosphere surrounding it, we live in quite an "état de grace" [state of grace] inside the international MSF movement: meetings and discussions are held in a very positive way, three additional serious candidatures applied for the International Council Presidency, etc.
>
> In general, participants were quite happy with the way the meetings went and the level of discussion we had. I share these views, despite not for all parts of the meeting.[38]

> MSF people are balanced between two different perceptions:
> —one is that we have achieved a lot, by agreeing on many things that separated us in the past (in conflicts and on access to health care), by accepting some common challenges (diversity, initiatives, innovation), by acknowledging the fact that we are so interdependent that we should give accounts to one another, and by being willing to change our identity by including much more "Southern" [national] staff as members.
> —the others estimate that there is really nothing new or bold in all of this. It either takes stock of existing agreements, or expresses some shy [sic] intentions to go forward in governance, while the point on [national] staff is [the] usual MSF bla-bla and will take a very long time to be implemented.
>
> In a way, bottle [is either] half full or half empty. . . .

While in the airplane flying back home [from the La Mancha conference], I was trying to recall in which field, which subject was there anything new announced or decided. All the main—and by definition controversial points—I had come to discuss, like typically . . . the impact of a new modus operandi linked with HIV/AIDS in MSF or else, creation of new MSF sections, a new international model—all of these had been diluted and watered down to vague consensus on non-essential matters and unprecise [*sic*] issues. The whole preparatory method was desperately turned towards consensus building . . . [rather] than open debate and self-criticism. . . .

La Mancha was a self-congratulatory exercise on how much—and rich and accountable—MSF was. . . . No surprise that it has contaminated the whole movement with a certain good mood. . . . MSF probably needed a bit of enthusiastic wind.

But total absence of ambition, of risk strategy . . . of perception of the external world and its challenges do not make me confident for the future.[39]

PART IV / In South Africa

CHAPTER SEVEN

Struggling with HIV/AIDS

HIV/AIDS is the greatest health crisis the world faces today. In two decades, the pandemic has claimed nearly 30 million lives. An estimated 40 million people are now living with HIV/AIDS, 93% of them in developing countries, and 14,000 new infections occur daily. . . .

There is currently no cure for HIV infection . . . yet the development of life-saving anti-retroviral drugs has brought new hope. . . .

Of the 6 million people who currently urgently need anti-retroviral therapy in developing countries, fewer than 8% are receiving it. Without rapid access to properly managed treatment, these millions of women, children and men will die.

WORLD HEALTH ORGANIZATION, *TREATING 1 MILLION BY 2005*

Who would have predicted that the end of the last millennium would see the emergence of new pathogens and epidemics, when the medical world thought it had it all under control . . . ?

PETER PIOT, *NO TIME TO LOSE*

A pestilence isn't a thing made to man's measure; therefore we tell ourselves that pestilence is a mere bogy of the mind, a bad dream that will pass away. But it doesn't pass away and, from one bad dream to another, it is men who pass away. . . .

Dr. Rieux knew . . . that the plague bacillus never dies or disappears for good . . . [H]e knew that the tale he had to tell could not be one of a final victory. It could only be the record of what had to be done, and what assuredly would have to be once again in the never ending fight . . . by all who, while unable to be saints, but refusing to bow down to pestilences, strive their utmost to be healers.

ALBERT CAMUS, *THE PLAGUE*

In 2000–2001, MSF began to integrate the treatment of HIV/AIDS with anti-retroviral drugs into its programs and to engage in intensive witnessing and advocacy to promote access, at affordable prices, to these medications, which are essential for treating the disease. The decision to do this was not arrived at quickly or easily. It was reached incrementally, movement-wide—preceded and accompanied by great hesitancy, strong resistance, and intense debate about the capacity of MSF to deal with an epidemic of this magnitude, which would entail undertaking the lifelong, intricate care of multitudes afflicted with a complex, chronic, and incurable disease, which was ultimately fatal, and about the feasibility of doing so in the characteristically resource-poor, economically and socially disadvantaged settings in which the disease was especially rampant.

The history of MSF has been coterminous with the global emergence of many new infectious diseases, and the reemergence of numerous old ones.[1] None, however, compared with the HIV/AIDS pandemic, which the medical scientist and public-health expert Helen Epstein has judged "the most serious health crisis of our time, and perhaps in all human history."[2] Moreover, MSF was not accustomed to dealing with long-term illnesses. It specialized in what one member called "a medicine of emergency" focused on "rescuing victims of conflict and the wounded of war," whose symbolic and substantive quintessence was epitomized by "the surgical act":

> Historically, MSF was not ready to battle head-on with AIDS when it occurred during the 1980s. It rapidly set into motion measures to counter the transmissible aspects of the epidemic. But its conception of humanitarian medicine remained rigid, and aspects of prevention and of public health, and therefore of access to care more generally were not yet integrated into it.[3]

It took a number of converging factors for MSF to break through what it described as its "ideological and sociological impermeability to any form of activism concerning HIV/AIDS," or even to recognize the potentially revolutionary implications of antiretroviral drugs for its treatment.[4]

One of these factors was the initiative taken by Paul Cawthorne, a nurse, and David Wilson, a physician, working for MSF in Thailand, which had one of the highest rates of HIV/AIDS in Southeast Asia during the 1990s. Partly because the early cases of HIV/AIDS there occurred primarily among men who had sexual relations with men, and partly because they were a gay couple, Cawthorne and Wilson became involved with the plight of homosexuals afflicted with AIDS. They went on to create a program of home-based care for AIDS patients that emphasized psychological and social support. Then, in collaboration with a network of local NGOs, they tackled issues associated with obtaining antiretroviral drugs and making them accessible to hospital and home patients in their care. Before MSF had decided to pay for antiretroviral treatment, they smuggled a small supply of these drugs into Thailand with the help of a sympathetic airline steward. In 1999, the first AIDS patients were put on treatment; and in 2000, an MSF antiretroviral treatment program was inaugurated.

Cawthorne's and Wilson's initiative had an impact on MSF that extended far beyond Thailand. The moment was opportune. Seeing "colleagues and friends" on the national staff of numerous missions "get sick and die from HIV/AIDS without being able to do anything" was an emotional experience, moving MSF members to make changes that enabled MSF to enter the fight against AIDS. As the head of the MSF mission in Rwanda wrote in 2001:

Wednesday, Georges, employed for years by MSF, hospitalized for three weeks without knowing why, telephoned me at the end of the afternoon, and told me in a quivering voice that he finally knew what he had, but did not wish to talk to me about it on the telephone.

The next day around six P.M., the co-med [medical coordinator] and I went to the hospital. I found [Georges] to be as feverish as he was a few days ago, but worse in every respect. He was much thinner, his face was sunken, his expression was sad, and he had difficulty breathing. . . . The physician in charge of his case confirmed that . . . Georges had AIDS. . . .

He is a friend whom I have known for eighteen months. I take his hands because words fail me. . . . I try to raise his morale, but I don't have the courage to come up with formulas like "as long as there is life . . . "

. . . I have had enough . . . of seeing my colleagues at work, my friends, waste away and die, while they work in a medical humanitarian organization. He is the fourth one in 12 months. Arthur, dead unexpectedly; Hervé, who took leave after leave, and then, died one week after we learned that he had AIDS; Marc, dead after a month of suffering in our view. . . . And now Georges who will die soon. . . . I have had enough. I cannot let Georges die without trying to do something. I feel miserable facing him and the national staff to whom I must say: "No, MSF does not take charge of [antiretroviral] triple therapy for its national staff." Why? "Because we cannot take care of everyone, we prefer to take care of no one?

Because we cannot privilege the national staff in relationship to the population? . . . Because MSF may not stay in this country, and so should it launch a treatment for life that it cannot ensure? Because it costs a lot? Because, because, because . . . " This is the discourse that we stick to, and as the [head of mission], I must convey it to the staff, while it revolts me. I understand this medical point of view, cold and sharp as a scalpel. But I cannot accept it! Isn't the role of a physician to prolong life? To give time to the sick person? It is possible here in this country to prolong Georges's life with triple therapy, or at least to try. Let's give him time![5]

As it became increasingly clear that countries in sub-Saharan Africa were the most drastically affected by AIDS, the emotional and moral pressure on MSF to confront the epidemic grew greater:

The latest UN AIDS report . . . gives an idea of the gravity of the situation [wrote Gorik Ooms, who had headed MSF Belgium missions in Burundi and in Mali]. The eight countries of the world most affected by AIDS are in southern Africa: Botswana comes first. If the risk of HIV transmission doesn't change, 85% of all boys of Botswana aged 15 today will sooner or later die of AIDS. In the year 2020, normally there would be 180,000 inhabitants in Botswana aged 35 to 40 years.

But because of AIDS, there will only be 60,000. Two-thirds of this age group, future farmers, merchants, doctors, nurses, teachers, but most of all parents, will have died. They will have died too young to have raised their children as independent adults, too young to have passed on their knowledge of how to work the land, or their modest businesses, too young to contribute their knowledge and experience fully to their community, too soon to help a next generation to accomplish higher studies. A decapitated society. . . .

No war, genocide, earthquake, flood or other epidemic has ever had an equally devastating impact on a nation [boldface in original]. . . . Calling AIDS a mega-atomic time-bomb would be an understatement.

"Botswana? Oh well, Botswana. That little country." In the classification of the countries most affected by AIDS, Botswana is followed by Swaziland, Lesotho, Zambia, South Africa, Namibia, and Malawi. Mozambique comes eleventh, after Kenya and the Central African Republic. . . .

We're not talking about a small country, we are talking about a subcontinent. More than a subcontinent, central Africa will follow.

"The year 2020? Oh well. Far away isn't it?" Sadly, but no, it isn't. . . .

Take a deep breath, close your eyes and try to imagine. Imagine this subcontinent as it is today, or rather as it was some years ago, focus on the people aged 35
to 40 years, and wipe half of them away. They will be dead! . . .

This is the future of southern Africa. This is our future! Our future? Indeed.
A medical relief agency that does not massively react against the worst medical
tragedy of our times, no longer deserves to exist! A medical relief agency that
accepts the challenge will be carried away in a maelstrom of infinite needs. We
can choose between denial or a big jump into the maelstrom. There isn't really a
choice, is there?[6]

Individuals like Gorik Ooms acted as catalysts in impelling MSF to commit
to treating AIDS. In the case of MSF Belgium, for example, the volition and the
synergistic relationship of Ooms, Alex Parisel, and Eric Goemaere, its executive director, galvanized the section into launching pilot projects offering a
full range of treatments for HIV/AIDS and helped forge a common policy integrating the HIV/AIDS programs incipiently developing throughout the movement.[7] The HIV/AIDS program that Goemaere inaugurated in the township
of Khayelitsha, in Cape Town, South Africa, was pathbreaking. It eventually
became an international model for dealing with HIV/AIDS in resource-poor
settings. But before it did, obstacles arising from within both MSF and South
African society itself had to be surmounted.

Eric Goemaere's Exploratory Trip to South Africa

From March to August 1999, Eric Goemaere had acted as the senior medical
advisor to MSF's Campaign for Access to Essential Medicines, of which Bernard
Pécoul, a member of MSF France, was executive director.[8] In concert with Alex
Parisel and Francine Matthys, then medical director of MSF Belgium, Pécoul
persuaded Goemaere to go to South Africa in August 1999 to explore developing an MSF HIV/AIDS project there. In their view, this undertaking had great
symbolic as well as empirical importance, not only because of the enormity
of the AIDS epidemic in South Africa, but also because of the obstacles in
that country to acknowledging its magnitude and causes, and to obtaining
the drugs needed to treat the disease and making them widely available. In
Parisel's opinion, Goemaere, a "man of experience, of the 1968 [radical po-
litical] generation," had the background to appraise the South African situa-

tion, which appeared to call for linking advocacy with medical humanitarian action.[9]

Goemaere arrived in Johannesburg in August 1999 with one suitcase and Lonely Planet's guidebook *South Africa, Lesotho & Swaziland*. Lacking a cell phone, he bought one after deplaning. His sole contact in the country was a former member of MSF France who had been a coordinator in South Africa for the assistance to refugees from Mozambique, which MSF had previously provided,[10] and had settled in Johannesburg after marrying a woman from Soweto, the city's most populous black residential area.

Goemaere began his exploration by paying visits to politically liberal physicians at clinics in the township of Alexandra who had fought against apartheid. Although they were interested in working with MSF, they did not have access to zidovudine (or azidothymidine—AZT), one of the first HIV/AIDS drugs approved, which was especially recommended to help prevent the transmission of the virus from mother to child.[11] "Naïvely," Goemaere remembers, "I next went to meet the director of the HIV programs in Pretoria, who blocked me from using any antiretroviral drugs. This was the first sign of a very serious problem." Subsequently, he made a futile attempt to obtain an appointment with the national minister of health, Dr. Mantombazana ("Manto") Tshabalala-Msimang, who declined to see him, signaling that she had never heard of MSF. The director for HIV/AIDS in the Health Ministry warned him that although it might be possible for him to proceed with plans to prevent transmission of HIV/AIDS from mother to child, the South African government prohibited his going forward with antiretroviral treatment for persons with AIDS.

Disappointed and discouraged, Goemaere telephoned Parisel at his MSF Belgium director's office and said the only sensible thing was for him to return to Brussels. At this critical juncture he received a message that led him to cancel his plane reservation for Europe. It was from Zackie Achmat, inviting Gormaere to meet with him in Cape Town.

Achmat was a former African National Congress–associated anti-apartheid activist, an engaged gay rights proponent, and an HIV-positive man. He was the charismatic leader of the Treatment Action Campaign (TAC), which he had founded on International Human Rights Day, December 10, 1998. TAC's goals included raising consciousness about the scale of the HIV/AIDS epidemic in South Africa and promoting openness about it. Its larger aim was to make treatment universally available. This could only be accomplished by breaking through the "denialist" stance toward AIDS adopted by South Africa's president, Thabo Mbeki, Minister of Health Tshabalala-Msimang, and the African National Congress (ANC) political party, of which Mbeki was the leader.

In December 1999, TAC was becoming a powerfully effective civil society movement. It was originally composed mainly of middle-class, urban white and "Coloured" members,[12] and very few black Africans. But it was beginning to attract young, urban black Africans with a secondary education and poor, unemployed black African women, many of whom were HIV-positive mothers. In January 1999, the Health Department of the Provincial Government of the Western Cape had initiated a program called Prevention of Mother to Child Transmission of HIV/AIDS in Khayelitsha, the poorest and largest township in the metropolitan area of Cape Town, where, out of an estimated population of between 350,000 and 400,000 persons, at least 40,000 adults were HIV-infected. Achmat told Goemaere that TAC was considering introducing treatment with antiretroviral drugs into the program. This ran counter to President Mbeki's obdurate refusal to recognize the gravity of the AIDS epidemic, or even that AIDS is caused by the human immunodeficiency virus (HIV), the skepticism about the effectiveness of antiretrovirals that he and the members of his government publicly expressed, and their emphasis on the toxicity of these drugs.

Immediately following the Goemaere–Achmat meeting, a tornado hit the Cape Flats. After seeing the devastation that the storm had left in its wake in Gugulethu, another Cape Town township, Goemaere telephoned MSF in Brussels to request emergency aid. Within a week, supplies (including five thousand blankets) arrived in Gugulethu, because as he wryly put it, "we are good at that kind of thing." Goemaere knew that "MSF [did] not dispute obvious emergency interventions," and so, "in a way," he later admitted, he had used the tornado to force MSF Belgium's headquarters in Brussels to "put a foot into the township" in order to "buy [himself] some time to further explore what meaningful work MSF could do there with AIDS." Neither Goemaere nor MSF was known in Gugulethu, but people were impressed with what he had made happen and began to ask, "Who is this guy?"[13]

Goemaere began to visit the Khayelitsha township every day. There he "tried to force the door" by speaking with the nurses and the few doctors who staffed its clinics. But he sensed that they had no interest in participating in an MSF HIV/AIDS program. One exception was Dr. Hermann Reuter, a young, white, politically radical activist physician, born in Namibia and raised in

South Africa. Reuter was a graduate of the medical school of the University of Stellenbosch in the Western Cape.[14] He had been recruited into TAC by Zackie Achmat and worked for TAC in Khayelitsha, where he was distributing condoms and circulating a petition for access to antiretroviral treatment. Both he and Achmat had once belonged to the Trotskyist Marxist Workers' Tendency of the African National Congress in the anti-apartheid struggle. Reuter said his involvement with HIV/AIDS through TAC gave him a chance to contribute to a movement as vital to the fight for human rights as the anti-apartheid struggle.[15]

Saadiq Karien, a physician affiliated with the provincial Ministry of Health, introduced Goemaere to the nurse-coordinator in charge of the Khayelitsha clinic where he was working. "I received only a 'lukewarm' reception from her," Goemaere said—adding with self-mocking MSF humor, "I was not welcomed as a savior from death!" "I was a problem for her, not a solution." She felt that what Goemaere wanted to do would give the overburdened nurses extra work by attracting fatally and inexorably ill AIDS sufferers to the clinic, where they would infect other patients with the disease. In Goemaere's view, she and most of her nurse-colleagues were "confusing" being HIV-positive with having terminal AIDS, and did not realize how many of their patients were already infected with HIV.[16]

A poignant indicator of the social isolation Goemaere experienced during this period occurred on December 10, 1999, the day MSF received the Nobel Prize in Oslo. Goemaere was in a shop in Cape Town where he was photocopying some papers. On the store's overhead television set, he saw an image of James Orbinski delivering the Nobel Prize acceptance speech on behalf of MSF. "Do you know that guy?" the proprietor asked Goemaere, who replied that he did. This was the only person in Cape Town with whom he had an opportunity to speak about MSF receiving the Nobel Peace Prize, or to mention his connection with it.

Goemaere vacillated between feeling very dispirited, on the one hand—as though he was continually "going back to square one"—and on the other, being tenaciously determined to go forward with creating an MSF-supported demonstration program in South Africa. When he traveled back to Brussels in mid-September for a brief visit, he reported to his colleagues that he thought he saw something promising in the contact with Zackie Achmat and TAC, and in the Prevention of Mother to Child Transmission (PMTCT) of HIV/AIDS program that the Western Cape Department of Health had begun in Khayelitsha, which he hoped might provide an opening for an MSF intervention. Although some staff members expressed concern about the political dangers for MSF of close relations with an activist group like TAC, Goemaere was given a "green light" by the Brussels office to proceed. His wife and two children moved to Cape Town at Christmastime in 1999 to join him—a decision that indicated a long-term commitment.

The Inception of the Khayelitsha Program

A breakthrough occurred in April 2000 when the Provincial Administration of the Western Cape permitted MSF to open government-run clinics for patients with HIV/AIDS in three of Khayelitsha's community health centers: Site C, Site B, and Michael Mapongwana (Michael M). Goemaere recruited Hermann Reuter to work as a physician in these clinics. The breakthrough never would have come to pass, Goemaere has testified, without Dr. Fareed Abdullah, who had initiated the Prevention of Mother to Child Transmission (PMTCT) program set up by the Western Cape Health Department in 1999 and directed the HIV/AIDS programs in the province. Among the first to welcome Goemaere to Khayelitsha, he "was key in sealing the [Provincial Government–MSF] agreement." This took courage, because Abdullah was also an African National Congress branch leader, and his support for the MSF clinics and their conception of dealing with HIV/AIDS was treated as a "sell-out" by the South African presidency. "If anyone, [Abdullah] deserves the credit for making this happen despite national politics," Goemaere says. Goemaere also had a more passive form of cooperation from the provincial minister of health, whom he described as "a very humble man—a bricklayer by training—who used to say to me, 'I do not understand much of what you are telling me, but do your job, and I will do mine, and everything will be sorted out.' "[17]

With relative alacrity, Goemaere was able to move the PMTCT program in the three community health centers into a new phase. This entailed collaborating with the School of Public Health and Family Medicine of the University of Cape Town to design a system for monitoring mothers and children postnatally and developing PMTCT training courses. But instituting a "feasible, affordable, and replicable" model program for AIDS treatment in those primary care clinics proved to be an impediment-ridden process.[18] Obtaining AIDS drugs at an affordably low cost and making them available to patients—with the cooperation, rather than the opposition of the multinational pharmaceutical industry and the South African government—called for advocacy. Chiefly in alliance with TAC, the MSF Khayelitsha project joined in public demonstrations and campaigns covered by the media to draw attention to milestone court cases that could make antiretroviral drugs more available, and ultimately universally accessible, in South Africa through its public-health system.

In 1998, the thirty-nine pharmaceutical companies grouped under the South African Pharmaceutical Manufacturers Association (PIASA) had sued the government of South Africa to prevent the implementation of a law to facilitate access to AIDS drugs at a low cost. The companies accused the government of violating patent protections guaranteed by international intellectual property rules. In 2001, in response to the "Drop the Case" press conferences and massive petitions mobilized by TAC, in which the MSF group took part, the pharmaceutical companies withdrew their lawsuit. And along with TAC, MSF also played a role in the South African Constitutional Court's July 2002 decision in the case of *Minister of Health and others v. Treatment Action Campaign and others*, which ordered the South African government to make an approved drug for the prevention of mother-to-child transmission of HIV available in the public-health sector, and to set a timetable for the rollout of a national PMTCT program.

The Khayelitsha project's advocacy was unprecedented in MSF's history. This was noted in the 2002 "consultancy report" on its operational research activities commissioned by MSF Belgium:

> MSF's antiretroviral care project in Khayelitsha is special in several respects. Whereas a simulation by M. Haacker of the IMF shows that economically speaking, South Africa probably would be able to provide ART nation-wide—if at a generic price level—political authorities have been notoriously resisting the concept of anti-retroviral drug use. In this context, MSF actively campaigns for access to anti-retroviral drugs in alliance with AIDS-activists from the South African Treatment Action Campaign (TAC) and other groups. Never before [has] MSF developed such a direct and sustained political action targeting national and international decision makers. Never before [has] MSF [gotten] in such a close alliance with an activist campaign to achieve this kind of political aim.[19]

Goemaere was aware of how this advocacy might violate MSF's commitment to the apolitical principles of independence, impartiality, and neutrality—all the more so because TAC was part of an alliance with the African

National Congress, the Congress of South African Trade Unions, and the South African Communist Party. This "raise[d] the question of political solidarity in the humanitarian field," he realized—"a border that MSF decided never to cross." He made sure that the relationship maintained with TAC was not "fusional," and that he recognized that "the mandates" of TAC and MSF were "different." For example, in the court cases against the government, MSF provided affidavits, but was not among the plaintiffs. And it refrained from being drawn into radical civil-society issues with which TAC was concerned (such as TAC's anti-eviction and anti-privatization campaigns). "At that time, we considered that MSF did not have added value on these issues, . . . not being part of South African civil society," Goemaere explained, and went on to say, "we avoided commenting on the 'daily news' to be able to justify, on the other hand, [being] . . . outspoken when it touched . . . our expertise field."[20]

Nevertheless, the Brussels headquarters of MSF Belgium continued to caution Goemaere about the danger of Khayelitsha's advocacy becoming politicized. At one point, an expert in health education sent to Khayelitsha by the Brussels office as a consultant drafted a report in which she charged that political intervention in Khayelitsha violated the axial humanitarian principles of MSF's Charter. Before she delivered the report to MSF Belgium's Brussels headquarters, Goemaere responded by writing a "counter-summary" to her conclusions, with the help of Hermann Reuter and Colwyn Poole, the local MSF Resource Center coordinator, a Coloured South African, and a TAC activist.

In May 2001, with the agreement of the Western Cape Provincial Department of Health, the MSF program in Khayelitsha began to provide a very small number of AIDS patients with HAART therapy—a three-drug regimen of high-acting antiretroviral drugs: Zidovudine, or azidothymidine (AZT), Lamivudine, and Nevirapine. The MSF group requested the technical assistance of the School of Public Health and Family Medicine at the University of Cape Town to support and evaluate the program.[21] The protocol of what was defined as this pilot, operational research project was approved by the Research Ethics Committee of the South African Medical Association. In September, MSF signed an agreement with the Fundação Oswaldo Cruz (Fiocruz), a public research body funded by the Brazilian government, which allowed MSF to purchase the generic forms of these antiretroviral drugs produced by Farmanguinhos, a Fiocruz pharmaceutical laboratory attached to the Brazilian Ministry of Health. In that same month, the South African Medicines Control Council authorized MSF to use the Brazilian generic versions of the antiretroviral drugs; and 177 patients had started antiretroviral/HAART drug therapy by May 2002.[22] Using the Brazilian-produced generic drugs reduced the price per patient per day from US$22.00 to US$1.55.[23]

I decided to make the Khayelitsha program a site of my firsthand field research into MSF. A number of factors influenced this choice. Foremost among them were the location of the program in Africa where such a large proportion of MSF's projects were situated; the devastating incidence of the HIV/AIDS pandemic in Africa south of the Sahara; the major transition and innovations it required of MSF to prevent and treat this incurable infectious disease; and the plethora of social, cultural, economic, and political issues, as well as the medical challenges, that such a commitment involved.

My professional history also contributed to my going to Khayelitsha—most particularly, the extensive research I had conducted throughout the 1960s and 1970s in Belgium and in the ex-Belgian Congo (later Zaïre, and now the Democratic Republic of Congo).[24] As a consequence, I felt a strong, positive identification with Africa; and I hoped that I could bring social and cultural knowledge acquired in another African society that would be relevant to my participant observation in South Africa. In addition, the Khayelitsha program operated under the aegis of MSF Belgium, with which I was familiar, and where I was known because of the professional and public notice that my research there had received. In fact, I had first met Eric Goemaere in Brussels during his term as executive director of MSF Belgium, before he became the head of MSF's Mission in South Africa. Our acquaintanceship emboldened me to contact him about the possibility of spending some time in Khayelitsha, and it played a role both in the access that he gave me to the program and in his willingness to act as my chief informant within it.

I made three successive trips to Khayelitsha, in 2002, 2003, and again in 2005, which allowed me to witness its HIV/AIDS program in action—how it had evolved from its inception, and how it was continuing to develop. What follows in the next chapter is an account, drawn from my field notes, of what I observed, learned, and experienced in that setting.

CHAPTER EIGHT

In Khayelitsha

With its sparkling and churning two oceans, rocky coastline, terraced hills dotted with white stucco and pastel-colored houses and villas, ancient mountains, luxuriant foliage, massive arrays of blooming flowers, and radiant light, Cape Town must be one of the most beautiful places on the face of the earth. During the early days of my initial trip here, I wondered where persons of more modest means, the underprivileged and the poor, and the majority of black and colored Africans lived. . . . But then I made my first visit to the township of Khayelitsha. . . .

The highway along which one drives to Khayelitsha is splendidly paved. . . . Nothing prepares you for the world you enter when your car crosses an overpass and turns into the streets of the township. The fact that these labyrinthine streets, like the highway, are smoothly paved seems incongruous—even ironic—in this crowded, poverty-stricken universe of corrugated iron shacks, most of which are without running water or electricity.

Nevertheless, Khayelitsha pulsates with vigorous activity. During the daylight hours, an unending procession of women, men, and children move swiftly and gracefully through its streets. Interspersed with all the people on foot are individuals riding bicycles, an occasional bus, and numerous cars that serve as taxis in this area where public transportation is scarce. The township contains schools, medical clinics, shops (many of them housed in shacks that are labeled with crudely painted, often amusing, promotional signs), an array of open-air stalls from which food and other merchandise is sold, a supermarket that does not seem to be operating, and a large number of churches and funeral parlors. I have been told that in this township . . . on Saturdays, the streets are filled with funeral processions, predominantly organized around commemorating, mourning, and burying those who have died from HIV/AIDS. And on Sundays, it is said, virtually "everyone goes to church."

The MSF Khayelitsha project offices are located in a worn concrete building, one floor above an arcade of shops, near police headquarters, and directly in front of a fruit stand from which cascades of oranges hang like curtains. Recorded African music blasts uninterruptedly from the stand at full volume, filling everything around it, including MSF headquarters, with its reverberations. . . .

The door to the MSF offices is locked and grilled. To enter, you have to be buzzed into its large anteroom, decorated with TAC [Treatment Action Campaign] as well as MSF posters, by a receptionist who is seated behind a plain, secondhand desk. MSF occupies office space on the left side of this reception area, and TAC on the right.

The MSF area is shabbily carpeted and consists of a series of doorless, cubicle-like working spaces demarcated by brightly colored painted partitions. It has a busy, unpretentious, highly social, pleasantly disordered ambience, with helter-skelter displays of posters and notices of various kinds, and a pell-mell of documents on its various desks. There is a central telephone line, but most of the incoming and outgoing calls are made via the cell phones that all the staff members carry with them. They work on laptop computers, which they bring to the office each day and take home at night.

The office closes at sundown. The prevailing rule is for all personnel to lock up the premises and leave at that time. It is strictly observed because when night falls, the violence that suffuses Khayelitsha intensifies.[1]

In 2002–2003, the HIV prevalence in Khayelitsha, measured by a mother-to-child transmission survey made in prenatal clinics, was estimated to be 25.5 percent; and as many as sixty percent of the persons who were HIV-positive were coinfected with tuberculosis. Each of the three Khayelitsha HIV/AIDS clinics (Site C, Site B, and Michael M) was leanly staffed with one permanent physician, one "sessional" physician, who worked there a day or two a week, two nurses, and two counselors. By the end of 2003, they were seeing more than eighteen hundred patients a month, including six hundred who were receiving antiretroviral (ARV) therapy. Nurses were the cornerstone of the clinic work. They were responsible for most of the continuing and follow-up care of both ARV and non-ARV patients. Physicians dealt primarily with desperately ill patients in advanced clinical stages of AIDS who were not receiving ARV medications. They also initiated ARV treatment and dealt with the side effects of the medications, and problems of resistance to the drugs that occurred. The counselors' work centered on preparing patients for ARV treatment, furthering their understanding of the disease, promoting their adherence to the drug regimen, and involving them in support groups. Plans were being made to increase the number of recipients of ARV therapy, but the main obstacle to doing so—even more than problems of funding, or of obtaining a sufficient supply of high-quality, low-cost ARV drugs—was the need to enlarge the health staff, and the difficulty of recruiting and retaining a sufficient number of well-trained nurses and physicians, who were motivated to care for, and work with, HIV/AIDS patients.

"HIV POSITIVE" T-Shirts

The buoyant impact of the growing availability of treatment and the collaborative activism of MSF and TAC on patients' outlook was one of the most striking things about the atmosphere pervading the three clinics that I observed in Khayelitsha. Many patients had not only broken through the silence and the sense of shame about their HIV status in which they had once been enveloped; they also wore T-shirts emblazoned with the affirmation that they were HIV-positive, and with exhortations to join the national struggle against AIDS, and for its treatment.

I was told that the first "HIV POSITIVE" T-shirts had been printed at the beginning of 1999, and that it was Zackie Achmat who had come up with the idea and their design. Allegedly he was influenced by the apocryphal story about the king of Denmark wearing a yellow star to publicly manifest his identification with Jews during the Nazi occupation of his country.[2] The underlying conception of the "HIV POSITIVE" T-shirts was that they could be worn by people of all backgrounds, whether or not they were HIV-positive, to show their solidarity with people who were. The shirts, which were originally issued by TAC, rapidly appeared on the South African scene in many colors, with different slogans and messages emblazoned on them. By the time that I made my field trips to Khayelitsha, tens of thousands of people were wearing these shirts, which had become iconic.

I was given two of them. One was bright green. "HIV POSITIVE" was printed in large black letters on its front, and on its back, the call for there to be "1000 People on ARVS in Khayelitsha 2004," and in this way to "Move with the times"—an exhortation identified as the goal of the MSF "Khayelitsha ARV Programme 2001–2004." The other T-shirt was bright yellow. Imprinted on its front, in very large black letters, was "HIV POSITIVE," and below it, in smaller print, the phrase "Issued By Treatment Action Campaign (TAC)." The entire back of the shirt was filled with an elaborately laid-out message printed in red and black:

Give women a
CHANCE
Give children a
CHANCE
TAC
Treatment Action Campaign
DEMANDS
a Treatment Plan
and a National
Mother-to-Child-
HIV Transmission
Prevention Programme
NOW

Khayelitsha Nurses

Clad in dark blue cotton dresses whose skirts fell well below their knees, wearing military-looking epaulettes on their shoulders,[3] and the silver and blue badge of the South African Nursing Council pinned to their uniforms, the Khayelitsha nurses with whom I conversed in September 2002 were committed to their HIV/AIDS-associated clinical activities. They expressed satisfaction with what they and their nurse-colleagues had accomplished working under the auspices of the Western Cape Health Department, MSF, and TAC.

Judith Z,[4] for example, the nurse-midwife who managed the mother-to-child transmission prenatal clinic, described the program she was supervising—which included testing mothers and children for HIV, the provision of pre- and postnatal antiretroviral treatment,[5] educating the mothers about feeding their babies,[6] and about the use of condoms, and follow-up care for mothers and babies over a period of twelve months. She also praised the support group that mothers had formed, through which they "educated and empower[ed] each other." This group of mothers teaching mothers-to-be, she said, were not only "doing wonders for themselves . . . but for everyone"— helping the nurses, as well as the mothers, she implied.

Judith Z reminisced about her initial reactions to the arrival of MSF in Khayelitsha in 1999. She had been working there since 1991, and she was "not keen" about it, she admitted, when rumors began to circulate that MSF was planning to conduct an HIV/AIDS program in Khayelitsha. She knew nothing about MSF. Why were they launching this in our community, she wondered. At that time, the nurses hardly knew anything about HIV/AIDS, she said, and yet MSF was "rushing" to begin a program there. The nurses were anxious about what this would entail when they already had so many patients to see and so much work to do. What would happen to our mothers, they worried, if and when they discovered they were HIV-positive. The atmosphere became one of "chaos" and "pandemonium," Judith Z said. Nevertheless, all the nurses stayed on; the program was started. "MSF has helped us a lot with education and medication," she affirmed. "All our troubles have been washed away." If mothers have a problem they say, "I have an appointment with MSF," or "I am going to TAC," and they are seen. "They feel confident and strong."

Victoria D,[7] who was trained as a psychiatric nurse, and was a senior member of the nursing staff at Khayalitsha's Site B clinic, described what it had been like to work on the medical and surgical trauma units of a Cape Town hospital before she became affiliated with this MSF HIV/AIDS unit. In the hospital, she had seen a considerable number of HIV/AIDS patients. Nurses did not know what to do for them. They viewed HIV/AIDS as a deadly disease—one from which patients would die in a few months. According to her account, these patients were neglected. Doctors did not even want to put their stethoscopes on such patients' chests; their diarrhea could not be stopped; and pharmacists did not order medications for their opportunistic infections. She considered this abandonment of persons with HIV/AIDS and discrimination against them to be "ungodly."

In April 2000, Victoria D noticed an advertisement for the position she now held at the Site B clinic, and came to Khayelitsha to be interviewed for it. "I felt that this was my work," she declared—"part of wanting to bring hope, and belief."[8] We started here in one room, she continued, and built our own resources. We didn't put up a sign at first. But people were curious, and they could see what we were doing. They saw that people could "disclose" their HIV status; that confidentiality was maintained; that doctors were spending time examining patients fully; and that they had medications available. "I say, 'Thank God' for MSF, and this pilot project,'" she exclaimed. "The [national] government has been so stubborn, I want to strangle them!"

At the close of our conversation, when I asked her to describe in more specific detail her current work, she replied that she did many procedures, which included treating opportunistic infections, and delivering antiretroviral treatment according to standard protocols. She laughingly described herself as "a half-doctor," and then more soberly affirmed, "I love my work—and yet I recognize that it is only a drop in the ocean."

The Ulwazi Project

On the morning of September 16, 2002, I attended a training session for a group of twelve women and two men who had volunteered to participate in a program called Ulwazi (the Xhosa word for "knowledge"), started in 2001, sponsored by MSF, and developed by TAC. Its aims were to advance education about HIV/AIDS, its prevention and treatment, and to destigmatize the disease by fostering openness about it and positive attitudes toward the HIV-positive.

Vuyiseka Dubula, a young South African woman, had played a cardinal role in the genesis of this program. Her involvement in HIV/AIDS-associated issues, she recounts,[9] began in March 2001, when she had a chance meeting with Eric Goemaere in a McDonald's restaurant in Cape Town where, at the time, she was employed as a waitress. Goemaere had taken his son and daughter there for a snack, and in the course of a conversation with her, Dubula learned that he was an "HIV doctor" connected with MSF who was based in Khayelitsha. His parting words to her as he left the restaurant were, "You don't belong here," intimating that she had the intelligence and ability to work other than as a waitress, and suggesting that she might consider working for MSF someday.

Dubula became curious about HIV, and in June, out of "sheer curiosity," she went to the MSF clinic in Khayelitsha to be tested for HIV. She discovered that she was HIV-positive. "Why did I go?" she lamented after she learned this, and for the first time she began to feel ill, "largely for psychological reasons," she supposed. It took a while for her to summon up the courage to begin to go as a patient to a clinic in Khayelitsha where MSF had started treating people with HIV/AIDS with antiretroviral therapy. There, she met a volunteer worker who talked knowledgeably about HIV, "as if she were a doctor," and who walked with her over to the MSF office, which was only two minutes away from the clinic, where she met Goemaere again. She was still employed at McDonald's, but as a consequence of her second meeting and conversation with Goemaere, she left her waitressing job there and began to work with a group of volunteers at the MSF Khayelitsha clinic. It was a small group at that point, supported by TAC, which placed special emphasis on "giving voice" to the many young women with HIV/AIDS, and "giving them hope" that in spite of their HIV-positive status, they could still have healthy children in the future who were HIV/AIDS-free. "Myself included," she added, because "I was twenty-two years old then." The group grew in size; it became more formalized; and its members were trained by physicians such as Goemaere, "like little doctors" (as Dubula put it), to educate and support others with HIV/AIDS. In turn, those whom they trained educated and supported still others, expanding their activities beyond the confines of Khayelitsha and health communities to other locales, and to prisons, churches, and schools.[10]

The Ulwazi group that met on the morning that I made my observations assembled around a large table in the conference room located in the suite of the MSF and TAC Khayelitsha offices. They were all HIV-positive, and wore T-shirts that announced their HIV status; and a number of them were patients in the Khayelitsha clinics.

The style of the meeting was testimonial, confessional, and affirmative. Its vocabulary and ambience seemed to me to be influenced by African oral tradition and praise poems, and also by African Christianity and churchgoing. The session began with the group leader asking the participants to write key details about themselves, their families, their education, and their relationship to HIV/AIDS on a slip of paper, saying how they had come to know of MSF and what they enjoyed and hoped for in life. Most of the morning was given over to oral presentations made by each of the volunteers (in English or Xhosa), based on their written notes. The leader went first. In essence, this is what she said:

I was born in 1973. I was brought up by my grandmother and grandfather. We experienced hardship. I had to go to the forest to fetch wood, and to the river to fetch water for washing and cooking. I went to a nearby school in the Eastern Cape. I became pregnant, and gave birth to a baby boy, who was brought up by my grandmother. I became pregnant once more, and this time I gave birth to a baby girl. She is ten years old now. I passed my matriculation in 1993 in a college of education. I began to teach in a private school. I had a brother and children to take care of. In 1999 I came to Cape Town. . . . That was my first time in a big city. I became pregnant and tested HIV-positive. The baby died, but not of AIDS. I joined TAC after I disclosed my status. That was in December 2001. Because I was HIV-positive I was discriminated against in the school where I was teaching. They ended my contract because they said I was a teacher who could infect others. I got angry. I said that I would take my case to court. I was very depressed. Then I saw a poster for TAC, and I joined. I am strong now. I speak about my status, and what to do to protect yourself against HIV/AIDS. I promote openness about HIV. . . . That's me, exactly me.[11]

All the women who spoke after her talked about the babies to whom they had given birth—with a "boyfriend" or an unspecified sexual partner as the father, and as the result of rape in one case. Several of the women discovered that they were HIV-positive during their pregnancies, and two of them gave birth to babies who were also HIV-positive. Everyone—the men, as well as the women—talked about the prejudice, discrimination, stigmatization, and rejection they had experienced from family members, employers, co-workers, and friends when it was revealed that they had HIV/AIDS. But now, they affirmed, through their contact with MSF and TAC, access to ARV medications, the support and gratification they were receiving from sharing their experiences, and reaching out to others with AIDS, they felt "strong." The declaration—"I feel strong"—made by every member of the assembled group did not only refer to their renewed physical and psychological strength. In a distinctively African way, it was also an affirmation of the sense of metaphysical security and well-being they felt they had regained.

The morning session ended with zestful statements, often accompanied by laughter, about what the participants found enjoyable in their daily lives (eating, singing, talking, being with people, going to church on Sunday . . .), and about their aspirations (a big house, a car, a job, more children, "being free in life").[12]

"We Live with HIV in Worcester":
An Ulwazi TAC Mobile Exhibition Trip

A week after I attended this meeting, I accompanied Colwyn Poole, the MSF Resource Center coordinator, on a day-long trip by automobile that he and two African women, trained by TAC, who were both HIV-positive, made to the town of Worcester. Their trip, and the teaching about HIV/AIDS in which they participated in a succession of clinic, school, and church settings, occurred in conjunction with an Ulwazi-constructed mobile exhibition called "We Live with AIDS in Worcester." Included in the exhibition were banners with pictures and the life stories of people infected with HIV, who were shown at home, at work, and performing other daily activities, as well as in hospital clinics. It took more than an hour, traveling over a splendid highway, through a spectacular mountain-ringed terrain, with extensive farms and picturesque vineyards, to reach Worcester, the largest town in the Western Cape's interior region.

En route, as he drove, Poole shared a bit of his biography with me. He came from working-class origins, he told me in impeccable English; he was "Coloured," and his first language was Afrikaans. He was currently taking lessons to improve his Xhosa. His grandfather ran a hardware store; his mother was a public-health nurse. He had been a medical student at the University of Cape Town; but before completing these studies, he had left the university to become a founding member of TAC. When Eric Goemaere had recruited him to work with MSF, he had done so on the condition that Poole would resume his medical studies after two years.[13]

Our first stop was at the Empilisweni Clinic, which operated under the auspices of the Western Cape Provincial Government Department of Health, and was located in Zwelethemba, a Worcester township. There, in the waiting room of its postnatal outpatient department, filled with many women and children, and some men, Poole and the two women joined a teaching and discussion session on HIV/AIDS conducted mainly in Xhosa.[14] In the midst of the hubbub of the waiting room, several TAC volunteers, wearing "HIV POSITIVE" T-shirts, who had arrived before us, were already instructing the assemblage on the advantages of formula feeding to prevent the transmission of HIV from mother to child, using a videotape shown on a TV screen to do so. When the videotape was over, everyone was invited to make comments and ask questions. Very little of the animated discussion that followed pertained to the passing on of HIV through the way that babies were fed. Rather, it centered around protection from becoming infected by the virus through sexual relations:

- Is a condom safe?
- If your boyfriend is HIV-positive, "sleeping around," and doesn't want to use a condom, what can you do?
- I stay at home. But my husband has lots of girlfriends. So I use a condom.
- If you have sex with a man, and you go for a test the next day, and you test negative, is it possible that if you get tested two months later, the results will be different?

Concern was also expressed about what could be done to inform people about HIV/AIDS in ways that would embolden and motivate them to protect themselves and others from contracting and transmitting it:

- TAC must do something abut people who are HIV-positive and are spreading the virus. It is a disaster! We have to educate people—go to the schools, educate the children. . . .
- I am HIV-positive. But I know a woman who is so scared that she won't go to TAC. What should I do about it?

The TAC volunteers and the group with whom I had traveled to Worcester responded to these questions and comments with factual information, practical advice, forthrightness—which included intimate autobiographical information—reassurance, and some moralizing:

Yes, a condom is safe—if you keep it in a cool place, and look for the expiration date. . . . You should take time putting on the condom before having sex. You don't have to rush. If you have a boyfriend, you have the right to ask him about his status, and to ask him to use a condom. . . . I myself am HIV-positive, and my boyfriend is HIV-negative. He uses a condom to protect his life.

HIV counselors are trained to help people. . . . When you go to be tested for HIV, the results remain confidential between you and the counselor. . . . And TAC does go to schools to educate the children about HIV/AIDS.

But you mustn't judge persons who are HIV-positive because they are HIV-positive. And you can live with HIV/AIDS for more than twenty years, if you take care of yourself. . . . You may die of something else. You can still own a house, buy furniture, take your children to school, and give them an education. And if you are HIV-positive, and not sick, you can go and look for a job. If you get one, you can tell your employer that you are HIV-positive. Our Constitution says everyone has rights, and it protects you.

From the clinic we moved on to the Esselen Park Primary School, located in the Worcester township of Roodewal, where the students were learning about HIV/AIDS, and receiving basic sex education with the assistance of TAC. The girls and boys assembled in the packed classroom appeared to be pre-teenagers. They were all Coloured, Afrikaans-speaking,[15] and dressed in school uniforms. They had already seen the "We Live in Worcester with AIDS" exhibition, and they were engaged in a remarkably open conversation with a TAC volunteer—a woman who was HIV-positive and told the students that she was. When they asked for more details about her history, she said that she had been sexually abused as a child, had married at age sixteen, and had subsequently divorced her husband because he "slept around." She became very sick, she continued, and discovered that she had HIV. "I don't want this to happen to you tomorrow," she said to the students. HIV causes AIDS, she explained, and it is dangerous because there is no cure. Your immune system becomes weak, and your body cannot protect itself against infection. It can be prevented if you abstain from sex. But if you engage in sex, then use condoms. She went on to say that she did not encourage them to have sex, but to wait until they were married. If your partner is HIV-positive it can be the cause of "heartbreaking pain," she declared. So it is best to abstain.

The students plied her with questions:

- How did you feel when you found out you were HIV-positive? a student asked. In response she admitted that at first both her family and her community had rejected her.
- Who abused you? asked another student. It was a family member, she revealed, and then declined to speak any further about it.
- How many children do you have? a student queried. She replied that she had three children, ranging from six to eighteen years of age. All of her children were HIV-negative, she said.
- Are you married? another student wanted to know. Yes, she said, I am married again to a man who is fifty-six years old. I am only thirty-five. I am very happy. He is HIV-negative.

- How does your husband feel about that? a student inquired.
  I explained to him, she said, and he gives me support.
- How do you feel physically? a student wondered. On certain days
  I am very healthy, she answered. On other days I am very sick. But I
  am a positive person, with a positive lifestyle. I help others, and I
  look after myself as well.

What followed were two presentations about how to use male and female condoms, made respectively by a male and a female TAC counselor. A ripple of classroom laughter accompanied a boy who volunteered to come forward and try putting the male condom on a brown pole and then removing it, in the way that students had been shown. When he succeeded in doing so, the class broke into laughing applause, and before he returned to his seat, in a gesture of appreciation, the TAC counselor formally shook his hand. A cascade of very specific, frank questions were asked by students following these presentations—for example: How does it feel to have sex? How does it feel for a boy? How does it feel for a girl? How were condoms discovered? Why are they so slippery? Is a female condom painful? Is sex more pleasurable for boys who are circumcised?—to which the TAC counselors gave outspoken answers. The most personally candid comment was spontaneously made by one of the primary-school teachers who, speaking from her seat in the back of the room, told the students that as a married woman she used a condom, and that it did not prevent her from enjoying sex.

After "Beat It, HIV and AIDS," a videotape about the immune system, was shown to the students, a final, short personal testimony was given in English by another male TAC volunteer. He described being "recognized" as having AIDS in 1998, the weight loss, diarrhea, and opportunistic infections he had experienced, and his current HIV/AIDS status (Stage 1), for which, he said, he was receiving antiretroviral medications.

Returning to Zwelethemba, another Worcester township, where we paid a visit to the St. Francis (Anglican) Church, housed in a small, rather shabby brick building, in front of which stood a signboard that read: "This Church is HIV/AIDS Friendly." We were welcomed by its pastor—a soft-spoken black African priest, wearing a purple tunic and a clerical collar—whom I had met earlier at the Empilisweni Clinic, where, I was told, he was very active in their HIV/AIDS program and support groups.

We had lunch in a bare wooden building on the grounds of the church, which looked as though it was ordinarily used as a meeting hall. Female members of the church, wearing long-skirted dresses, aprons, and bandanas on their heads, led the saying of grace, before they served a simple meal that consisted of fish, bread, chips, orange juice, and water. The pastor's wife, dressed in the same fashion as the other church women, joined us at the large, wooden picnic-style table. While we ate, colored photographs were passed around that elicited much enthusiastic conversation. They were snapshots taken at a demonstration that had occurred on April 8, 2002: a march staged by the church's Sinethemba Support Group, demanding HIV/AIDS services that people were not receiving—especially antiretroviral medications.

After lunch, we attended a meeting of this support group, which was held in a room adjacent to the church's place of worship and its sanctuary. A major item on its agenda was evaluating the impact of the "We Live with HIV in Worcester" Mobile Exhibition. The sentiments expressed were approving. It was the general opinion that the exhibition, coupled with TAC's teaching and their own activities as a support group. raised people's consciousness about HIV/AIDS and its "challenges"; changed some of their attitudes toward it for the better; educated people in valuable ways about HIV/AIDS—its disclosure, transmission, prevention, and treatment; and enlightened them about the importance of "condoming." There was also some discussion about what was happening at the Empilisweni Clinic. When someone reported that another full-time HIV/AIDS counselor would be appointed at the clinic, and that an additional room there would be provided for such counseling, the group responded with applause.

Colwyn Poole then made a long, impassioned speech about the work their support group had accomplished, and all that still remained to be done. He referred to the case of one man with HIV whom they had helped. Previously this man had been so short of breath that he could barely talk; but now he could speak, he was mobile, and he was "free." His "spirit" had been lifted by TAC. Poole commended the Sinethemba Support Group for their participation in the April demonstration-march, demanding services for others that had assisted a man like this, for their help in creating a counselor's post that had been filled by someone able to speak in several languages (Xhosa, Afrikaans, and English), and for the quality of their decisions and decision-makers. He underscored the need to teach the people who they counseled about tuberculosis, and the frequency with which it accompanied HIV. Both an HIV service and antiretroviral (ARV) therapy were needed at the clinic, he continued. But

ARV was not enough. What would the community do to take these advances forward? He suggested that TAC groups like theirs go to prisons to visit and teach about HIV/AIDS. Make noises about social services! he exhorted the group. Organize workshops! The mother-to-child transmission program that you started in April does not have enough help, he commented. Put pressure on to get at least a few more people for that job. Representatives of TAC should be present each and every day in the clinic, in educational institutions, and in the churches. Go wherever you can in the community, preaching, "No More AIDS for Our Children." Making reference to the national government's "denialist" outlook on AIDS, Poole declared that AIDS caused poverty, not only the reverse, as President Mbeki had insinuated, and that their partnership in the fight against AIDS was based on truth and the saving of lives, not on lies and denial. He closed his talk by informing the Sinethemba group about a forthcoming meeting of TAC members from the entire Western Cape that was being planned. It would be held in a stadium, he told them, and organized around the fight for making AIDS treatment available and affordable by taking drug companies to court to oblige them to lower the prices of their antiretroviral drugs, and to allow less expensive generic forms of these drugs to be produced and sold. We are saying we cannot wait for their patents on these drugs to expire in twenty years, because hundreds of thousands of persons all over the world who cannot afford those drugs at their current prices will die of AIDS by then, he declared.

At the end of Poole's motivational talk, the pastor brought the meeting to a close, in what he called this "place of hope." After some amiable, parting chatter with him standing outside the church in the hot mid-afternoon sun, we took our leave and drove back to Cape Town and Khayelitsha.

A TAC Rally

On September 27, 2003, I had a chance to attend a TAC "Mass Rally for Treatment" in the Sports Complex of Gugulethu, a township fifteen kilometers from the center of Cape Town. As stated in a TAC Newsletter communication,[16] the rally had multiple aims:

- To "welcome and show support" for the decision that had been made on August 10, 2003, by the South African government to develop an "operational antiretroviral treatment plan"—after TAC had staged a march of almost ten thousand people at the opening of Parliament on February 14, 2003, to demand a national HIV/AIDS prevention and treatment plan that included antiretroviral therapy for all people in South Africa who needed it (in which MSF had joined), followed the next month by the launching of a civil disobedience campaign to put pressure on the government to take steps to meet this demand.

- To "urge the task team" just appointed to draft the plan for the nationwide treatment of "HIV-positive people" with antiretroviral (ARV) drugs to "hand their report to the Cabinet by September 30."
- To insist that ARV treatment "begin as soon as possible," and that "dates and targets for rolling out" treatment . . . be published."
- To "propose a target of 280,000 people on treatment by March 2005" [out of the 500,000 people who, it was asserted, needed treatment now].
- And to affirm that TAC was willing to suspend its civil disobedience campaign, and "ready to work with government to make treatment a success" through a "people-centered ARV program" in which there was "active and expanding community involvement and mobilization—particularly the involvement of people living with HIV/AIDS and people already taking ARV treatment"—and that "treatment literacy training in communities . . . with health care workers to promote openness, adherence to treatment, and treatment literacy" be a core part of this program.

The "key messages" of the rally and of TAC's conception of the treatment plan around which it was organized also included choosing rural sites in the "roll-out" in order to address the "inequity" that existed between urban and rural areas; government measures to make medicines more affordable by issuing compulsory licenses for the manufacture of generic versions of them; breaking the patent-holding and the drug-pricing monopolies of pharmaceutical companies; the encouragement of voluntary HIV counseling and testing by clinics; and more effective treatment of opportunistic infections.

It was estimated that some eight hundred people attended the rally, despite torrential rain and strong winds. Participants included members of religious and of women's organizations, health-care personnel, hospice staff members, and a striking number of children and young people, whose presence, a TAC member explained to me, was attributable to the effort that TAC was making to raise youngsters' personal and civic consciousness about AIDS. Zackie Achmat and Eric Goemaere were key speakers at the rally.

The atmosphere of the rally was energetically enthusiastic and festive. Short pep talks, delivered by people seated in rows of plastic chairs in front of the audience-participants who filled the stands of the Sports Complex's basketball stadium, were interspersed with group cheers, outbursts of choral singing (including hymns), and dazzling dancing (some of it Michael Jackson–like) to the music of CDs, amplified by loudspeakers. Although the level of attentiveness was high, a great deal of moving about and social visiting between those assembled took place. Almost everyone present—women and men, boys and girls—was dressed in blue jeans or slacks, and T-shirts imprinted with HIV/AIDS slogans:

- "HIV Positive"
- "Stand Up for Our Lives"
- "Two Pills a Day Saves Lives"
- "Treat the People"
- "Prevent New Infections"
- "End Stigma"
- "Health Care Workers Support"

On some of the T-shirts a smiling image of Nelson Mandela was printed alongside the phrase "HIV Positive."

Eric Goemaere gave one of the closing speeches (in English). Together we have won a battle, he said, but the war is not over. To have 280,000 people treated by 2005 is a worthy goal. But so far the treatment plan exists only on paper. More than ever TAC will have to keep the pressure on the government to ensure that it lives up to its promises. The officials of hospitals will also have to be approached to make certain that they follow the plan. Yesterday, he continued, I was called to see a patient at Clinic Site B in Khayelitsha. She was a woman with HIV/AIDS who was making her first visit to the clinic, and she was close to death. Yet she lives in Khayelitsha, near the clinic. You all have the responsibility to patrol the area where you are living, making sure that people are not afraid to come out because of the stigma associated with AIDS. All of us have this responsibility. There is a lot of work to be done to implement the plan—to make the dream reality. If it does become reality, it will be one of the biggest treatment plans in the world.

Goemaere's speech evoked strong applause. A black African Protestant pastor, who said a few quiet words to the gathering in Xhosa and then led them in prayer, followed him. The rally closed with everyone rising to sing the South African national anthem in thrilling polyphonic harmony, followed by a mass cheer, which, to my ears, sounded like, "*Viva!*"

Unfortunately, I had arrived at the rally after Zackie Achmat had given the opening speech, but Eric Goemaere introduced me to him after the rally was over. He was a handsome, intelligent-looking, light-skinned man, with neatly barbered hair and glasses, dressed in a silk zippered jacket, worn over an "HIV POSITIVE" T-shirt, and well-pressed trousers. He appeared to be in good health. One of the featured events of the rally had been the announcement that Achmat, who was HIV-positive, had begun antiretroviral treatment. Before this, he had publicly refused to take these drugs until a national treatment plan was put in place. He had even resisted an appeal made to him by Nelson Mandela to start treatment. And although he testified that the ARV medication was making him feel better than he had for many years, he had told the rally that it continued to be painful for him to be taking the drugs when so many people who could not afford them were still dying. In turn, Achmat introduced me to a broadly smiling, darker-skinned man, who he said had been his "comrade" for more than twenty years. Their association, he informed me, went back to the days of their mutual involvement in the anti-apartheid struggle.

Several weeks after this rally took place, TAC received the Nelson Mandela Award for Health and Human Rights. The selection of TAC for the award, which bore his name, had been personally approved by Mandela. Graça Machel, Mandela's wife, presented the award to Zackie Achmat at a ceremony in Johannesburg. "We are here today to celebrate the efforts of an extraordinary group of people and an organization that in less than five years has moved a nation, shifted government policy and advanced the rights of people with HIV/AIDS," she said in the speech that she delivered on this occasion. "Civil society helped win the victory over apartheid. . . . The Treatment Action Campaign's struggle grows out of the best traditions of the anti-apartheid movement."[17]

Enter Nelson Mandela

Eric Goemaere told me that the colored photo of Mandela printed on the "HIV POSITIVE" T-shirts worn by some of the participants in the TAC rally had been taken on the day in December 2002 on which Mandela had "honored

Khayelitsha's HIV program" by paying a visit to it. The impact of his visit on the project was described to me in an e-mail from a member of its staff:

> Mandela's visit was of great reach and weight. He came and sprinkled the dust of hope and humanity on a sometimes rather lost and sad place. You can imagine the pleasure of all those working near and far to the project. On the day of [his] visit, when he was offered [an "HIV POSITIVE"] T-shirt, he immediately took off his shirt, and slipped on the T-shirt. As he did this, I saw explosions of joy in people's eyes. . . . An instant of pure, pure joy.

A photo of Mandela donning the T-shirt was transmitted all over the world.

This visit resulted from a prior meeting that Goemaere had had with Mandela in August 2002 at his home, along with Maria Ramos, who was then director-general of the South African Treasury. (Dr. Ayenda Ntsaluba, director-general of the national Department of Health, had been invited to be present as well, but to Mandela's displeasure, had been kept from doing so by Minister of Health Tshabalala-Msimang.) At this meeting, Mandela had asked Goemaere to develop an HIV/AIDS program in the Eastern Cape in collaboration with the Nelson Mandela Foundation. Goemaere had agreed to do so, and in exchange, he had requested that Mandela make a visit to the MSF HIV/AIDS Program in Khayelitsha, and thereby help to "rescue it" politically from the "vociferous attacks" to which it was being subjected by the national government, which at that time was strongly opposed to antiretroviral treatment for HIV/AIDS, to TAC's role in campaigning for it, and to what it construed as MSF's "manipulation" and funding of TAC.

The fact that Mandela's son had died from AIDS probably contributed to his decision to become actively involved in the battle against the disease. Inaugurated in person by Mandela on December 12, 2003, the program was called "Siyaphila La" (Xhosa for "We are alive"), and located in Lusikisiki, in one of the poorest, most remote rural parts of South Africa—the former Transkei homeland in the Eastern Cape Province. This was not only the area of Mandela's birthplace, but also President Thabo Mbeki's, and the place from which many of the inhabitants of Khayelitsha had migrated. An inadequate health infrastructure existed in the region, with only one provincial hospital, and a sparse number of health personnel, for a scattered population of some 200,000, among whom there was estimated to be an adult HIV/AIDS prevalence rate of between thirty and thirty-five percent. The goal of this project was to develop a model that would demonstrate how comprehensive HIV/

AIDS care, prevention, and treatment could be successfully carried out under these circumstances, and therefore virtually anywhere in the country—contrary to the claim of the South African government that such conditions posed insuperable barriers. The approach taken was derived and adapted from the Khayelitsha experience. It was set up as a community-impelled program, managed by nurses, which stressed primary care, using simplified regimens, with education about HIV/AIDS integrated into its clinical services. Hermann Reuter became the coordinator of the Lusikisiki program.[18]

AIDS "Denialism"

On each of my field trips to Khayelitsha, in 2002, 2003, and 2005, members of the MSF and TAC staffs expressed great indignation about what they termed the "denialist" attitudes and behavior of the South African government under the presidency of Thabo Mbeki with regard to the AIDS epidemic, and the prolonged delay in rolling out a national program for the prevention and treatment of HIV/AIDS that included antiretroviral therapy. The consequences of this delay, MSF wrote in a February 12, 2003, open letter to the government, were catastrophic:

> Today, five million South Africans are infected with HIV, and nearly 1,000 are dying every day of AIDS-related complications. The 600,000 South Africans who clinically require ARV treatment now to stay alive do not have time to wait. Their families do not have time to wait. . . .
>
> For the past four years, MSF has witnessed first-hand the daily devastation caused by the AIDS epidemic in South Africa and the extraordinary clinical benefits—and hope—that the availability of ARV treatment brings to the community. Our work in Khayelitsha in the Western Cape . . . clearly demonstrates the feasibility of ARV treatment in resource-poor settings; there is no longer any question that it is possible. Our new program in a rural remote setting in the Eastern Cape explores the specific challenges of providing ARV treatment [in such settings]. . . . But, despite their success, such programs cannot become a substitute for what is ultimately the responsibility of the South African government.[19]

The obstructive AIDS denialism of the government was expressed in a number of ways, which included playing down the gravity and extensiveness of the incidence of AIDS in South Africa and maintaining that it was only one among many medical and public-health problems in the society; voicing doubts about whether the human immunodeficiency virus (HIV) actually existed, and if it did, whether it was an infectious virus and the crucial causative agent of AIDS; challenging the role that heterosexual relations might have in the transmission of the disease; questioning the efficacy of antiretroviral drugs, and emphasizing their potentially toxic, even poisonous effects; promoting nutritional remedies and traditional African medicine in lieu of these drugs; and likening the ideas about the etiology, prevention, and treatment of AIDS being set forth by the Western scientific community to notions that had supported the apartheid regime. Minister of Health Tshabalala-Msimang, who served in the Mbeki government from 1999 to 2008, was a key figure in publicly espousing and promoting these denialist claims, recommending, in international as well as national forums, the benefits of treating AIDS with substances such as garlic, beetroot, and lemon juice, rather than with antiretroviral medicines.

In addition, Tshabalala-Msimang and the Mbeki government seemed to support the claims made by Matthias Rath, a highly controversial German physician and businessman, that a program of nutritional supplements—particularly high-dose vitamin C pills that he manufactured and sold—could reverse the course of AIDS. Rath contrasted the therapeutic power of his "natural remedy" with what he characterized as the "poisonous" properties of antiretroviral drugs. He had managed to infiltrate Khayelitsha, where employees of his Rath Health Foundation not only distributed vitamins that resembled one of the antiretroviral pills, but also recruited persons with AIDS to participate in what he called a clinical pilot study that entailed substituting his vitamins for antiretroviral therapy. It was reported that some of the participants in this trial, who were in advanced stages of AIDS, had died because of this ineffective medication. The national Health Ministry and government stood passively by. It was not until the Treatment Action Campaign and the South African Medical Association took the Rath Foundation to court, with the support of MSF, that he was legally stopped from conducting any further trials and claiming that vitamins could prevent and cure HIV/AIDS.

"Why Has AIDS Happened in Our Country?"

I wondered if the stance that President Mbeki and the members of his government had taken with regard to AIDS was based on what they genuinely believed about it, to what extent it was politically and economically motivated,[20] and why they supposed that South Africans would find their allegations credible. An October (2003) morning that I spent in the Khayelitsha MSF office with eight black South Africans was illuminating to me in these regards.

The group, which was composed of four women and four men, was engaged in pre-testing an HIV/AIDS survey research questionnaire about the relevant attitudes, beliefs, and behavior of a large, random sample of Khayelitsha inhabitants. I had been invited to meet with them to offer any suggestions I might have about improving the penultimate, trial version of the questionnaire that they were evaluating.[21] The most extensive and revealing discussion that I ended up having with the group stemmed from our consideration of the items on the questionnaire that asked respondents to state why they thought a person might become infected with HIV/AIDS. A checklist of potential causes of HIV/AIDS was provided by the questionnaire—one of which was "witchcraft." I expressed the tentative opinion that people might be reluctant to respond to this question if it was stated in such a forthright way. Perhaps, I suggested, it might be more fruitful if respondents were asked a series of more indirect questions about some of the components of witchcraft—for example, "if they believe that persons can get HIV/AIDS because of the jealous, resentful, or angry feelings about them that are harbored by significant others; because they themselves have engaged in wrong-doing or broken important taboos; or because someone has solicited the services of a magico-religious practitioner to cause this harm to befall them."[22]

At first, the group dealt evasively with my remarks about witchcraft. But then, initiated by the person who seemed to be the most highly respected among them because of his heroic actions in the anti-apartheid struggle, they began to speak freely about the beliefs that people had about what causes AIDS. Those that they mentioned included punishment by the ancestors; punishment by God; both black and white "foreigners" who had migrated to South Africa, either legally or illegally, in recent years; the malevolence of some of the whites who promoted the use of condoms because they did not want to see the black population grow too greatly; the evil intentions of some of the advocates of antiretroviral drugs—Western medicines that could do harm as well as supposed good; and the belief that the dissemination of HIV was part of American biological warfare being waged to destroy Africa. Underlying the beliefs that they identified, I recognized elements of a traditional African cosmic view, in which:

[A]ll experiences and goals that human beings consider desirable and good are part of the natural order of things. . . . [But] the universe also throbs with malevolent forces and presences that fall outside the natural order. All that is evil is caused by them, through the malignant thoughts and feelings of significant other persons. . . . Thoughts and feelings of a malefactor have the capacity to cause harm, either directly or indirectly through harnessing one of the powers of the spirits present in the cosmos. Illness, sterility, failure, impoverishment, dissension, corruption, destruction, death—all the negative, disappointing experiences of life—are caused by witchcraft or sorcery.[23]

Intermixed with these latent metaphysical assumptions about the causes of AIDS that the group reported were the xenophobic apprehensions that they identified, which seemed to be vestiges of unhealed wounds associated with South African colonial and apartheid experiences. And overarching all of these beliefs was a plaintive question of meaning voiced by one of my interlocutors: "Why, in our free and beautiful country" had it come to pass that HIV/AIDS had spread like a plague and caused so many people to sicken and die?

What the members of the group did not make clear was whether they shared some of the beliefs that they attributed to unnamed others. It seemed to me likely that they did. Furthermore, as I wrote in a personal e-mail to a European member of the MSF Khayelitsha staff, "I would not be surprised if Minister of Health Manto Tshabalala-Msimang, and even President Thabo Mbeki, held some of these beliefs, too."

"Patient Selection" in Khayelitsha

On each of the field trips that I made to Khayelitsha, I attended a meeting of one of what they called their "selection committees." The purpose of these meetings was to consider prospective candidates for admission to the antiretroviral treatment program. Even long after the South African government had finally set into motion a national treatment and care plan to progressively make free antiretroviral medication available to all citizens of the country with HIV/AIDS, coverage remained far from universal. The slow and fitful implementation of the plan in response to the massive number of persons in the population who were HIV-positive or had full-blown AIDS, continually augmented by the scores of individuals to whom the virus was newly transmitted, necessitated deciding who would receive the medication, and who would not, in a country that had the highest incidence of HIV/AIDS in the world.

During the period of 2002–2005 in which I made my visits to Khayelitsha, the project succeeded in gradually increasing its patient enrollment for HIV/AIDS care.[24] As a consequence, it altered its patient selection procedure from a monthly meeting of one central selection committee for the entire Khayelitsha site to fortnightly meetings of the individual selection committees that had been established for each of the three HIV clinics. These were composed of doctors, nurses, and counselors on the clinical staff, and at least one patient, identified as an "external witness." At the time, some thirty to forty patients were reviewed by each clinic each month. The meetings characteristically began with short reports from the nurse in charge of the home visits made to the patients who were being considered as potential recipients of antiretroviral treatment.

A set of medical, social, and "adherence" criteria were used to evaluate the patient-candidates, all of which, in principle, they were required to fulfill in order to be eligible for antiretroviral treatment. Medically, patients had to have undergone two tests to confirm their HIV serostatus and had to be in stage 4 of the disease, or in stages 1, 2, or 3 if the CD4 count (the number of T lymphocytes, blood cells that fight infection) in a sample of the patient's blood was less than 200 CD4. Socially, patients were required to have a record of regular clinic attendance (at least four scheduled visits to the HIV clinic); to reside in Khayelitsha, and to have promised not to move away from the township for at least six months; to be committed to long-term antiretroviral treatment and to be practicing safe sex; to be willing to disclose their HIV status to a person in their confidence (older than eighteen years of age) who had agreed to act as their treatment assistant; and to have manifested readiness to attend a support group for persons on antiretroviral treatment at least once a month during the first year of treatment. Alcoholism, other forms of substance abuse, and untreated depression were considered to be social contraindications for initiating antiretroviral therapy. Counselors—who were responsible for long-term patient adherence—had the final word in the decisions regarding the start of treatment.

The most striking characteristic of the selection committees' actions that I observed was that in almost every instance, they decided to accept the patients proposed for treatment. Even when patients did not meet some of the social and adherence criteria—such as readiness to "condomize," faithful and punctual keeping of clinic appointments, disclosure of their HIV/AIDS status, or participation in a support group—the committees' inclination was to assume that both before and after the initiation of treatment, with the help of counselors and fellow patients, the candidates could be successfully prepared to fulfill them. The reluctance of the committee members to refuse anyone treatment and their tendency to find extenuating reasons to explain and override indications that a patient had not met the selection criteria were rooted in their commitment to making antiretroviral medication available to all who might benefit from it—especially the most disadvantaged. Above all, in the words of one committee member, they did not want to act as a "tribunal" that assumed it had the knowledge, the wisdom, or the right to make life-or-death judgments about who received antiretroviral medication and who did not. He suggested in all seriousness, although with a tinge of humor, that it might be more appropriate to call the "selection" committee the "eligibility" or "preparation" committee, or even to rename it the "approval" or "acceptance" committee.[25]

"Queue-Jumping," the "Lazarus" Phenomenon, and Transformed Hospices

Committee members were likely to circumvent the system of selection criteria by "fast-tracking" patients in a very advanced, rapidly evolving stage of HIV/AIDS whose death appeared to be imminent, allowing them to "jump the queue" to begin antiretroviral treatment. This was impelled by the overriding dedication of the project and its staff to prolong the lives of patients with HIV/AIDS, no matter how low their CD count, how sick they were, or in how many ways they diverged or "defaulted" from the selection criteria. As a physician working in the Khayelitsha clinics vividly put it, "Once you've seen Lazarus coming back," after starting a desperately ill patient on antiretroviral therapy, you find it almost impossible to decide to withhold or withdraw it from anyone with AIDS.

This outlook also played a significant role in the way the Khayelitsha program looked at hospice care and the influence that it had on the ethos of the two hospices to which it referred patients who were too sick to be cared for at home. One of these institutions was run by the Missionaries of Charity, the Roman Catholic religious congregation established by Mother Teresa of

Calcutta; the other functioned under the auspices of a less-renowned group of nuns, the Sisters of Nazareth. Originally, Eric Goemaere said, although he admired the two groups of nuns, their commitment, and their ability to cope with death, these hospices constituted "a step into the grave." Prior to Goemaere's establishment of relations with the Missionaries of Charity, their hospice was what he characterized as a "one-way path to death"—an "antechamber to Paradise," he mischievously remarked, supported by the sisters' conviction that "it would be better to be in Paradise." It was consistent, he said, with the "fatalistic attitude towards people dying with infectious disease" that had "shocked" him when he visited the Missionaries of Charity headquarters in Calcutta in 1978. He considered this attitude to be "the antithesis of the spirit of MSF." However, he felt that the Khayelitsha program had succeeded in "slowly instilling" into the sisters its "ideology of diagnosis and treatment," which not only involved giving patients the best possible nursing care, but "fighting for their well-being" with the goal of sufficiently increasing their strength and improving their health so that they could return home and be started on a regimen of antiretroviral treatment. The conversion of the Sisters to this outlook, Goemaere said, was partly attributable to the invitation that was extended to several of them to attend the regular HIV training sessions that MSF organized for nurses in Khayelitsha, to which they had responded with enthusiasm.

On November 8, 2005, I visited the hospice of the Missionaries of Charity.[26] In front of the small house where the five sisters resided, and in which their chapel was located, they had somehow managed to cultivate a little rose garden despite the windswept aridness of the terrain. The sisters had also erected a grotto adjacent to the garden, in which a statue of the Virgin Mary was enshrined. A neat, red-brick walk led to their house, which was attached to several pavilion-style, one-story buildings, constructed around courtyards, in which those for whom they cared were housed. I was greeted warmly and cheerfully at the front door by two of the five sisters, dressed in the traditional white saris with three blue stripes and the sandals of their congregation, who took me on a tour of the facilities. Religious images, texts of prayers, and pictures of Mother Teresa hung on many of the walls. In the sisters' recreation room, a framed chart listed the 113 countries in which the Congregation had missions, to which was affixed special mention of sisters martyred in Yemen and Sierra Leone. Everything was immaculate. The wardlike rooms occupied by the patients were painted in bright colors, and each bed was made up with a colorful quilt. The relatively new pediatric ward, for whose construction MSF had contributed funds, was not only gaily painted but also festooned with toys, and through its windows a rudimentary playground with several swings was visible. We stopped at a crib occupied by a nine-month-old child with an exquisite face and beautiful eyes, framed by long lashes, who had a huge hydrocephalic head, on which surgeons at Cape Town's illustrious Groote Schuur Hospital had operated several times, but to no avail. In a recreation room through which we passed, an overhead television set was turned on, although no one was watching it. All the patient-residents of the hospice who I saw were neatly dressed. Those who were ambulatory or in wheelchairs wore street clothes. The number who seemed to be severely spastic or mentally retarded was striking. The atmosphere felt serene, and responsively open to anyone in any condition in need of care. But a patient to whom I spoke—an American man, a musician who had lived in South Africa for many years—made me conscious of the fact that there was no reading matter anywhere in the hospice other than prayer books, and that there was what he considered to be a dearth of anything to do, or anyone to whom he could talk. For him, the degree to which the hospice was sealed off from the outside world was disturbing.

After making these rounds, the sisters invited me to their recreation room, where, over soft drinks and cake, we conversed. They did not think of their establishment as a hospice, they said, but rather as a "home," to which the Hindi words *nirmal hrday* ("pure heart") applied. They were currently caring for forty men, thirty-eight women, and sixteen children. Assisting them were a group of persons whom they called "helpers." These were very poor people from the local community, who received wages and two meals a day—lunch and dinner—for their work. It was "not unusual" for deaths to take place among the patients, the sisters quietly stated; but they noted that the number who were dying each year seemed progressively to be going down. I ventured to ask them whether they thought that the care they were currently giving persons with HIV/AIDS, with the goal of helping to improve their health and prolong their lives, constituted a modification in Mother Teresa's founding vision of caring for the incurably ill, the extremely disabled, and the dying. The sisters vigorously responded that they had not changed "Mother's mission"; rather, they declared, they were following and fulfilling her mandate.

The sisters told me a little about their way of life. They prayed five times a day, they said, and also attended morning mass, celebrated by an old Irish priest, to which patients were welcome to come. They did not choose their assignments, but were sent to each mission for a period of ten years, at the end of which they went home to visit their families for three weeks, before departing for their next mission. It was very easy for them to move on any time they were summoned to do so, they explained smilingly, because their only possessions were three saris (one to wear, one to launder, and one to mend), a pair of sandals, a crucifix, a rosary, a prayer book, a plate and a metal spoon, and a canvas bag.

When I took leave of them, the sisters accompanied me to the front door of their house. There, they bid me farewell in the traditional Indian way—with their hands pressed together, palms touching and fingers pointed upward in front of their chests, near their hearts—accompanied by a slight bow.

Later that same day, I joined Eric Goemaere when he made a short visit to the hospice directed by the Sisters of Nazareth to examine several patients who the head nurse there had asked him to see. This facility was less hospicelike than the home run by the Missionaries of Charity. In both its appearance, and in the way that it functioned, it resembled a small hospital or a skilled nursing facility. Its religious auspices were only discernible in one icon of a Byzantine Madonna that hung on a corridor wall, a discreet cross, and a small photo of the foundress of the Sisters of Nazareth, dressed in black-and-white, pre–Vatican II nun's garb. Apparently, the only Nazareth sister who was presently a member of its staff was its nurse-director. Her picture was displayed on a bulletin board, along with those of several registered nurses who were laywomen and of a number of male and female black African paramedical personnel. Prominent among these photos was one of a European physician associated with the Khayelitsha program, who made regular visits to the hospice and was warmly referred to as "Doctor Peter."

The facility was spotless. It smelled clean and fresh. Talcum powder was intentionally sprinkled at various places on its floor. The glass doors of its several wards were open; and patients' beds were covered with attractive quilts. We were accompanied by a pleasant and competent black nurse to the bedsides of the three patients Goemaere had been asked to examine. She was able to give him the details of each of the cases without consulting their charts.

The first patient was a young woman with a staring gaze and a bewildered expression, whom the nurse described as "confused," and who had marked problems of balance when Goemaere helped her out of bed and tested her equilibrium and ability to walk. His working clinical diagnosis was that she had meningitis, along with HIV/AIDS and tuberculosis. He expressed optimism about her improvement and her eventual recovery once antiretroviral treatment could be begun. The second patient was an emaciated-looking older woman with HIV/AIDS and tuberculosis, who seemed to be quite sick, although she asked both the nurse and Goemaere if she could go home. They told her that she was not yet ready to do so. In the bed next to hers was the third patient who Goemaere examined: a younger woman, who also had both HIV/AIDS and tuberculosis. The main reason why she was being cared for here was because of the social and emotional disorganization of her family. After she told Goemare that she had spent the last weekend at home, and found that her family situation had greatly improved, he gave his permission for her to be discharged from the hospice at the end of the week.

We appreciatively accepted the glasses of juice that the nurse offered us, which we drank standing up, exchanged a few professional and personal words with her and with the head nurse, and then exited less ceremoniously than I had earlier in the day from the community of the Missionaries of Charity.

The Entwined Epidemics of HIV/AIDS and Tuberculosis

An exploding individual and public-health problem confronting Khayelitsha was reflected in the fact that all three of the patients at the Sisters of Nazareth hospice whom Eric Goemaere had been asked to evaluate were coinfected with HIV/AIDS and tuberculosis (TB). Entwined epidemics of the two diseases had spread throughout South Africa following the appearance of a multi-drug-resistant form of TB (MDR-TB), with the specter of an even deadlier strain, called XDR-TB, looming on the horizon.

Khayelitsha not only had one of the highest HIV prevalence rates in Cape Town and its environs, but also the highest TB incidence. The two diseases were overlapping. HIV makes people more susceptible to *Myobacterium tuberculosis*, which in turn accelerates the progression of HIV. Consequently, a large percentage of Khayelitsha patients were afflicted with both diseases.

During the period that I spent in Khayelitsha in 2005, I had the chance to see the pilot project that had recently been created to integrate the care of people living with TB and HIV/AIDS. It had been launched by MSF in co-operation with the Provincial Administration of the Western Cape and the City of Cape Town, and it was located in the Site B Ubuntu clinic, which had previously been one of Khayelitsha's HIV clinics. Historically, the treatment of each of these illnesses had been provided by separate programs in the Western Cape region and run by different health authorities. This meant that patients with both HIV/AIDS and TB were cared for in several different health centers. Not only did they have to move from clinic to clinic, often from a considerable distance, and with transportation difficulties, but as a result of their uncoordinated care, many patients who were found to have one disease were not diagnosed as also having the other. In this connection, for example, TB in HIV-positive patients was frequently missed by tuberculosis clinics, whose staffs were trained to make a definitive diagnosis on the basis of positive sputum tests. However, persons with HIV/AIDS who also have tuberculosis tend to contract less common types of TB, which are difficult to detect with sputum tests, and thus are more likely to be "sputum negative."

Patients were quickly attracted to the new "one-stop" clinic, where the examinations, tests, consultations, medications and their monitoring, and surveillance of opportunistic infections significant for both illnesses were available and jointly managed in the same place. On the several days that I visited the integrated clinic, its spacious waiting room—which had been designed with natural ventilation to reduce the risk of further person-to-person TB contamination—was full of patients, who had begun to arrive there as early as 8 A.M. The nurses and physicians working in the clinic reported that they were seeing more than two hundred patients each day. Among the most audacious features of the integrated clinic was its commitment to the same kind of decentralized, patient-and-community-centered care for tuberculosis as for HIV/AIDS. Patients with TB were not being isolated, hospitalized, or having their prescribed TB medications overseen on a daily basis by a health worker. Rather, after several weeks of being educated about their disease, and observed taking their medications by a health-care provider, patients were given responsibility for taking these (five or six) pills a day at home, and for making regular visits, at spaced intervals, to monitor how they were reacting to and faring with the drugs.[27] The same methods for reinforcing adherence to this TB regimen that Khayelitsha was using in connection with antiretroviral medications for HIV/AIDS were being applied here—particularly, requiring patients to select a member of their family or an unrelated person in their entourage to act as a "treatment assistant," who would help them to comply with these conditions, which were not only important for the successful outcome of their therapy, but also for helping to prevent the development and spread of drug-resistant forms of the disease.

Several of the Khayelitsha nurses with whom I spoke expressed uneasiness about the integrated clinic. They were concerned about the added workload and greater complexity that dealing with two grave diseases and their interconnection entailed, and anxious about how adequately they, as well as the patients, were protected by infection-control measures at the clinic. Counterbalancing their anxiety, however, was their appreciation that the purpose of the integrated clinic was to provide more competent and effective care for the growing number of patients coinfected with the two diseases, and thereby to reduce the many deaths taking place of HIV/AIDS patients from TB, and of TB patients from HIV/AIDS.

The Simelela Rape Survivors' Centre

The orbit of the Khayelitsha program extended beyond the prevention and treatment of HIV/AIDS, TB, and their interrelated occurrence. In mid-September 2003, MSF opened the Simelela Rape Survivors' Centre in Khayelitsha, which, in conjunction with a special clinic located in the nearby Site B Day Hospital, was created to provide counseling, medical, and forensic services to the escalating number of women, and children of both genders, who were victims of rape. In addition, it aimed to reach a better understanding of the reasons for the extraordinarily high incidence of this form of sexual violence, and to develop ways of forestalling its occurrence.[28]

In November 2005, I made two successive visits to the Simelela Centre, where I spent time with its coordinator, the nurse Emma O,[29] learning from her about the cases of rape that the center was seeing, and how it was handling them. Our conversations took place in what was designated as the Centre's "interview room": a small room, sparsely furnished, with a number of relatively new, adult-sized chairs, and a special smaller chair for children, in which two black rag dolls—one female, the other male—were seated.

Emma O detailed for me the steps that the Centre took to help a woman when she came to report a rape and seek assistance. Encouraging her to talk about what happened and listening attentively and supportively to her story was fundamental. This was followed up by counseling. All the women underwent several medical examinations, and also a forensic examination to identify the rapist through his DNA. In addition to antibiotics to prevent sexually transmitted infections, those who were seen within seventy-two hours after being raped were given a morning-after pill to prevent pregnancy. They were also tested for HIV infection, and if they were not already HIV-positive, and gave their consent, they received a medically monitored, twenty-eight day course of prophylactic antiretroviral treatment. Women who were found to be pregnant, and who sought an abortion, might be helped to obtain one, after counseling. However, twelve weeks into a pregnancy was the limit for an abortion, because "in our culture, abortion is not right," Emma O declared in a rather moralistic tone of voice. If a woman became pregnant through being raped by "a stranger," she went on to say, she was more likely to want an abortion. But if she knew the person who was the father, although there was shame attached to this, she would be more inclined to go through with the pregnancy, and ask him to support the child. If the rapist was a family member, a social worker would be called in to deal with what was defined as a "social problem."

The Centre worked collaboratively with the Khayelitsha police, as well as with social services. In Emma O's opinion, however, most members of the police force were not very knowledgeable about rape, and many of them were disinclined to believe a victim when she reported having been raped. Perhaps this was because most of the police were men, she acerbically remarked. But she expressed appreciation for the director of the Khayelitsha police, whom she described as a very well-trained man, who had helped with the planning and organization of the Centre. In the end, she went on to say, very few reported rapes were prosecuted; and although depending on the evidence available, a perpetrator might receive five years' imprisonment or more as punishment, she did not think that this "made much difference," because, by and large, rapists "g[ot] out of jail before you know it" and were likely to rape again.

Over the course of the past weekend, Emma O told me during my first visit to the Centre, they had handled sixteen cases of rape. Rapes seemed to occur more frequently over weekends, she commented, and a number of these were "date rapes," or associated with alcohol or drugs. But several small children—she exclaimed that they were "four years old, seven years old, nine years old!"—had been among the rape victims seen by the Centre over the past weekend. Children are often raped, she informed me—boys as well as girls—and usually by persons known to them, frequently members of their own family. "Why does this happen?" she asked with a mixture of anguish and indignation. This was the aspect of her work that she found the most stressful, she said, especially because she had a child who was the same age as some of the child victims. What flashed through my mind as she talked was a flyer issued by the Simelela Rape Centre that I had seen, featuring a colored photo of a robust, maternal-looking young African woman, with a kindly expression on her face, dressed simply in a striped, sleeveless tank top and blue jeans. Behind her, in the near distance, one could glimpse the corrugated-iron and cinder-block walls of typical Khayelitsha houses. In front of one of these walls, with his/her back turned to the viewer, and out of the range of the mother-figure's vision, stood a scrawny, vulnerable-looking child. Whether the child was a girl or a boy was not discernible. "Mother speak out, our children are being abused," read the caption on the flyer. "My child is your child."

One of the last things that Emma O said to me as I was leaving the Centre on my second visit was that she was grateful that she now had a chance to go for personal counseling, as well as to get training in counseling rape victims. She hoped that it would help her to better understand "why men do this"—what could conceivably be "in their minds."[30]

The Zip Zap Circus School Show

For all children on treatment
Come See **ZIP ZAP Circus School**
Oliver Tambo Hall, Khayelitsha
Thursday, 1st December
Show Starts 2pm
FREE ENTRY
Bring Hospital Appointment Card

One of my most enduring memories of the time that I spent at Khayelitsha was attending a performance of the Zip Zap Circus on December 1, 2005, the date of the annual observance of World AIDS Day. The show took place in Oliver Tambo Hall, a big community center, with a spacious basketball court, a large stage, and a multitiered spectator balcony. When I entered the hall, the rows of green plastic chairs that covered its entire main floor were rapidly being filled with excited children—mainly black African children from Khayelitsha, many of whom were HIV-positive. Most of them came as whole classes from schools in the Khayelitsha township, dressed in their school uniforms, and accompanied by their teachers. Music blared from enormous loudspeakers. Cameramen, readying themselves to take photographs and to videotape the pending performance, were rushing about. More and more people arrived, many wearing "HIV POSITIVE" T-shirts, and greeted one another warmly.

As the excitement mounted, I turned around in my seat to look at the audience, which now included at least a thousand high-spirited children, filled with energy and expectation. And then, with musical fanfare, the Zip Zap Circus show began. It was initiated by the appearance on the stage of two young men, comically play acting, with pantomimed gestures, two elderly men engaged in an animated conversation. The essence of their discussion (in Xhosa)—"We used to have a big problem of relations between blacks and whites; but now we have the problem of HIV/AIDS"—drew gales of laughter from the audience.

What followed, accompanied by very loud throbbing music that changed to suit each performance, was one fast-paced act after another of floor acrobatics, trapeze artistry, tightrope walking, trampoline bouncing, juggling, jump-roping, unicycling, dancing, drumming, and clowning. Twenty-five Khayelitsha children who were HIV-positive participated in some of the acts, along with Zip Zap Circus professionals. These children had attended weekly workshops run in conjunction with MSF where they had learned circus skills. The delighted applause, cheers, and laughter of the children in the audience mounted higher and higher—especially when they recognized children whom they knew from the township on the stage.

Toward the end of the show, when the song "I Feel Good" boomed out over the loudspeakers, and the children who were dancing to it on the stage were joined by others from the audience, I wept. I wept because of the exuberant, affirmative joy of the children that I was witnessing, and my knowledge of their lives in the shacks of Khayelitsha, in the midst of poverty, unemployment, crime, rape, violence, and HIV/AIDS and TB—diseases with which so many of them, along with their parents, other members of their families, inhabitants of their township, and citizens of their society were infected. The juxtaposition of the life force that emanated from these children, and the deadly medical and social plagues with which they were surrounded was profoundly moving—both tragic and inspiring.

Achievements, Limitations, and Dilemmas of the Khayelitsha Project

S. Africa marks milestone in AIDS fight
Associated Press / June 4, 2011

Cape Town, South Africa—AIDS patients and government officials yesterday celebrated the 10th anniversary of a pioneering program that brought AIDS drugs to impoverished South Africans, a program that patients credited for saving their lives.

Patients and officials danced and sang in Cape Town's gritty Khayelitsha area to mark the establishment of a Médecins Sans Frontières program that showed sophisticated treatment could work—and people would stick to schedules for taking a cocktail of drugs—in impoverished areas. International specialists had questioned that at the time. . . .

South Africa, a country of 50 million people, has more people living with HIV than anywhere in the world, with 5.7 million infected.[31]

Looking back ten years ago when we first arrived in Khayelitsha, it was striking to see that people were dying everywhere, from a disease [that it] was forbidden to name at the time, because no solution existed for it. There was such intense community denial about it all. . . . Ten years down the line, over 55,000 people test for HIV a year; people understand that HIV is no longer a death sentence. . . . Khayelitsha is proof that with concerted efforts, despite limited resources, universal coverage can be achieved. The challenge ahead will be to reduce HIV transmission, although some early signs of this are seen in Khayelitsha. We are still lagging behind in making a major impact in this area. . . . We have our work cut out for us.[32]

When I made my third and last visit to the Khayelitsha project in 2005, it was well on its way to achieving what it celebrated six years later on the tenth anniversary of the creation of its HIV/AIDS program. MSF was even taking steps toward handing that program over to the Provincial Department of Health—notwithstanding the anxiety among the staff about whether with this transfer of responsibility, the quality of HIV/AIDS care would be maintained.

At the same time, MSF was contemplating expanding some of the HIV prevention services that it offered at Khayelitsha by opening several youth clinics, where, in a setting responsive to their attitudes and needs, the sexually transmitted infections of young persons could be diagnosed and treated, and they could be tested for HIV and counseled about HIV/AIDS. It was also planning to locate a male walk-in clinic in the area of Khayelitsha's busiest taxi rank, to which it was hoped more men would come for the early diagnosis and management of sexually transmitted diseases and HIV/AIDS.

The most ambitious new project that the MSF Khayelitsha group was about to undertake was located in another African society—in Lesotho, a small, extremely poor country completely surrounded by South Africa, with the second-highest HIV prevalence in the world and the fourth-highest TB incidence, where the majority of HIV/AIDS-related deaths were due to TB. An unofficial moratorium on launching new HIV/AIDS programs had been called by MSF, "due in part to concerns about the ethical (and also financial) implications of having started tens of thousands of people on antiretroviral therapy (ART) without necessarily having any 'exit strategy' or a solid plan for guaranteeing long-term continuity of care independent of MSF."[33] But as a consequence of the intensive lobbying with MSF Belgium's Brussels headquarters that Eric Goemaere and several of his colleagues in South Africa conducted, an exploratory HIV/AIDS project mission in Lesotho had been authorized. It was designed as a joint pilot program with the Lesotho government's Ministry of Health and Social Welfare, which would provide free primary HIV/AIDS care and treatment to the entire population of the rural catchment area of the Scott Hospital of the Lesotho Evangelical Church in Morija, just south of Maseru, the country's capital. Its local partners included the Christian Health Association of Lesotho. Drawing on MSF's Khayelitsha and Lusikisiki models and experiences, it was to be a decentralized program that would bring the care and treatment of HIV/AIDS and TB as close as possible to people's homes; train nurses to initiate and manage antiretroviral therapy; and recruit "lay counselors" from the community (including persons living with AIDS), who would play an important (remunerated) role in supporting HIV/AIDS and TB patients and following them through the continuum of their care. The project was planned for a three-year period (from 2006 through 2008), after which, supposedly, MSF would gradually transfer full responsibility for it to the Lesotho Ministry of Heath and Social Welfare.

In addition, what Goemaere had defined as one of his long-range "dreams"[34] —the creation of MSF South Africa as an association recognized by MSF's international organization, with the hope of eventually becoming a full partner section—seemed to be gradually moving toward becoming a reality.

Since the discovery of HIV in the 1980s we had all implicitly hoped that AIDS would go away one fine day and that technology—a vaccine, perhaps a cure— would eliminate HIV. No such luck. HIV is firmly embedded in both human cells and societies.—Peter Piot, *No Time to Lose*[35]

Despite all that it had accomplished, and the responsibilities that it had turned over to national and local authorities and personnel, the MSF mission based in Khayelitsha was not planning to take definitive leave of South Africa. Rather, given its conviction that it had not yet had enough "impact," and that there was vital "work cut out" for it to do, which might not be accomplished otherwise, it intended to remain on the scene.

Notwithstanding the establishment of the South African National AIDS Council (SANAC) in 2000, which was supposed to provide leadership, over- sight, and continual assessment and monitoring for the country's response to AIDS and tuberculosis, all signs already indicated that it would not be organi- zationally competent to do so.[36] South Africa continued to have "5.7 million HIV-infected people, more than any other country; the highest rate of TB per capita; and, after Russia, the second highest reported number of MDR [multi- drug-resistant] TB cases."[37] The number of persons newly infected with HIV was still high, and the incidence of rape, a significant source of new infections, had mounted. Although the donning and collective display of "HIV POSI- TIVE" T-shirts publicly showed that the stigma associated with HIV/AIDS had diminished, it had not been expunged. Despite the success of decentralizing and "task-shifting" the treatment and care of HIV/AIDS to nurses and com- munity workers piloted by MSF, there continued to be a dearth of needed staff for managing the increasing numbers of persons on treatment. National and international funding were still insufficient to make antiretroviral drugs available to everyone who needed them, or to put everyone who suffered from severe side effects of the standard regimen of these drugs, or had become resistant to them, on new, more expensive second-line ones. Furthermore, because of the international economic crisis, donor countries were making large budgetary cuts in their contributions to the Global Fund to Fight AIDS, Tuberculosis and Malaria, which was threatening the financial situation of the agency that is the greatest source of support for HIV treatment in the world.

The economic, social, and political problems with which South Africa con- tinued to be fraught contributed to the persistence of the high incidence of HIV/AIDS in the country, to the difficulties and deficiencies in how it was being societally handled, and to the ways in which rape and other forms of violent and criminal behavior were connected with it. The official national unemployment rate was twenty-five percent, the unofficial, "real" rate, over forty percent; and the jobless rate among youths was estimated to have reached the staggering level of seventy percent.[38] Approximately forty percent of South Africans were living in poverty, with the poorest fifteen percent among them subsisting on less than two dollars a day. Furthermore, South Africa had one of the most unequal income distributions in the world, with the chief divide now between rich blacks and poor blacks, rather than between blacks and whites, as had been the case during apartheid.[39] Although government per capita expenditures for education were substantial, by and large, the quality of education that students were receiving was poor; and the public universities were so overstretched and inundated by applicants that they were able to admit fewer than half of those seeking admission. Even among college graduates, it had been reported, as many as six hundred thousand were unemployed.[40] The African National Congress (ANC), which had begun as a liberation movement, had played a historic role in defeating white minority rule, and had come to power in 1994, in South Africa's first nonracial elections, remained the country's ruling political party. Notwithstanding its important role in the establishment of stable, liberal democratic institutions, and in ensuring civil and social as well as political rights, it had tenaciously held on to political power, and was inclined to allocate positions in the government to its members who had been actively involved in the struggle against apartheid, or had demonstrated strong loyalty to the party. Increasingly (with foundation in fact), the top echelons of the ANC were being critically perceived as engaging in self-promoting and self-enriching forms of corruption (including graft, bribery, and ostentatious displays of wealth acquired from business backers), and as embroiled in vicious power struggles. And yet it was highly likely that the majority of black Africans, who constituted seventy-nine percent of the country's population, would continue to emotionally support the ANC and vote for its candidates because of its historical and symbolic anti-apartheid role.

A medical humanitarian organization like MSF had neither the international mandate nor the ability to alter or ameliorate any of these socioeconomic and political conditions in South Africa in which the festering of HIV/AIDS was embedded. Would South Africa ever become an "AIDS-free" society? Would MSF only then be able to feel that its work there was done, and that the time for its departure had arrived? Or would it have to be acknowledged (to invoke Albert Camus's allegorical conception of a plague) that HIV/AIDS was a pestilence "not made to man's measure," that "never disappears for good," but entails a "never ending fight," over which there is "no final victory"?[41]

During the time that I spent in Khayelitsha in 2002, 2003, and 2005, questions about when MSF might definitively withdraw from the activities in which it was engaged in South Africa were not overtly raised. What appeared to be its implicit guiding intent was to remain there, building on the progress that had been made and disseminating the model of HIV/AIDS prevention, treatment, and care on which it was based, in diversified projects and roles.

And yet Eric Goemaere, who was then head of the mission in Khayelitsha, was not unaware of the fact that this stance opened onto important, dilemma-ridden questions about MSF's medical humanitarian commitments, which were not confined to its presence in Khayelitsha and South Africa, or to its involvement with HIV/AIDS. "[H]anding over large cohorts of patients [with long-term pandemic diseases] to vertical national programs brings with it huge dilemmas around issues of [the] continuum of quality care, absence of integrated approaches to co-infection, [the] need for second- and . . . third-line affordable treatments and [the] specific needs of children," an MSF study noted.[42] On a larger scale, how should MSF allocate its material and human resources between all "the victims of natural or man-made disasters [and of] armed conflict" in the world, and all the "populations in distress" to which it is committed by its Charter to respond? When can it be said that MSF has sufficiently attained the goals it has set for a particular mission to justify taking leave of it, and allocating the resources it had designated for it, elsewhere? And how should MSF deal with the limitations, and with the finitude of humanitarian action—with what it cannot ultimately accomplish?

Global Fund cuts spell more AIDS deaths, more HIV infections, & rationing life-saving treatment, South Africa's Budget Expenditure Monitoring Forum warns

JOHANNESBURG, 25 November [2011]—The shock announcement by the Board of the Global Fund to Fight AIDS, TB, and Malaria that financial shortfalls forced the cancellation of its Round 11 of new grants threatens to run back the clock on the gains made in the fight against HIV. The Global Fund financial deficit is primarily the result of donors scaling back commitments, and not releasing already-promised funds. It will have severe repercussions for millions of people who are in urgent need of life-saving antiretroviral therapy (ART) in Southern Africa.

The Global Fund is the largest multilateral funder of HIV treatment, financing more than 70% of antiretroviral drugs in the developing world and approximately 85% of TB programming in Africa. . . .

Since Round 11 will not be launched, in countries where program disruptions are expected, yet-to-be-secured emergency monies are meant to be made available to continue HIV treatment for those already receiving it through a Transitional Funding Mechanism. . . .

Canceling Round 11 is devastating. With no new patients able to be initiated on treatment in some countries, already unacceptable long treatment wait lists will become even longer. Treatment rationing may also be on the horizon, with doctors having to select patients to give treatment to rather than providing it to all those who seek it. In Southern Africa, we know treatment rationing all too well, having battled for programs that are robust enough to provide care to all of those who need it. People living with HIV who are in urgent need of life-saving treatment cannot afford to go back to the dark days we experienced years ago. . . .

Funding shortfalls [have] also meant that despite commendable efforts to scale-up HIV programs across southern Africa, some countries have been unable to fully implement the most recent World Health Organization HIV guidelines. These guidelines call for earlier ART initiation . . . and with better first-line drugs. Earlier ART is more important now than ever given landmark scientific evidence released this year which showed that HIV treatment not only saves lives but also prevents new infections. This proves that we can end AIDS if we place more people on HIV treatment earlier. . . .

The international community must recognize that we are at a critical crossroads: we either use the science, tools, and policies already at our disposal to save lives and prevent new infections; or see the hard-fought gains of the last decade lost. It is criminal that at the time when we can truly make an impact on the epidemic by ensuring that more people are placed on treatment, we are instead witnessing a massive funding retreat which threatens to push us back by years.[43]

For Goemaere, the cancellation of Round 11 of the Global Fund to Fight AIDS, Tuberculosis and Malaria grants meant a potential return to what he called "the graveyards' scenario" of AIDS. In response, he immediately sprang into "a flurry" of witnessing action—alerting MSF to the "terrible consequences this might have," asking its secretary-general to put it on the agenda of an international meeting scheduled to be held in Paris on December 16–18, 2011, and bringing its gravity to the attention of the media.[44] Because of this new set of circumstances, the continuing physical presence of MSF in Khayelitsha and other areas of South Africa, in active engagement with HIV/AIDS and its concomitants, seemed more likely, more intensive, and more extensive than ever.[45]

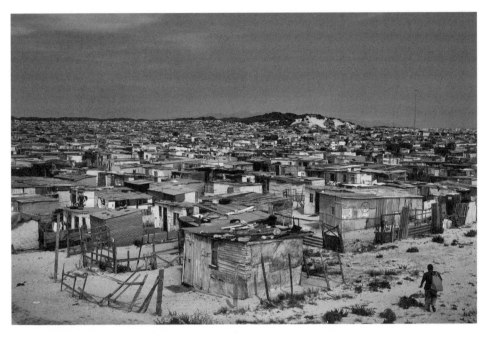

Khayelitsha, Cape Town. "That these labyrinthine streets are smoothly paved like the highway seems incongruous—even ironic—in this crowded, poverty-stricken universe of corrugated iron shacks, most of which are without running water or electricity." Photographer: José Cendón. Reproduced by permission of Eric Goemaere.

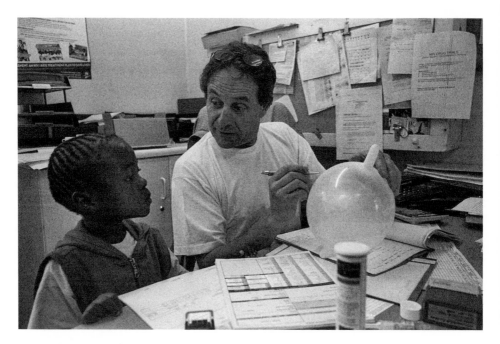

As they recover from life-threatening illnesses such as HIV/AIDS, if they do, the emerging brightness in children's faces helps restore their MSF caregivers' hope, reassuring them that their work matters. Photographer: Francesco Zizola. Reproduced by permission of Eric Goemaere.

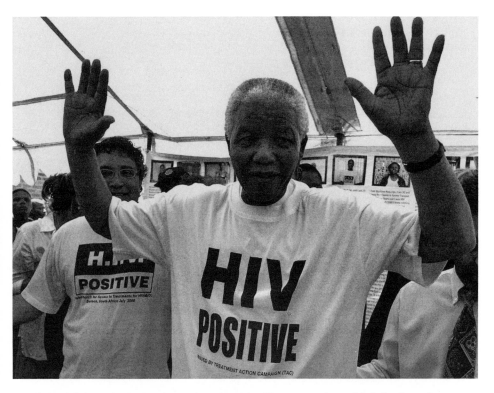

"Mandela's visit was of great reach and weight. He came and sprinkled the dust of hope and humanity on a sometimes rather lost and sad place. You can imagine the pleasure of all those working near and far to the project. On the day of [his] visit, when he was offered [an "HIV POSITIVE"] T-shirt, he immediately took off his shirt, and slipped on the T-shirt. As he did this, I saw explosions of joy in people's eyes. . . . An instant of pure, pure joy." Photographer: Eric Miller. Reproduced by permission of Eric Goemaere.

MSF members stood in the midst of an MSF General Assembly (2008) with microphones in hand, making spirited contributions to the ongoing discussion. Reproduced by permission of MSF, South African office.

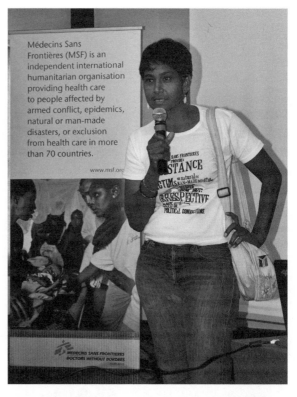

MSF General Assembly attendees in 2008 beating traditional African drums, led by three professional drummers. The language of the drums touched everyone, deeply connecting them. Reproduced by permission of MSF, South African office.

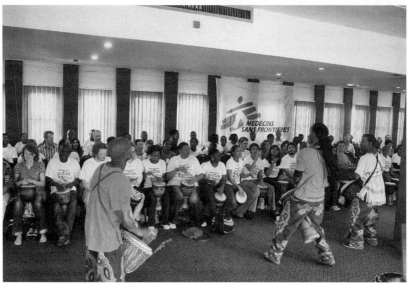

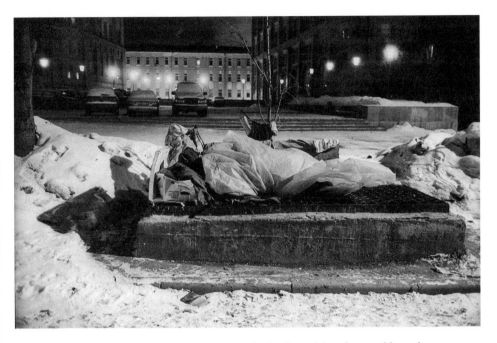

When MSF began its work in 1992, Moscow had at least thirty thousand homeless living and sleeping on its streets or in improvised digs. Photographer: Alexander Glyadelov.

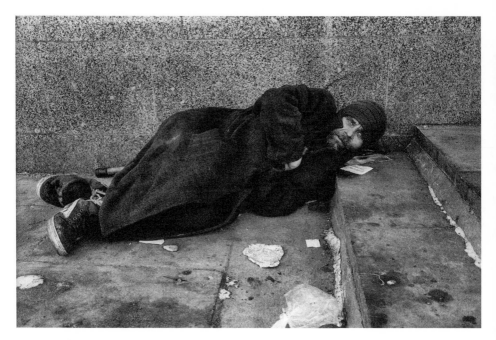

An MSF survey among 22,513 of its Moscow patients between 1995 and 2000 revealed that the majority (ninety percent) of the homeless persons were men between the ages of twenty and fifty. One in ten had a college education, and one in five, vocational training. Most were law-abiding citizens with no criminal record, were fit to work, and were looking for a job. Photographer: Alexander Glyadelov.

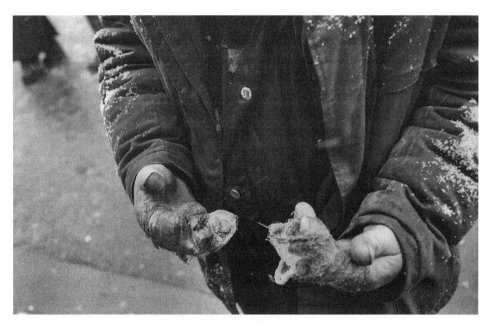

The most common medical conditions from which Moscow's homeless suffered were not infectious diseases, but ulcers and infected wounds due to exposure to the elements, poor living conditions, and lack of access to medical care. Photographer: Alexander Glyadelov.

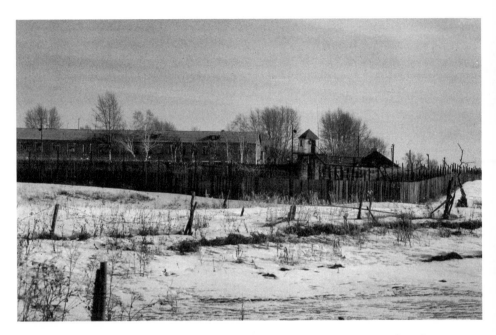

Penal Colony No. 33—a referral colony for the tuberculosis patients sent there from the twenty-six penal colonies in the Kemerovo region of Siberia—where MSF Belgium began to work in 1996. Image from the MSF archives by unknown MSF photographer. Obtained from Natalia Vezhnina and reproduced with her permission.

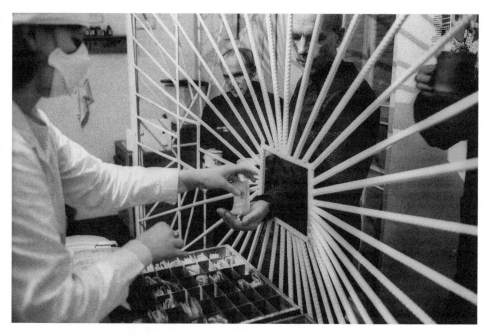

DOTS, "directly observed treatment, short-course" with a standardized group of antibiotic anti-TB drugs, gave promise of curing as many as 85 percent of TB patients. Photographer: Alexander Glyadelov.

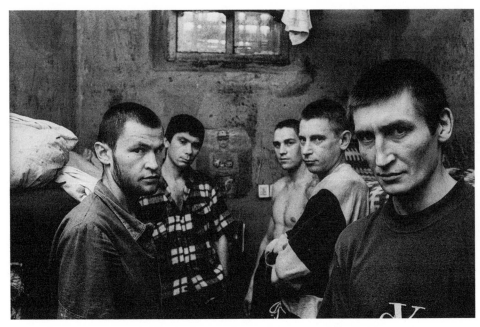

Initially, a suspicious fear circulated among the prisoners that the MSF "foreign doctors" had entered Penal Colony No. 33 to experiment on them with unproven drugs. The most powerful "thief in law" among the prisoners told them not to accept the drugs from these foreigners and, at first, almost all of them followed his instructions. Doctors spent hours with this prisoner-leader, explaining MSF's principles and intentions, the medical characteristics of tuberculosis, and the optimal way to treat it, before he gave permission to his fellow prisoners to accede to the DOTS regimen. After that, prisoners no longer refused to be treated by DOTS, and those who received the treatment fully complied with its strict protocol. Photographer: Alexander Glyadelov.

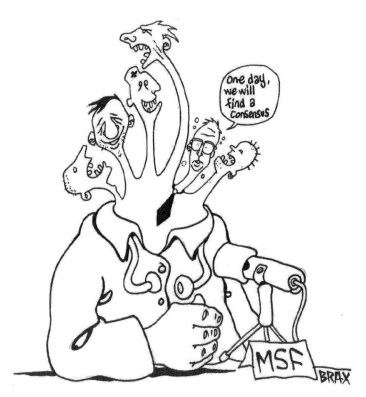

MSF has been constantly preoccupied with these questions: What kinds of "compromises" ought to be made to stay in the field? When, in the face of what conditions, should MSF depart from an area or country where it is embedded and engaged in committee work? And although MSF's Charter states that its workers should be "aware of the risks and dangers of the missions they undertake," when do these become so great that an organizational decision to leave the field is both necessary and justified? Reproduced by permission of Samuel Hanryon, a.k.a. "Brax," Rash Brax.

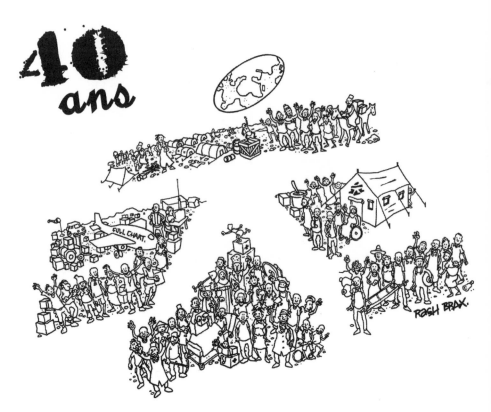

In 2011, MSF celebrated its fortieth anniversary and held the first meeting of its newly created International General Assembly. Reproduced by permission of Samuel Hanryon, a.k.a. "Brax," Rash Brax.

CHAPTER NINE

A "Non-Western Entity" Is Born

> Informed and active associations and their representatives are crucial to assuring the relevance of our actions and the maintenance of a strong MSF international movement. Invigorating participation . . . at all levels of MSF is essential to building and maintaining credible, competent and relevant international governance.
>
> DOCTORS WITHOUT BORDERS / MÉDECINS SANS FRONTIÈRES,
>
> "LA MANCHA AGREEMENT" (2006)

MSF South Africa officially became a new MSF "association" on December 16, 2011, the first day of MSF's first International General Assembly in Paris, France, and of the simultaneous fortieth anniversary celebration of the movement's foundation.[1]

Discussions at MSF's international "La Mancha" conference in 2004 had catalyzed the recognition of MSF South Africa, bringing home to members that as many as ninety percent of the field positions in the countries where MSF had missions were filled by indigenous "national" personnel, and that over seventy percent of its projects were situated in Africa. Notwithstanding its "without borders" vision and commitment, MSF was still mainly run by western Europeans, however, and in many contexts where it worked, it was perceived as a predominantly foreign and white, if "international," organization.[2]

"New Entities": Initiatives and Deterrents

Within the post–La Mancha framework, questions arose about how to deal with MSF's extraordinary growth. The challenge was to fuse furthering MSF's internationalization and its social mission with the "desire for a compact and dynamic movement, cautious of being headquarters-heavy and eager to engage the great growth that MSF had undergone over time."[3] New "entities" were developing around MSF in countries where it was in the field—including Argentina, Brazil, the Czech Republic, India, Ireland, Kenya, Mexico, Portugal, South Africa, Turkey, and the United Arab Emirates—and a number of these had asked for formal status in MSF. They wanted to be recognized at least as something akin to a branch office, but perhaps hoped, as was true of the group that had coalesced in South Africa, to be eventually recognized as a "real MSF section."

As the vagueness and generality of the term "entities" suggests, it was not at all clear what such units ought to be—or what they should be called, or how to go about creating them, or what criteria they would have to meet to be approved, presumably by MSF's International Council. This uncertainty is apparent in a 2007 memorandum concerning "new entities in Brazil and South Africa" that Gorik Ooms, then the director-general of the Brussels Operational Center (OCB), sent to the OCB board and the International Office's committee of direction. In this memo, Ooms spoke of his perplexity about what to advise the groups in Brazil and South Africa about the necessary next steps toward becoming MSF affiliates:

> I personally informed the MSF International Office about the intention to create MSF entities in Brazil and South Africa, and asked which procedure I needed to follow to obtain permission. I was told that there is no procedure for new entities as long as they don't become independent sections (as long as they are controlled by one of the 19 sections). . . . We can only guess which criteria the International Council will use to accept or reject the demand coming from the new MSF entities to become a real MSF section.[4]

The two most important of these criteria would probably be "the existence of a solid associative basis,"[5] he conjectured, consisting of "a majority of field staff or former field staff members . . . to make sure that [these entities] can develop an independent position on all [the] dilemmas MSF is confronted with" and "financial independence." The latter seemed "almost impossible" for South Africa, he stated. "This is a bit of a headache," he pointed out, "because as long as MSF South Africa is not accepted as a real MSF section, it must be under the control of an existing MSF section or operational center. It is a 'catch 22' situation":

- As long as MSF South Africa cannot achieve financial independence, it will not be accepted as an MSF section;
- As long as MSF South Africa is not accepted as an MSF section, it cannot have a formal associative structure.

What Ooms proposed was "creating a formal associative structure, with a board of which at least 50% of the members are appointed by the OCB board. It fits with the rules of MSF (controlled by an existing MSF operational center) and it fits with South African law."[6]

In the concluding section of his memorandum, Ooms gave vent to the frustration he was experiencing in dealing with his own and other MSF operational centers and their boards about matters that were not confined to new MSF entities issues:

> The whole idea of creating an OCB Board was to simplify and improve the governance of the OCB. I cannot do the job you want me to do, if for every decision I need to discuss with ten directors in Brussels, six general directors outside of Brussels, and seven national boards (in total: about 100 people to be convinced.) And that does not even include the international MSF platforms, which increasingly decide what MSF operational centers are allowed to do, and what they're not allowed to do.[7]

Notwithstanding MSF's commitment to defining itself as a movement rather than an organization, and its wariness about becoming overly institutionalized, dealing with questions about new entities entangled it in what critical members called "structural navel-gazing," and the assumption that "designing [and redesigning] structures" would resolve issues and "fix problems." In November 2006, MSF South Africa was officially recognized by the International Council as a "branch office" that would function under the Brussels Operational Center. This was partly a consequence of a three-month-long "feasibility study," involving interviewing a wide variety of "stakeholders" in South Africa, mandated by the International Council.

The study concluded that creating an MSF entity in South Africa would be a win-win situation, good for both MSF and South Africa:

> There is clearly willingness and a momentum to start an entity of MSF in South Africa. . . . a momentum to grasp. This willingness is not only manifested among members of the MSF team in South Africa, but also among . . . South African partners . . . (many triggered by the HIV/AIDS fight) . . . [who have been] discussing

the idea of MSF [for] some time. . . . A strong network exists made up of individuals and organizations that favor and support the initiative. They represent a source of legitimacy to start. . . . The capacity and the environment to open an MSF entity are present and look inviting.[8]

MSF veterans like Ooms and Goemaere regarded designating MSF South Africa a branch office under the control of the Brussels Operational Center, rather than making it an independent new section, as a "half-baked solution" at best.[9]

MSF South Africa

MSF South Africa's office is located in Johannesburg, where, at its inception, it was run by its founding director-general, Sharon Ekambaram, a dynamic, astutely intelligent woman.[10] Ekambaram's family came to South Africa from a Tamil-speaking area of India. She was raised in South Africa by her parents in what she describes as "a very British manner"; but her involvement in "the struggle against apartheid," she says, "gave me a black identity." She defines herself as "a Marxist" and a "committed activist," dedicated to socioeconomic equality, "passionate in [her] outrage against any form of injustice," and "an organizer in building movements."[11]

Ekambaram was propelled toward involvement with MSF by her "burnout" from dealing with all the people dying from HIV/AIDS whom she had come to know through her work for the AIDS Consortium ("a network organisation primarily concerned with servicing people infected and affected by HIV and AIDS"),[12] at a time when few South Africans had access to antiretroviral drugs. Eric Goemaere, with whom she had had some contact since the early 2000s, was her chief link with MSF. She admired his firsthand knowledge of the HIV/AIDS situation in South Africa gained through field experience, the cogency of the data he had gathered based on that experience, and above all, the role that the presentation of these data to South African officials had played in the passage of legislation supporting universal access to antiretroviral therapy. Goemaere is one of the persons inside of MSF to whom she feels the most indebted for the international organization's recognition of MSF South Africa.

Because she was "intrigued by, and in awe of an organization [like MSF] that . . . delivers and does not [just] churn out rhetoric" like other NGOs, she felt that it was "worth being part of a battle to change it."[13] A crucial change, in her view, was to avoid duplicating how MSF's five operational centers in Europe were "entrenched," in a way conducive to "empire building." She was convinced that MSF South Africa should neither be nationally "Afrocentric" nor "based on narrow geographic reasoning." Thus, from the beginning, she, as director, along with its board, had "conceptualized" the branch office as regional, rather than national in scope—as MSF Southern Africa, not just MSF South Africa—"with members from across the Southern Africa region, encompassing Malawi, Mozambique, Lesotho, Swaziland, Zambia, and Zimbabwe," as well as South Africa. "MSF SA did not want to give the impression that it represents the entire continent, or that it would be defined by national boundaries," Ekambaram explained.[14]

> Given the current role of the South African state in the rest of Africa . . . [with] its potential . . . of being the richest country . . . or one of the richest in Africa . . . it is often described as having imperialist intentions. Many surrounding countries are nervous [about this]. . . . So the structure that is developing is based on working in the region on issues relevant to the operations that are within the proximity of the office. . . . [It has a] cross-operational center character.

MAMELA!

"The spirit with which MSF SA is being built is strongly influenced by the spirit of 'struggle' from which South Africa is emerging," Ekambaram asserts. "The central logic behind the MSF South Africa office" is, however, to "enable MSF to look at Africa—where two-thirds of MSF's work is done—from an African perspective."[15]

What Ekambaram refers to as MSF South Africa's spirit of "struggle" and "activism," with its passionate indignation about social injustice and social suffering, and its "vibrant, . . . almost celebrat[ory]" ambiance,[16] pervades the e-newsletter that MSF SA inaugurated in August 2008, *MAMELA!*[17] *Mamela*, a Sesotho word, means "listen." Ekambaram chose it as the title of the editorial that she wrote for the first issue, which began by asking: "What does South Africa have to offer the MSF international movement?" It answered the question thus:

> As a movement, MSF has a rich history of using the oral concept of *témoignage* or witnessing, which has strong resonance in South Africa. South Africans spoke out and resisted apartheid. This rich tradition is still very much in the fabric of

our society. We experienced this again with the struggle for access to treatment for people living with HIV and more recently the rallying of forces to support refugees violently kicked out of their makeshift shelters in various communities. This spirit of collaboration and solidarity is what MSF SA wants to bring to the MSF international movement.

"To mark this first edition of *MAMELA!*" the editorial continued, "I want to inform you of the work done by MSF as part of its medical humanitarian support: Addressing the plight of vulnerable women. This, as we celebrate this month, on August 9, the role played by brave women in the struggle against apartheid, and to inspire you as we feel anger thinking about the way many, many poor oppressed women are treated all over the world":

> In December 2006 MSF related the stories of 10 Congolese women who were brave enough to tell their stories. These testimonies were used [by MSF] as a tool to try and end the sexual violence against women who cross the border from the Democratic Republic of Congo into Angola, then only to be expelled by the perpetrators . . . of this sexual abuse . . . many of whom [are] soldiers in the Angolan army. By MSF medical staff working in the field, speaking out and confirming the stories of otherwise voiceless women, MSF legitimized their experience and brought the attention of the world to witness this crime, forcing a reaction from the authorities concerned.

In its conclusion, the editorial dedicated the first edition of *MAMELA!* to "the memory of Promise Sanelisiwe Tshiloane, who worked as a supply assistant in the co-ordination office in the MSF project in Khayelitsha":

> On Friday, 4 July, around 15:00, Promise's body was discovered by the police in her flat in Parklands, Cape Town. She was killed by her husband who afterwards committed suicide. . . . Promise was a young and beautiful woman, struggling to deal with everyday challenges that women are faced with. Hate crimes of this nature are witnessed on a daily basis, often adversely affecting those most vulnerable. Speaking out about this restores dignity to women facing violent crimes and hopefully will force more people to commit to addressing this horrible blight on the human race.

Subsequent issues inveighed against the "xenophobic violence" unleashed on "foreign nationals" from neighboring African countries seeking refuge and asylum in South Africa.[18] A fervent article commemorated the attacks by "marauding mobs" in the Alexandra township of Johannesburg in May 2008, when 62 foreigners had been killed and 100,000 displaced. *MAMELA!* described how MSF SA responded. In the immediate wake of the attacks, it treated "nearly 4,000 people for gunshot and stab wounds, diarrhea, respiratory infections, and trauma related illnesses"; it distribute[d] "thousands of blankets, hygiene kits, and other goods, while conducting approximately 11,000 medical consultations among traumatized foreigners in numerous makeshift camps" in the South African province of Gauteng; it spoke out in protest, and along with others, through court action, prevented Gauteng authorities from "moving approximately 1700 displaced foreigners from a makeshift camp to a formalized camp which was set in a veritable lion's den—between aggressive hostel dwellers and a dusty mine dump"; and it worked in the camps housing foreign nationals "left helpless and homeless," who were now "living in conditions that resembled incarceration."[19]

A number of newsletter articles recounted some of the humanitarian crises "across borders" to which MSF was responding. These included the devastating earthquake that struck Haiti; catastrophic floods that occurred in Pakistan; the "alarmingly high" incidence of leishmaniasis, a life-threatening protozoan disease, in a village in southern Sudan; and caring for the sick and the wounded in a region of the Democratic Republic of Congo that was ravaged by terrorist conflict and the raping of women.[20]

MSF workers' outrage at the poverty, hunger, disease, and violence they saw in such field situations also came through in *MAMELA!*

> I've been working as a nurse for MSF in southern Sudan since the beginning of 2010. The security situation in the region remains precarious and the people suffer from malnutrition, which has grown worse due to a late harvest. Leishmaniasis . . . is common here. . . . Without treatment, the majority of patients die. Because leishmaniasis mainly occurs in poorer countries where patients can't afford medicine, there are very few therapies available. The pharmaceutical industry doesn't invest in treatments as there's no profit to be had. We treat almost all our patients with a combination of drugs through intramuscular injections over 17 days, which causes them a great deal of pain. . . .
>
> In mid August I left Lankien for Pagli, a small village . . . where leishmaniasis is a particularly serious problem. The nearest health clinics are about three days' walk away. The rainy season has made the region inaccessible to vehicles. . . . [T]here are no medical personnel and we have to provide the treatment ourselves.[21]

I've been working for more than a year now in the DRC [Democratic Republic of Congo]. . . . North Kivu is a large region, full of hills and narrow valleys, there are villages (and people) everywhere, and while doing mobile clinics or transferring patients, we inevitably meet armed groups. Most of them respect us—we also cure them when they are sick or wounded, we treat their families like anyone else's. Although we never know when it is the case, because we never ask anything, we treat all people equally, but they let you know. . . . So somehow they say thanks, and they let us pass. But then one week later you hear there was some shooting in that area, and some villages in the neighborhood were ransacked and burned, people fled. That night you imagine that they were the same fighters that you met on the road. . . .

. . . warriors and terrorized population all in the same patch of territory, all of them close to each other, separated by just a few kilometers. . . .

But fighting can start everywhere, and violence occurs even without shooting: There's rape and threats and looting, all the time, and we only know it when people come to seek shelter or are wounded and brought to the hospital. . . .

All of this [is] so sad, this has gone on for years but seems never ending. Difficult to keep the hope [sic] in these circumstances. But as they say in the Eastern Congo, every day may bring new hope, as long as we're alive.[22]

With a mixture of candor and intrepidness, some of the notices in *MAMELA!* addressed to potential MSF recruits alluded to the hardships that they should be prepared for:

In addition to the required medical skills, MSF SA invites applications from persons who wish to work in places such as the desolated [sic] deserts of Sudan or humid Liberia; people who are able to cope with the isolation of Mali and the complexity of Chad. Above all, MSF needs applicants who are willing to work in an environment avoided by most.[23]

Not a Western European NGO

Over the course of the years 2006–2011, MSF South Africa evolved dynamically, growing in size, membership, diversity, dedication, and fund-raising capacity. At the governance level, it elected a multinational board and convened annual general assemblies, which served as forums for discussion and for its collective decision-making.

As the South Africa office became more integrated into the overarching organization of MSF, some of the South Africans became more outspokenly critical of how "Western" and "European" MSF, seen as a whole, continued to be in its outlook, "institutional architecture," and functioning. These sentiments were vigorously presented in an internal paper by Jonathan Whittall and Ekambaram, "Genuine Reform: Adapting to a Changing Global Environment,"[24] which declared:

> We can acknowledge our Western roots, but it is time to internationalize and accept that Europe is no longer the center of the universe. . . . Being of Western origin is not the problem, but functioning in the current world as a Western organization is. . . .
>
> MSF is not keeping up with a changing global environment. [T]he West's influence is declining relative to the rising economic powers of Brazil, China, South Africa, and India. States affected by "humanitarian crises" are increasingly taking a more proactive stance in delivering services, and occupying powers—such as the US in Iraq—are offering "humanitarian assistance" to achieve the goal of stabilization and state building. . . . This requires MSF to navigate [the] newly emerging framework. Considering that the international humanitarian framework, traditionally the reference point for all of MSF's work, is increasingly being co-opted by a state-led moral humanitarian imperative, where does that leave us?

"In this context, how can we ensure continued access to vulnerable populations and independence to operate and speak out?" the paper asks. "[W]e cannot expect to fall back on the quality of our medical operations, as the only way of gaining acceptance," it asserts:

> Our ability to respond effectively to emergencies will be more based on our existing presence and our acceptance by communities rather than on our arrogance around principles which are increasingly associated with a Western industry of double standards.
>
> We have to become more aware and distance ourselves from a number of different factors, not least of all the organic links between MSF and its European mother-ship (such as in Haiti where Al Jazeera continually referred to us as the "French NGO," reinforcing this perception.) In addition to this, we have to distance ourselves from [the] humanitarian circus.

But, this "need for change cannot happen with multiple MSF sections working in one context," the paper contends. "There is an inherent tendency within this environment for each section to retreat into a nationalist logic—informed by their specific (European-based) national analysis—which entrenches the very perceptions that reduce our legitimacy."

At various points the paper refers to the colonialist and missionary-like attitudes and behavior that persist in MSF:

> There needs to be a thorough understanding of the societies within which MSF international expats work. For example, many countries in Africa are regaining [their] sense of dignity and independent selfhood after decades of colonial oppression. Instead of lamenting the good old days when governments were weak and aid agencies could do whatever they wanted, MSF has to work to open itself up to establishing networks or building necessary links with progressive elements of civil society on an issue by issue basis.
>
> . . . Western expats often see people in communities where we work as "beneficiaries"—passive recipients of humanitarian aid—and not as active agents capable of changing the conditions that lead to their vulnerability or at least participating in the process. At worst the role of MSF in parts of Africa cannot be distinguished from that of the missionary.
>
> . . . Ask yourself how our interlocutors perceive us when another [European] "boss" arrives from headquarters. Try to explain to people outside MSF that we really are an international organization, even though all our operational centers are in Europe.

The paper ends with what it terms "the obvious conclusion" that "there is a need for an integration of the voice of the 'non-Western' entities within MSF. . . . New entities should be acknowledged as offering a solution to some of the biggest challenges facing MSF today and should be given the space and support to . . . address those challenges. . . . It is time to move beyond tokenism," it declares. The "roadmap for change" that it proposes envisions "an equal MSF" in which a "conscious move" is made "away from the distinction and unbalanced power dynamics between 'expat' and 'national' staff, and towards valuing all staff based on their skill sets, experience, contextual understanding and analysis, and [their] . . . independent voice in certain contexts"; and "a more democratic process of decision making [is] established that ensures . . . it is not only the European sections with the most financial resources that control the decisions taken at the International Council."

Joyous Assemblies

The militant ardor that surrounded MSF South Africa's commitment to the MSF movement takes a joyous form at its yearly general assemblies. Serious business is transacted at these annual meetings in an effervescent atmosphere of camaraderie, which at times erupts into revelry.

Photographs of the MSF SA's 2008 General Assembly capture this ambiance, portraying lively gatherings of black, brown, and white women and men of European and American, as well as South African and other regional African origins. Many wear T-shirts with the MSF logo or "I AM POSITIVE" HIV/AIDS T-shirts. Others are clad in T-shirts with a universalistic message on the front:

REFUGEE OR **MIGRANT**

BLACK OR WHITE

CHRISTIAN OR **MUSLIM**

MILITARY OR **ARMED OPPOSITION**

MALE OR FEMALE

FOREIGNER OR **CITIZEN**[25]

On the backs the shirts is an affirmation taken from the MSF Charter: "MSF provides medical assistance irrespective of race, religion, creed, or political convictions." Both statements are framed by schematic, gray, left and right footprints. Displayed in white letters on the black T-shirts of some other attendees is the word KWEREKWERE—a derogatory, xenophobic term meaning "a foreign visitor to a township"/"a foreign outsider," which was being widely applied to immigrants and refugees in South Africa at the time.[26]

Included among the photos are a number of shots of different MSF members standing in the midst of the assemblage with microphones in hand, making spirited contributions to the ongoing discussion. In several instances, the enthusiastic, broadly smiling commentator, whose arms are dramatically upraised, appears to be mocking his own grandiloquence.

An especially animated group of photographs depicts the act of voting at the assemblies. The resolutions proposed were affirmed by raising yellow signs reading, "Member Voting Card." Other photos show lines of broadly smiling people with yellow or red cards making their way toward ballot boxes.

The most celebratory of the photos are those showing General Assembly attendees beating in synchrony on traditional African drums. Each person in the room has a drum and the entire assemblage is being led in collective drum music by three professional African drummers in bright orange tops and trousers fashioned of multicolored African fabrics. The language of the drums touched everyone, deeply connecting them.

From "Branch Office," to "Delegate Office," to "Association"

In November 2009, MSF South Africa was recognized by the International Council as a delegate office, and thereby moved one step further toward the goal of becoming a section, fully integrated into the movement, on a par with MSF's European operational sections.

Two years later, in December 2011, when it applied to MSF's newly formed International General Assembly to become an association, MSF South Africa had what it described as two hundred "dedicated members," from different sections of MSF's five Operational Centers, most of whom were "spread across the South Africa region, encompassing Malawi, Mozambique, Lesotho, South Africa, Swaziland, Zambia, and Zimbabwe." Eighty-four percent of these members were "national staff," sixteen percent "present and former international staff," forty-five percent "medical and para-medical," and fifty-five percent "non-medical." MSF South Africa also had what it characterized as "a fully functional board," comprised of three members delegated by the Operational Center in Brussels, five so-called "co-opted" members, and five members elected at its General Assembly. The composition of the board—four South Africans, three Belgians, two Zimbabweans, one Malawian, one Mozambican, one Zambian, and one American—was deemed "multinational." And although MSF South Africa frankly stated that it continued to be funded by the OCB, it proudly reported that it now had a very active fund-raising unit, which had so far raised 8,989,775 rands from 2009 to 2011.[27] "We hail from South Africa," "We are Dedicated and Diverse," We are Young and Vibrant," MSF SA proclaimed at the December 16–18 meeting of the International General Assembly in Paris, where it was formally recognized as an accredited MSF association. It would now be a more visible presence and have a vote at the international level.

MSF South Africa still has not been accorded the status of a full-blown section, although it was considered to be closer to being granted this status. Rather anomalously, it continues to be defined as a delegate office, even though this status had supposedly been abolished by the International General Assembly and International Board. There was some concern among its members about this but, like Ekambaram, they were more focused on recent changes in MSF's international organization. These were changes to which MSF South Africa felt it had made a significant, movement-wide contribution through its formation of "a structure that [had] direct influence over operations in the region"; its building of a regional association that was acting "like a magnet for predominantly national staff"; its "development of a different relationship with MSF other than of employee/employer"; "the [networking] relations [it had] forged across operational centers"; and its firsthand "proximity" to fields in which MSF was operating.[28]

MSF South Africa's ultimate goal, Ekambaram attested, was to have a board "elected from a cadre of MSF associate members, irrespective of their 'status' as national or international members, but based on the quality of their input and insight into operational experience and analysis," which would further the evolution of MSF into "a truly international movement," with "no association to any specific geographic location." "This is what the world needs now," she declared— a world that is "very different from the one that MSF was born into." In her view, MSF still had a long road to travel to realize that vision.[29]

PART V / In Postsocialist Russia

CHAPTER TEN

Reaching Out to the Homeless and Street Children of Moscow

with Olga Shevchenko

My interest in seeing MSF's work in Russia firsthand had several personal sources. Both my maternal and paternal grandparents came to the United States from Russia in the early years of the twentieth century as part of the great wave of East European Jewish migration to the United States between 1880 and 1914. Determined that their children and grandchildren would be "one hundred percent American," they conveyed to us no personal memories of the country that they had forever left behind. I had often wondered what their lives in Russia had been like in the Jewish shtetl community of my maternal grandparents, which they never identified by name, and in the urban Jewish milieu of Odessa, where my paternal grandparents had lived. And during my years as a graduate student in the Harvard Department of Social Relations, my curiosity about Russia was ignited in a quite different way by an exciting course in the history and sociology of the Soviet Union given by the sociologist Alex Inkeles.[1]

When choosing Russia as one of the sites of my research inside MSF became a possibility, my biography fueled my interest in traveling to that country for the first time—although I did not expect to find even vestiges of the long-ago worlds of my grandparents there, or the continued existence of the USSR.[2] In fact, one of the major reasons for which I eventually decided to undertake field research in Russia in 2000 was to learn about Russia's problems in the wake of the social changes of the past decade, and about MSF's response to these problems. Postsocialist Russia is neither a so-called developing nor a resource-poor country like so many of the societies in which MSF operates, and so I surmised that the issues MSF faced in Russia, and the ways it dealt with them, would be quite different from those in most other settings. This turned out to be only partially true.

Without the collaboration of Olga Shevchenko, a Russian-born associate professor of sociology at Williams College, I would not have had the knowledge and understanding of Russian society and culture, not to speak of fluency in the Russian language, to qualify me to make MSF in Russia one of my case studies—or the temerity to consider doing so. Olga Shevchenko received a BA at Moscow State University and an MA from the Central European University in Budapest, then earned a PhD in sociology from the University of Pennsylvania. At the core of her doctoral dissertation,[3] and her book based upon it—Crisis and the Everyday in Postsocialist Moscow—are 103 in-depth interviews that she conducted recurrently with a sample of thirty-three "Muscovites from various walks of life, and of various ages and political persuasions," and her participant observation among them between 1998 and 2000.[4] As one of her teachers in the Sociology Department at the University of Pennsylvania, and a member of her dissertation committee, I had privileged access to her firsthand data, and to her thinking about the subject. In addition, a warm collegial relationship developed between us, and our many conversations came to include discussions about my ongoing MSF research. Eventually, it occurred to me to ask her if she would be willing to conduct field research with me on MSF in Russia, and she graciously—even enthusiastically—accepted my invitation.

Our observational, interview, and documentary research unfolded between 2000 and 2005. It involved two successive field visits together to Moscow (in May–June 2000 and June 2001). There, using MSF Belgium's Moscow office as our base, we extended our research into some of its projects, with site visits to the Moscow offices of MSF France, MSF Holland, and MSF Switzerland.[5] Subsequently, during the summers of 2002, 2003, 2004, and 2005, Olga updated and supplemented our data by conducting additional interviews in Moscow—chiefly with the Russian staff of MSF Belgium and with Russian physicians who had worked in its tuberculosis project. Although I remained in Philadelphia during those summers, Olga and I were in constant communication via e-mail, telephone, and postal mail, so there was a "long distance" sense in which I participated in her fieldwork. Nonetheless, throughout the 2002–2005 period, she was the primary field researcher. Her role in collecting, translating, and analyzing the data presented in the following two chapters on "MSF in Postsocialist Russia" was indispensable.

Before I went to Moscow, I had a rather limited view of MSF's activities in Russia. I had been told that MSF Belgium was the chief section on the Russian scene; that its major local project was its work with homeless people on the streets of Moscow; and that it was a key participant in a program treating prisoners afflicted with tuberculosis in a number of penal colonies in Western Siberia. But it was not until Olga and I made our first visits to MSF Belgium's shabby offices, in a dilapidated two-story building in the center of Moscow, that we learned how complicated the situation of MSF in Russia was.

MSF Belgium, France, Holland, and Switzerland had all participated in MSF's "Caucasus Project" in Chechnya, Dagestan, and Ingushetia. In those high-risk settings, MSF had been providing shelter, food, water and sanitation programs, medicines, medical equipment, medical care, and psychosocial support for the thousands internally displaced by the two successive wars that had been waged between Russia and Chechnya in 1994 and 1999.[6] The wars were officially over when we arrived in Moscow in the summer of 2000 to begin our research, but conflict persisted. And life-threatening security problems for humanitarian workers in the area had escalated to the point where MSF had reluctantly withdrawn all its foreign and Russian personnel from the Caucasus region, replacing them with a "remote control system of intervention" through Chechens and Ingushs.[7]

For pragmatic reasons, Olga and I decided to focus our research on MSF Belgium's programs in Moscow for homeless people and for children living in the city's streets, and its tuberculosis project in the prisons of Siberia.[8] These important MSF undertakings were accessible to us, and their personnel were not at risk. However, although the TB program in Siberia was not physically imperiled, its ongoing existence hung by a thread—something we did not realize at the time.

In December 1988, a devastating earthquake took place in Armenia, then a republic of the Soviet Union.[9] Soviet leader Mikhail Gorbachev called for outside foreign aid from a number of countries and humanitarian organizations. MSF responded to his appeal. Provision of emergency medical care for victims of the earthquake constituted its first action in the region. Subsequently, in 1991, after the fall of the Soviet Union, MSF Belgium became aware of a humanitarian crisis in the environs of its Moscow office: the thousands of homeless persons in Moscow who were totally excluded from outpatient medical care.

Several MSF reports describe the predicament of the Moscow homeless, and how they fell into this social abyss:

> In order to strengthen the totalitarian regime [in the USSR], homelessness was declared illegal. In a country where socialism was "victorious," there were not supposed to be any homeless or vagrants. And so this "became reality."[10] During the 1930s, persecution of people living without proper documents and official work (for men of working age) began, in accordance with the existing Criminal Code. Structures for providing assistance to homeless people created before the Revolution were outlawed. Hidden homelessness existed, but officially, it was not mentioned.
>
> In 1991, articles 198 and 209, which made homeless persons criminals . . . were removed from the Criminal Code of the Soviet Socialist Republic of the Russian Federation. In connection with the beginning of reforms in the society, the situation changed drastically in all areas of life. . . . During [this] period of the collapse of the Soviet Union, in the context of the country's worsening social and economic situation . . . the conditions were established for a dramatic increase in the number of homeless.
>
> Since there were no shelters or any other type of housing, all these unlucky people ended up on the streets.[11]

> Whether sick or injured they are turned down when they want to see a doctor at a polyclinic because they have no medical insurance. Although decree # 535 of the city of Moscow theoretically grants them access to polyclinics, in practice the decree is not followed—partly due to human rejection of the homeless, and partly due to a lack of financial resources allocated to cover these consultations.[12]

These were the circumstances that in May 1992 impelled MSF Belgium to launch a program of medical assistance for the estimated thirty thousand homeless of Moscow.

The Coordinators of the Program

We were introduced to the program by Hedwige Jeanmart, head coordinator of MSF's Assistance Program for Homeless People in Russia, and Dr. Alexei Nikolaevich Nikiforov, who worked as a coordinator under her direction.

Jeanmart grew up in Namur, in the Walloon, French-speaking region of Belgium. At the University of Brussels, she studied journalism and became interested in Russia. She wrote her thesis on the magazine *Ogoniok*, focusing on the "revisionist way" it presented the literary testimonies of Russian veterans of the 1979–1989 war in Afghanistan. In 1992, she traveled to Russia for six months, where she conducted research in the Moscow State University Library. After her graduation, she took a position in the library at the University of Brussels and worked for a particular professor; but she was eager to return to Russia to "do something useful"—especially in the field of international development.

From a French friend she heard that MSF was running a program for homeless people in Russia. She applied to MSF Belgium's recruitment office, asking explicitly to be assigned to that project. She never heard from them about that request, but six months later they asked her to go on a short mission to the North Caucasian region of Russia to help transfer some vehicles from Brussels. Subsequently, several positions that MSF proposed to her—one in Abidjan, in the Ivory Coast, and the other in Goma, in the Democratic Republic of Congo—failed to materialize for reasons internal to MSF. Finally, after she had decided to take a two-year, unpaid leave of absence from the university, MSF contacted her again, this time with an assignment in Grozny, the Chechen capital. MSF's work there included rehabilitating the water supply and improving sanitation; providing medicine and medical care for the main hospital, polyclinics, and maternity clinics; running a canteen for older people; and assisting refugees in the North Caucasus Republic of Dagestan. The security situation in Grozny proved to be so menacing that she and her colleagues were evacuated several times—the last time to Moscow after an administrator from their mission had been kidnapped and held in captivity.[13]

When MSF asked Hedwige to undertake another mission—this time to Liberia—she turned it down because she felt that after only two post-Grozny months, it was too soon for her to go back into the field. In July 1996, however, she accepted the post of financial administrator in MSF Belgium's Moscow office, a position that she held for two years. In July 1998, she left Russia and embarked on a long trip with her partner, who had been working since 1994 with Action Contre la Faim (Action Against Hunger), an international humanitarian organization committed to ending world hunger. After traveling to Central Asia, China, Pakistan, and India with her partner, she returned to Russia again, where for five months she taught French in a school in Moscow. Once more she petitioned the MSF office in Brussels to be assigned to work with the homeless program. This time, in July 1999, she achieved her goal, becoming the coordinator of its Assistance Program for Homeless People.

Dr. Alexei Nikolaevich Nikiforov, who worked in MSF's homeless program, began his conversation with us by displaying several traditional Russian *matryoshkas* ("nested" dolls) carved by a homeless person on his desk. These sets of painted wooden dolls of decreasing size, placed one inside the other, successively depicted a homeless man who begins to sell bottles on the street, is apprehended by the police, is rescued by a humanitarian NGO, starts to cultivate a garden, obtains a job and a home, and begins a "new life" (those last words printed in English). The dolls were being sold for one hundred rubles apiece (about US$3 at the time) for the benefit of those who made them.

Dr. Nikiforov—who was thirty-eight when we first met him—is a Muscovite who graduated from the Moscow Medical Institute in 1986. His original desire was to become a medical scientist, doing research in molecular biology and genetics. While the Soviet Union was still in existence, he worked for three years on a genetics project connected with a cardiology laboratory. Like many young people, he said with a smile, he "wanted to change the world." Originally, he thought he could do this through genetic research, but he came to believe that the time was not ripe for genetically based medicine with a significant therapeutic potential. In his laboratory, he came into contact with a famous Russian cardiologist Dr. Evgeny Chazov, renowned as a medical practitioner, medical scientist, and manager of health-care systems, who made it plain that what came first with him was caring for patients. Dr. Chazov's example awakened in Alexei the desire to practice medicine, rather than to pursue a career as a medical researcher.[14]

After completing specialized training in cardiology, Dr. Nikiforov became the chief of the Therapeutic Department in a Moscow city hospital, where one-third of the patients were homeless. In this setting, a social worker associated with MSF's program for the homeless sought his advice and the help of his department in dealing with the problems of the homeless individuals she was trying to assist. He was the first chief of a department and one of the only physicians who was willing to talk with her. Because they had such negative feelings about the homeless, the other doctors ignored her. In September 1994, she had Alexei meet with the head of MSF Belgium's mission in Moscow. An invitation to join MSF's homeless program followed, confronting Alexei with a difficult decision. He was drawn to the prospect of working full-time with the homeless, whom he already "carried in [his] heart," and to treat them socially and medically "in one cup," in close collaboration with MSF's social workers, nurses, and physicians. However, MSF was a foreign NGO, and he had always worked in a government-supported Russian organization. Although modest, his MSF salary would be greater than what he earned as the head of a medical department under government auspices. But both he and his wife (who was also a physician) were worried about how long his employment with MSF would last. If and when the homeless program achieved its goals, MSF might move on, and he would have to look for another job, which might not be easy to find. Still, in the end, with the support of his wife, he agreed to join the MSF project.

From the very first day that he began to work with MSF, he said, there was a "very different spirit from a state organization":

> The doctors, nurses, and social workers work together with a friendly team spirit. It is not like a state organization in which I am the chief and you are only a worker. We work together. We discuss all problems and proposals together. They are my friends, not my workers. These people have close contact with their patients. They know who they are. They know that they are not dirty drunkards, but rather that they themselves are the same people as those in the streets. . . . Our motto is that "anyone can become homeless," that it is "a disease of society," and that there are large holes in this society in which people fall.

The Scorned *Bomzhi*

When MSF began its work in 1992, Moscow had at least thirty thousand homeless living and sleeping on its streets or in improvised digs. At first, MSF provided emergency medical consultations for homeless persons in train stations. In January 1993, the municipal health department and the railway station administration gave permission for it to use rooms for night consultations in two stations where, for a while, MSF members were joined by some members of the Nezavisimye Vrachi [Independent Doctors] organization. In September 1993, when a diphtheria epidemic broke out in Moscow, the city's Center of Epidemiology and Sanitation asked MSF to organize a vaccination campaign for the homeless. Nonetheless, eighteen months later, in December 1993, MSF was expelled from the train stations. The railway administration felt that they were attracting too many *bomji* (homeless persons).[15]

Bomzh (*bomzhi* in the plural) is an acronym in Russian. Its literal meaning is "without a fixed place of residence." Originating in police reports, it made its way into everyday colloquial language as a derogatory term for the homeless, connoting that they were vagabonds, beggars, drunkards, thieves, criminals, and disease-spreaders—"good for nothings" who deserved their lot. An MSF survey among 22,513 of its patients between 1995 and 2000 challenged this image of the homeless. It revealed that the majority (ninety percent) of the homeless persons were men between the ages of twenty and fifty. One in ten had a college education, and one in five vocational training. Most were law-abiding citizens with no criminal record, were fit to work, and were looking for a job. About three-quarters were Russian-born, of whom only twenty percent were from Moscow. Many had come to the capital from other regions of the country and from other former republics of the Soviet Union in search of employment. Thousands had lost their domiciles as a consequence of the waves of privatization and housing fraud that had swept Russia during the early and mid-1990s in the wake of the dissolution of the USSR, and the social and economic chaos that accompanied it. That ex-prisoners composed thirty to forty percent of the homeless was largely attributable to an old Soviet law still in effect that made it easy for such persons to lose their housing registration. Once released, these former prisoners no longer had the right to move back into their apartments. Furthermore, in violation of existing laws, the state would not issue internal passports to them—documents without which it was legally impossible for them to find a new home or earn a living. The MSF survey also found that the homeless were not the public-health menaces portrayed by the *bomzhi* stereotype. The most common medical conditions from which they suffered were not infectious diseases, but trophic ulcers and infected wounds due to exposure to the elements, poor living conditions, and lack of access to medical care. Untreated, these initially minor pathologies could lead to physical disability.

In February 1994, the Moscow Center for Epidemiology and Sanitation made available three rooms in the city's Disinfection Station No. 1, where MSF opened a free medical dispensary for the homeless.[16] MSF also began to conduct medical consultations for the homeless from two mobile buses that operated in the vicinity of four Moscow train stations.

In April 1996, MSF received an honorary award from the Moscow Health Department for its work with the homeless. However, by this time, their number was estimated to have risen from thirty thousand to one hundred thousand, and negative prejudice about the homeless persisted among city officials, who did little to aid them. For example, although the city of Moscow created eight night shelters between 1996 and 2001, they were reserved for

Muscovites, or ex-inhabitants of the Moscow region, who constituted only one-third of the city's homeless population.[17]

MSF concluded that a strictly medical approach to the problems of the homeless was not sufficient. If people MSF was helping were to be reintegrated into society, they needed social assistance as well; and so MSF incorporated social workers into its team.[18] Their role was to inform homeless persons about their housing and pension rights, to help them to obtain food and clothing,[19] and, above all, to assist them in acquiring identification papers or an internal passport, which was the most basic hurdle they had to surmount in order to be eligible for housing or a job.

In June 1999, MSF ceased running its mobile clinics near Moscow train stations, and centered all of its medical and social assistance efforts in its dispensary. In addition, it began to intensify its lobbying and advocacy on behalf of the homeless, unleashing a barrage of appeals to the public and to local government officials.

One appeal took the form of a poster campaign in Moscow's metro stations with reproductions of the photographs of homeless persons that MSF had previously exhibited in the lobby of a theater showing *The Lower Depths: Scenes from a Russian Life* by Maxim Gorky, a classic play about the denizens of a Russian shelter. As the severe winter approached, during which hypothermia killed hundreds yearly in Moscow's streets, MSF put posters up captioned, "And you, without a home, could you survive?" They also exploited the media—for example, helping to produce a professional film about the homeless entitled *Who Are These People?* (which was run on the Kultura television channel and shown in schools and universities in Moscow and other Russian cities).

MSF's appeals to government officials were relentless. They were focused on persuading Moscow's bureaucrats to build, finance, and run a municipal center, modeled on MSF's dispensary, that would provide free medical and social assistance to the homeless. Initially, the stream of letters was addressed to what Nikiforov referred to as lower-level functionaries. However, this was not effective. "MSF may have won a Nobel Prize, and be well-known in the world," Alexei said, "but here in Moscow it was no different in the eyes of those government bureaucrats than any other NGO. They looked at us as little children who didn't understand." Spearheaded by him, in collaboration with Hedwige Jeanmart and with MSF Belgium's head of mission and medical coordinator, MSF changed its strategy. It addressed its letters to higher-echelon officials, including the chiefs of the Social Protection Committee, Sanitary

Service, and Militia, and to thirty-three deputy-members of the Moscow City Duma (council). Based on a calculated premise that, as Alexei quipped, "one general can speak with another general in the same language," each letter contained supportive opinions about MSF obtained from other high officials.[20]

Finally, MSF was invited to present its homeless program before the Moscow Duma. The Duma deputies unanimously voted to create a municipal center that would combine medical and social assistance to the homeless modeled on the MSF dispensary. Unlike other city services, it would be accessible, not only to Muscovites, but to all homeless persons. The plan was to begin construction in the winter of 2000, with the expectation that the center would open its doors in August 2001. "This is our greatest victory in nine years!" Nikiforov exclaimed when we interviewed him in June 2001. "We'll see if it works or not," he added.

Two years later, in June 2003, when Olga revisited him in his MSF Belgium Moscow office, Alexei reported that although the new municipal Medical-Social Center for the homeless was physically equipped and had officially opened a month earlier, it was not yet operating. Its "staffing schedule" had not yet been approved by the municipal Health Department. Without this schedule, the center could not begin to hire people. The main deterrent was the social-work component. The framework for cooperation between medical and social-work personnel, which was integral to the MSF conception of the center, had been accepted by municipal authorities, and was expressed in the title of the new organization—the Medical Social Center. Nevertheless, the final version of the project issued by the Moscow Department of Health did not include social work. In Alexei's opinion, this omission was not attributable to the ill will of the Health Department; rather, there was virtually no precedent in Russia for medical and social workers to collaborate. The department bureaucrats did not know how to deal administratively with the social workers, who, they assumed, would have to report to a different set of people from the medical staff, and to be paid from a different budget source. Unsure how to resolve this difficulty, the Health Department bureaucrats chose to exclude the social worker positions from the staffing schedule altogether. For Alexei, this demonstrated how important MSF's oversight would continue to be even after the Center began to function. There was also much work to be done to normalize the legal status of the homeless, he told us. MSF was collaborating with Nochlezhka, a Russian NGO based in Saint Petersburg, in drafting a federal law that would recognize homelessness as a social, rather

than criminal, problem, establish the right to ambulatory and hospital services for homeless persons, and include measures pertaining to their employment, housing, and education.

Children of the Street

In addition, Alexei was now actively involved in a new project called "Children
of the Street," which he and Hedwige had jointly proposed to MSF Belgium's
headquarters in Brussels.[21] The project grew directly out of MSF's work with the
homeless. MSF's personnel had observed thousands of children on the streets
of Moscow—predominantly boys, but an increasing number of girls—whose
health was often compromised by injuries, the side effects of drug usage, and
sexually transmitted diseases. These children were wary about making contact
with unknown persons and entities, and they were subject to a "policeman-
hospital-shelter" trajectory that increased their alienation, failed to address
their problems, and in the end, often returned them to the streets.

The MSF project envisioned the psychological and social rehabilitation of
street children through a two-step process. In the first step, an outreach team
of social workers would contact homeless children where they tended to con-
gregate (mainly train stations), and establish rapport with them. In the second
step, operating out of a day-care center, a twelve-person team composed of an
MSF physician, a psychologist, and several social workers and teachers would
interact with the children over a longer period of time, and help them with
their medical, psychological, and social problems. The goal was to reintegrate
them into a more normal life—in their families, if possible.

Olga's last visit with Alexei came during the summer of 2005. At that time,
he sounded pleased about the progress made by the Medical Social Center for
the homeless. It was functioning well under the auspices of Moscow municipal
authorities, he said, with a staff of Russian personnel, including social workers.
The majority had previously worked in MSF's homeless program. Although
earning less than when they were employed by MSF, their wages were still
several times higher than those of comparable employees in other state institutions. Of course, things were not perfect, Alexei remarked. But, he mused
philosophically, you have to have the wisdom to not demand too much.

Alexei was vigorously lobbying to change the legal status of the homeless
on the federal level of the Russian government—especially to systematize their
employment status and to make their registration easier. During the past six

months, he had traveled to six cities of the Russian Federation, giving lectures and seminars about this to medical professionals, government functionaries, and police officials; and he had also sent a copy of MSF's legal proposals to Social Protection Departments in eighty-six regions of the Russian Federation. So far, the results of these efforts had been disappointing. Formerly operated under the aegis of the Ministry of Labor and Social Protection, homeless shelters had recently been moved to the jurisdiction of the Ministry of the Interior. This was problematic, he explained, not only because the Labor and Social Protection Ministry was more knowledgeable about homeless matters, but also because the Ministry of the Interior reported directly to the president of Russia, which made lobbying more difficult.

Alexei conducted most of his lobbying via e-mail, allowing him to devote ninety percent of his workday to the Street Children project. As its coordinator, he was overseeing the work of two psychologists (one of them Belgian, the other Russian) who were working on the streets, trying to gain homeless children's trust. But the project had yet to find a place for a day-care center. Locating it within the Garden Ring of Moscow, where most of the children could be found, was expensive, and there were onerous fire and safety regulations to comply with. Further complicating the search for a locale were the repercussions of the "Indifference Is Murder" campaign that MSF had waged during the previous year to raise public consciousness about the homeless who died on the streets of Moscow each winter. The campaign helped reduce the number of victims to some 140 fewer persons than had died during the previous winter. However, the vociferousness of the campaign had made official organizations wary about helping MSF obtain space for a day-care center, and more prone to place obstacles in its way. Although mindful of the price that MSF had paid for "witnessing" for the homeless, Alexei had no regrets about it. The campaign was "entirely worth it," he affirmed.

Assessing the Ambiguous Progress of the Homeless and Street Children Programs

"Ten years is a long time," Hedwige Jeanmart told an interviewer in 2002, on the tenth anniversary of MSF's work with Moscow's homeless:

> When MSF began its [homeless] program in May 1992 the number of homeless persons in Moscow was about 30,000. At that time, they did not have any medical

or social services. MSF decided to provide emergency medical consultations in the capital's train stations.

Ten years later, MSF is still here. . . .

Are there reasons to celebrate this anniversary? The mere fact that our program has been running for ten years is a sad sign that the problem still exists, that solutions continue to be ignored, that we are up against the inertia of authorities. But there are also positive results—signs that our daily refusal of the unacceptable has borne its fruits. And though they may not be as big or as ripe as we would have liked them to be, these are the fruits that we have decided to put on the table, the day of our tenth anniversary.[22]

It is "hard to assess" the results of the programs for homeless adults and for the children on the streets of Moscow, according to those who initiated them and participated in them. There have been observable positive consequences, they say, but the tenacity of the problems associated with homelessness in Russia is daunting. Tackling them has involved dealing with characteristics and institutional structures of the Soviet regime that persist in postsocialist Russia. MSF has had to try to alter the disdainful attitudes of the public, the police, and government officials toward the homeless, and to work to change laws that adversely affect their rights and well-being.

Some of its activities have brought the MSF Belgium office in Moscow closer to politics, straining the movement's principles of "independence," "impartiality," and "neutrality." The threat that this political engagement could pose to its work on behalf of the homeless and street children was increased by a law passed by the Russian national Duma in 2006. The law charges the so-called Rosregistratsia, a powerful agency with a staff of several thousand members within the Ministry of Justice, with seeking information about the activities of the more than forty thousand NGOs operating in Russia, including the sources of their funding, with attending their organized events, and with shutting them down if they are found to be unsatisfactory.

"[T]he day we can close our program because it's not useful anymore— that's the day we will really celebrate," Jeanmart declared when she was the coordinator of MSF's homeless program.[23] But "[t]he problem is here to stay," said the president of Samusocial Moscow, an NGO that has worked closely with MSF on the predicament of the street children.[24] "With a population of 150 million and an area of 17 million sq. kms, Russia is 32 times bigger [than] France [and] 560 times [bigger than] Belgium. The sheer size of Russia implies how difficult it is to cover the needs of the whole country. MSF will never cover the whole needs in the country even if we focus only on one theme," a member of MSF wrote at the close of his term as head of MSF Belgium's mission in Russia.[25] The juxtaposition of these statements encapsulates a cluster of questions that have constantly confronted MSF. When can it say that its programs have been fruitful enough to close them and depart? How can it tell what will go forward once it is gone? Are some problems so vast, enduring, or recurrent that there seems to be no end to them? This is suggested by the fact that MSF has been working in some societies for more than twenty or thirty years.[26] Should MSF stay on indefinitely in such places? Or should it decide, through a process of evaluation and self-evaluation, discernment, and accountability, that it has accomplished all that it can, and that, however regrettably, its work there is done?

The last time (in 2005) that we checked in on MSF's mission to Moscow, they were still facing such dilemma-infused questions. As Alexei Nikiforov recounted to Olga, the Medical Social Center for the homeless, which MSF had created, subsidized, staffed, and run, was now being funded and administered by local government authorities, and it was functioning effectively with all-Russian personnel. However, MSF continued to keep an eye on it, and to be actively engaged in lobbying for federal legislation to help the homeless on a national scale. The program for street children had not progressed sufficiently for it to be uncoupled from MSF. In addition, partly in retaliation for its "Indifference Is Murder" campaign, MSF was confronting renewed hostility from Moscow's city government. Meanwhile, the national government was exerting more centralized authority over many spheres of Russian life, including the activities of NGOs. Although for the time being MSF Belgium in Moscow had decided to be relatively quiescent about what it was trying to do for street children, it was clear that it intended to persist, buoyed by the sense that it had the strong support of the operations desk in its Brussels headquarters.

CHAPTER ELEVEN

Confronting TB in Siberian Prisons

with Olga Shevchenko

The Medical-Historical Context

During the nineteenth and early twentieth centuries, there were more deaths from tuberculosis (TB) in Western industrialized societies than from any other disease. It was not until 1882, when Robert Koch discovered *Mycobacterium tuberculosis*, the bacterium causing TB, that it was understood to be a disease produced by an airborne infectious agent, and one that was highly contagious. Sixty-one years later, in 1943, the antibiotic streptomycin, the first effective agent against the tuberculosis bacterium, was isolated. The discovery of streptomycin, and subsequently of two other antibiotics—isoniazid in 1952 and rifampin in 1959—were revolutionary breakthroughs in the therapeutic management of individual cases of tuberculosis and the ability to cure them. They were considered to have the capacity to significantly reduce the incidence of TB cases, to forestall their reaching epidemic proportions, and, beyond that, to hold forth the promise of totally eliminating the disease.

In 1979, the World Health Organization (WHO) officially certified that smallpox had been eradicated. Tuberculosis, however, still flourishes. In 1993,

WHO declared that some two million deaths from TB occurred each year; that one-third of the world's population was infected with *Myobacteriuum tuberculosis*; and that the global incidence of TB constituted a public-health emergency. It called on the governments of the world to make the "scaling up" of TB control an immediate priority, and it strongly recommended a strategy to combat TB. So-called "directly observed treatment, short-course" (DOTS) of a standardized group of antibiotic anti-TB drugs gave promise of curing as many as eighty-five percent of TB patients. The factors identified as driving the TB epidemic included the lack of access in poor countries to the diagnosis and treatment of the disease, and inadequate laboratory facilities and shortages of appropriately trained health personnel in numerous societies with a high incidence of TB. Somewhat later, it was recognized that the TB epidemic was also being fueled by the worldwide HIV/AIDS epidemic, and the pronounced risk that persons living with HIV had of developing TB; and by the emergence of multi-drug-resistant tuberculosis (MDR-TB) and of extensively drug-resistant tuberculosis (XDR-TB), primarily due to previous ignorant or careless drug treatment.[1]

In 1997, WHO classified Russia as one of the ten countries in the world with the highest prevalence of TB; the death rate from the disease there surpassed that in any other European society.[2] In 1999, "at the end of a decade of explosive growth in TB . . . Russia reported over 120,000 new cases of tuberculosis and nearly 30,000 deaths," which "probably underestimate[d] the true numbers."[3] TB in Russia had also become virtually "synonymous with multi-drug-resistant tuberculosis."[4] Russia's prisons were epicenters of this major TB epidemic. "Fully one in ten of the country's more than 1 million prisoners [was] sick with TB," and "[m]any reports suggest[ed] that TB ha[d] again become the leading cause of death in Russia's prisons."[5]

This state of affairs constituted a dramatic reversal of the steady progress made in Russia during the Soviet period in controlling the incidence of tuberculosis. The highly centralized Soviet system of preventing and treating TB that had been erected had included mass yearly chest radiography to detect active cases of TB; prolonged hospital stays, in isolation, for TB patients; dependence on surgery as a primary mode of treatment; and the use of free, long-term, multi-drug regimens administered on an individual, case-by-case basis, which were prescribed "more on disease site, severity/activity of disease and the presence of complications . . . than the likelihood of resistance."[6] In addition, under the aegis of the Soviet system, a TB patient "was entitled to a separate apartment, complimentary trips to seaside resorts, and an excuse from work for at least a year."[7]

This system became financially untenable after the political and economic collapse of the Soviet Union, which contributed significantly to the resurgence of tuberculosis. Nowhere was the disease more virulent than in the overcrowded, poorly ventilated, and unsanitary Russian prisons, whose malnourished, inadequately clothed inmates constituted a third of Russia's new tuberculosis cases. These conditions emanated from what Yuri Ivanovich Kalinin, head of the Russian Prison Administration (GUIN/Chief Directorate of the Execution of Punishment) from 1992 to 1997, and an advocate of penal reform in Russia, characterized as an "excessively harsh criminal system, [which] had given rise to an unjustifiably wide use of restrictive measures."[8] The system "locked away more than 700,000 people every year" and "held 45,000 people . . . in investigation confinement cells longer than the terms set by law." In a 1998 interview, not long after he became deputy minister of justice, Kalinin exclaimed: "We have created a kind of incubator for breeding Koch's bacilli."[9]

Notwithstanding the epidemic conditions and the dearth of funds, equipment, and supplies available to them in postsocialist Russia, prison physicians clung to the customary mode of treating tuberculosis. With only one out of four recommended drugs on hand, or with not enough drugs for all patients, this often meant "sharing" the available medicines among the prisoners. This improvised regimen worsened their condition and contributed to the proliferation of multi-drug-resistant forms of tuberculosis throughout the penal system.

It was under these circumstances that in 1996, MSF Belgium began to work in Penal Colony No. 33—a referral colony for tuberculosis patients sent there from the twenty-six penal colonies in the Kemerovo oblast (region) of Siberia.[10]

Penal Colony 33

Nicolas Cantau, then head of MSF Belgium's mission in Russia, described its program in Colony 33 as follows:

In early 1996, MSF began a program to combat tuberculosis in the prison hospital of Mariinsk in the Kemerovo region of Siberia. This prison colony [Colony 33], with a capacity of 750 prisoners, lodges an average of 1,800 inmates. It is the referral institution for all the prisoners suffering from TB in the region of Kemerovo, of which the total incarcerated population is around 30,000 persons. [This is] the Russian region that has the third largest number of prisoners. The lack of medications, the unsuitable treatment protocols, [and] the extreme life conditions of the prisoners prompted MSF to launch a program. As a matter of fact, in 1995, none of the prisoners who left Colony 33 were cured; on the contrary, . . . a form of tuberculosis resistant to classic antibiotics . . . developed, and the freed prisoners are a significant source of contagion in the region. . . .

Penetrating what were the gulags of mythic Siberia was a real challenge that MSF was able to undertake thanks to the opening of the system, but above all thanks to the dynamism and the proactive intervention of the medical director of the TB hospital of Colony No. 33 of Mariinsk. Refusing to be resigned in the face of the dramatic problems with which the colony was faced, [she] contacted MSF in the hope of obtaining assistance. After carrying out several evaluations, MSF decided to begin a program, in spite of the difficulties envisaged, and without possessing real expertise with regard to combating TB in a prison milieu, in particular in Russia. . . .

Target population: The inmates of Colony 33 (1,790 persons in December 1997) as well as 1,250 prisoners with TB in the other colonies of the region. . . .

General Objective (1998): Treat and cure the detainees of Colony 33 using the protocols, and the treatments advocated by WHO, and from the angle of technical aid. Introduce the DOTS method [directly observed treatment, short-course], and in this way try to interrupt the chain of transmission of the disease in the prisons and in the general population.[11]

The medical director who invited MSF to Colony 33, and made their entrée into it possible, was Dr. Natalia Nikolayevna Vezhnina. A native of Siberia, whose distant forefathers had been deported there in tsarist times, Dr. Vezhnina graduated from Kemerovo State Medical Institute in 1977, with special training in phthisiatry (the study and treatment of tuberculosis).[12] Following her graduation, she began to work in the penitentiary system of the Kemerovo region, which, she discovered, still retained many of the notorious characteristics of the Stalinist Gulag. She later described it as a depository of all that was wrong with totalitarianism, in which punitive logic ruled and obsessive discipline, secrecy, and repression were endemic.[13]

From 1989 to 1992, Dr. Vezhnina undertook graduate study at the Moscow TB Research Institute. During those years she also worked as a freelance correspondent for a professional journal, *Human Formation, Law and Order*, publishing several articles describing the deplorable TB situation in the prisons. This antedated Russia's entry into the Council of Europe in 1996, which required its penal system to become more transparent, especially regarding its adherence to international norms of human rights. Its prisons were not yet open to the kind of scrutiny and reform that Dr. Vezhnina proposed.

In 1993 after completing her graduate studies, she was promoted to the directorship of Colony 33's TB hospital. In November of that same year, in Moscow, at the First International Conference on Prison Reform, she made a powerful presentation about conditions in Colony 33, with its soaring rates of morbidity and mortality from TB, the absence of basic drugs to treat prisoner-patients, and its inhuman detention policies. Members of MSF present in the audience were deeply impressed by her talk.

In September 1994, as a consequence of Dr. Vezhnina's influence, Valerii Abramkin, a former Soviet dissident, who was then the head of the Moscow Center for Prison Reform and also a Duma deputy, asked MSF Belgium's office in Moscow to assess TB in Russian prisons. Christopher Stokes, MSF's head of mission, and Nadine Delamotte, its medical coordinator, accordingly made exploratory assessment visits to prisons in Moscow and Saratov that September, and to Colony 33 in October. In November, they sent a situation report to the Brussels headquarters of MSF Belgium requesting the opening of a long-term MSF TB project in Colony 33, using WHO's recommended DOTS tuberculosis control strategy. If this test project proved to be successful, as indicated by an increase in TB cures, MSF proposed that the DOTS protocol be extended to other TB prison colonies in Russia, and subsequently to the treatment of TB in the civil, extra-prison population as well.[14] In early 1996, MSF Belgium and the penitentiary administration of the Kemerovo region (GUIN) agreed to sign a five-year contract to collaboratively develop a TB control program in the Kemerovo penal institutions.

It was with trepidation that Dr. Vezhnina's chief—Lieutenant General Vladimir Semenyuk, the Kemerovo Region director of the Department of the Execution of Punishments—gave her permission to open the colony for the first time to foreign personnel from a Western NGO. It was unprecedented, and Semenyuk had what Dr. Vezhnina acknowledged were many legitimate concerns. He was worried that the "thieves in law,"[15] who had high status in the social system of prisoners in the penal colony, might take a foreigner hostage. He was especially anxious about what would happen if MSF "trumpeted around the world" what they saw firsthand in Colony 33.[16] In this latter regard, there was a tacit agreement between the colony administration and MSF that as a prerequisite for their entry into the prison and their access to patients, the organization would not make public comments on the living conditions that its staff observed in the prison. Although it was never formulated in writing, in effect this agreement meant that MSF personnel had to compromise their principles-based commitment to bear witness and speak out about deficiencies they observe in aid systems, about human rights abuses, and about the divergence of humanitarian assistance for political reasons. It was a compromise that evoked controversy and great discomfort among MSF staff, especially when they encountered the dire conditions to which prisoners were subject.

In May 1996, the first MSF expatriate staff members arrived on the scene. Before they could even begin a TB treatment program, they had to supply all the basic necessities lacked by the prison. Although as many as forty Russian physicians and forty Russian nurses worked in the colony, when Dr. Vezhnina opened the doors of its warehouse to the MSF team, all they saw on its shelves were some containers of aspirin. MSF had to supply everything, not just drugs, but soap, clothing, footwear, bed linens, and food for the prisoners, and even such basic construction materials as nails and paint.

The social organization of the Russian penal system also challenged the team. To begin with, the authority structure of the prisons was military. Most of its administrators were military officers—including Dr. Vezhnina, who was thus subject to hierarchical pressures and commands from her military superiors in the colony.

Furthermore, when MSF began work in Colony 33, the penal system operated under the jurisdiction of the Russian Ministry of the Interior, charged with upholding public order and suppressing crime. Other matters regarding the prisons were of no more than secondary significance to this ministry. Not until 1998, when the penal system was transferred from the Interior Ministry to the Ministry of Justice, were reforms introduced to bring it into closer compliance with the rule of law and with fundamental human rights and freedoms—including its progressive "demilitarization." Although these reforms were compatible with MSF's values and with the goals of its TB program, the Justice Ministry moved slowly to implement them. Along with reducing the number of prisoners in the penal colonies,[17] the Chief Penitentiary Directorate of the Ministry of Justice was trying to change conditions in "the catastrophically overcrowded" pre-detention centers called SIZOs ("Isolators for Investigation"),[18] where tens of thousands of detainees were confined for periods ranging from a few weeks to more than two years while awaiting trial and sentencing. Tuberculosis was rampant in these SIZOs. Upon admission to a SIZO, all detainees underwent fluorographic screening for TB, and a large number of active TB cases were found among them. Because of the overcrowding, those diagnosed with TB were not usually physically separated from other detainees. If drugs were available, detainees with TB were started on treatment, which at best was erratic. This was the case with regard to the anti-TB drugs used, their source (the detainees' families were often encouraged to supply the drugs),[19] and the irregularity with which the detainee patients received them. During a detainee's stay in a SIZO, he or she might be moved to a jail called an "Isolator for Temporary Detention." If convicted and sentenced, the prisoner was then moved once more to either a general or a TB penal colony. During their transfer from one institution to another, although accompanied by a file identifying their medical condition, those with TB were not separated from those who—at least for the time being—were uninfected.[20]

As the MSF team were eventually to learn, the treatment in the SIZOs was not only a major source of the dissemination of the disease, but also of its mutation into multi-drug-resistant forms.

The Introduction of DOTS

The core intent of the MSF Belgium TB Siberian project was to introduce the "directly observed treatment, short-course" (DOTS) protocol, based on a standardized regimen of five first-line drugs,[21] into the prison system—initially into Colony 33.

Although Dr. Vezhnina responded enthusiastically to the premises and procedures of the DOTS strategy, a number of other physicians in Colony 33 were not convinced. The DOTS approach differed markedly from the TB treatment practices of the Soviet era, in which they took considerable pride. These included "long-course chemotherapy," "individualized dosing schedules," "monotherapy for active disease in some cases,"[22] and also fluoroscopy for diagnosing, evaluating, and following a patient's condition,[23] rather than the bacteriology-based sputum-smear microscopy method for detecting acid-fast tuberculosis bacilli (AFB) employed by DOTS. For the Russian physicians skeptical about DOTS, or resistant to it, a "diagnosis of tuberculosis based on bacteriology [was] a diagnosis made too late"; the notion of "standard" treatment" had "negative connotations," which were associated with "limiting a doctor's right" and duty "to take an individual approach to patient care"; and the concept of "short course" treatment was felt to be inadequate, given the much longer period of therapy to which they were accustomed.[24] In addition, some physicians reacted with indignation to being asked to adopt the DOTS strategy, because they felt that it lowered Russia to the level of African countries where it had been pioneered. "'Russia is not Tanzania, so DOTS won't work [here],'" they contended.[25]

Initially, a suspicious fear circulated among the prisoners that the MSF "foreign doctors" had entered the colony to experiment on them with unproven drugs. The most powerful "thief in law" among the prisoners told them not to accept the drugs from these foreigners and, at first, almost all of them followed his instructions. Dr. Vezhnina, along with Dr. Hans Kluge, the MSF physician who was then the project's coordinator, spent hours with this prisoner-leader, explaining MSF's principles and intentions, the medical characteristics of tuberculosis, and the optimal way to treat it, before he gave permission to his fellow prisoners to accede to the DOTS regimen. After that, prisoners no longer refused to be treated by DOTS, and those who received the treatment fully complied with its strict protocol.[26]

Concretely, the procedure consisted of the following: Every morning at 7 A.M., the prisoner-patients receiving DOTS treatment lined up to receive the medications. Along with the drugs, they were given a food supplement of five hundred milligrams of high-energy milk with oil and sugar, and three protein biscuits.[27] Their intake of the drugs was strictly monitored by members of the prison medical staff and the MSF medical team. The prisoners were made to open their mouths after ingesting the pills to show that they had been swallowed, and each prisoner's personal DOTS card was then marked to indicate that the doses had been punctually and properly taken. Recorded on these cards as well were the results of the sputum-smear microscopy analyses given at fixed intervals during the course of the treatment—at its inception, two months into its intensive phase, one month before its end, and at its termination. These data were used to assess the status of the tuberculosis bacilli, manage the patients' program and condition, and evaluate the treatment's effectiveness.

The "first measured impact after the introduction of DOTS prison-wide" was very encouraging. A "rapid" and "dramatic" reduction in deaths occurred— "395 in 1996, 316 in 1997 and 50 in 1998."[28] In later years, Dr. Vezhnina looked back on this interlude in MSF's program as a "golden" period—one, as she remembered it, characterized by an atmosphere in which the members of MSF and the Russian doctors and nurses on the prison staff related to each other "like brothers." Two marriages even occurred during this time—one between a Belgian MSF doctor and the daughter of a Russian colony physician, and the other between a French logistician and an Italian nurse.[29]

However, a cloud hovered over these bright days of the project. Notwithstanding the decline in deaths, and the rise in the effectiveness of treatment from sixteen to seventy percent, "using WHO definitions of cure based on sputum examination," the cure rates "did not meet international standards," and "treatment failures remained unacceptably high."[30]

Expansion of Tuberculosis Control

Mobilized by Dr. Vezhnina, MSF Belgium extended its DOTS-centered TB control activities to Colony 16, where prisoners under strict terms of detention were held, and to Colony 35, the only women's colony. Colony 21 and Colony 35 were developed as dispensaries for treated TB cases that had supposedly been cured, and equipped with laboratories to identify relapses by smear microscopy. In 1998, case-finding by sputum examination was decentralized. Laboratories were installed in nine colonies where sputum-smear analyses were carried out on a routine basis. "Regular," non-TB colonies in the northern, southern, and central "clusters" of the penitentiary system that did not have clinical laboratory facilities were assigned to one of these nine laboratories, and arrangements were made for a mobile team from Colony 33 or Colony 16 to be sent to such peripheral colonies to collect sputum samples whenever more than thirty suspected TB cases were identified there. Mycobacteriological laboratories were opened in Colonies 33 and 16 in order to survey the emergence of drug resistance. Colony 33 became the referral center for the training of nurses, laboratory technicians, and doctors working in the penitentiary system.

But it was not until late in 2000 that the DOTS program was extended to the three pre-detention centers (SIZOs), acknowledged "breeding sites" for TB. GUIN accepted Dr. Vezhnina's recommendation that TB-infected inmates be transferred from SIZOs to prisons and back only with the permission of a physician, and without interruption of their ongoing treatment.

The additional protocol for SIZOs was needed because, unlike the penal colonies, which were under the full control of GUIN, SIZOs operated under the aegis of a number of different ministries—including the Ministry of Justice, the Ministry of Internal Affairs, and the Ministry of Health. (Among themselves, with ironic humor, MSF staff members referred to the SIZO agreement as the "Protocol of the Seven Generals.") In the face of the numerous government officials and agencies that it involved, the MSF project regarded the agreement concerning the continuity of care of patients who were moving between all these bureaucratic structures to be a considerable achievement.

In 1999, in recognition of her role in these developments, Dr. Vezhnina was promoted to colonel ahead of schedule and appointed assistant head of the Medical Division of GUIN. In addition, she received several awards for her work during 2000, including one for her "dedicated and selfless devotion" from George Soros's Open Society Institute. But despite all this, 2000 was a negative turning point in the history of the TB project. It ushered in a period of complications, emanating from the Russian prison staff, local, regional, and national authorities, and from within MSF itself, that three years later led MSF to end its participation in TB control in the Kemerovo region. Trouble centered on the incidence of so-called multi-drug-resistant forms of tuberculosis in the prison system.

Multi-Drug-Resistant Tuberculosis and DOTS-Plus

Despite the fundamental role that the DOTS treatment regimen had played, and continued to play in TB control, clinical resistance to the first-line anti-TB drugs used by DOTS emerged almost simultaneously with their introduction. A 1997 survey conducted by WHO and the International Union Against Tuberculosis and Lung Disease found that drug-resistant tuberculosis had become ubiquitous, and existed in several forms: TB resistant to only one first-line anti-TB drug; TB resistant to two or more first-line drugs; and XDR-TB, resistant at least to isoniazid and rifampicin, the two main first-line drugs, and, in addition, to any fluoroquinolone drug in the group of broad-spectrum antibiotics among the second-line drugs, and at least one of the three second-line injectable drugs. The survey identified particular geographical "hot spots" of MDR-TB. Russia, where fifteen percent of new TB infections were multi-drug-resistant, was considered to be one of them. Within Russia, such drug resistance was especially rampant in the prison system.

Paul Farmer and Jim Yong Kim, two young physicians specializing in the treatment of infectious diseases, particularly tuberculosis, were prominent among those who raised the alarm about the serious outbreaks of MDR-TB. They had received both their MDs and their PhDs in medical anthropology at Harvard, under the auspices of the Medical School's Department of Social Medicine,[31] where they subsequently became faculty members and heads of its newly created Program in Infectious Disease and Social Change.

In 1987, Farmer and Kim (with Ophelia Dahl) co-founded Partners in Health (PIH), a nonprofit NGO committed to providing health care in partnership with the poor. In 1994, PIH established a program in shantytown areas of Lima, Peru, to treat patients with MDR-TB. "Ironically, perhaps it is the globalizing economy that brings into relief the flabby relativism of the public health *realpolitik* that leaves us with a double standard of therapy—prompt effective MDR-TB treatment for those with resources, and no treatment at all for prisoners and the poor," Farmer wrote. "The only good news, for those ardently opposed to such double standards, is that transnational TB epidemics will at least remind the affluent few that no one is really safe if these epidemics are not brought into check."[32]

The community-based therapy program that PIH initiated in Peru significantly influenced WHO's development of operational protocols for case management of MDR-TB, standardized regimens of second-line drugs called DOTS-Plus, and guidelines for DOTS-Plus feasibility studies. As will be seen, it also had serious implications for the way MSF responded to MDR-TB in the Siberian penal colonies.

The patients enrolled in the PIH Peruvian program, mostly relatively young residents of the designated slum districts of Lima, had undergone at least one course of DOTS therapy that had failed to work, and had developed MDR-TB that in most cases resisted all of the DOTS drugs. Out of the sixty-six patients who completed four or more months of treatment with second-line drugs that were practically the same as those subsequently adopted by WHO as DOTS-Plus therapy, fifty-five (eighty-three percent) had "probable cures."[33] For Farmer and Kim, this program demonstrated how MDR-TB could be successfully treated in resource-poor countries, with high cure rates, and prevented from spreading, at lower costs, even under adverse field conditions.

The conclusions that Farmer and Kim drew from PIH's work in Lima became the springboard for a landmark meeting in Cambridge, Massachusetts, convened in April 1998 by the Harvard Program in Infectious Disease and Social Change, and cosponsored by the American Academy of Arts and Sciences,

WHO's global tuberculosis program, and Partners in Health. It was attended by fifty invited experts in tuberculosis and public health, and by some representatives from foundations, aid agencies, and the pharmaceutical industry. One of its key participants was Dr. Arata Kochi, who headed WHO's TB program at the time and was a forcefully influential international promoter of DOTS. In Kochi's opening remarks he used the term "DOTS-Plus" to refer to treatment of MDR-TB, coinage that was enthusiastically embraced by Farmer and Kim.

The resolutions forthcoming from this important meeting were fundamental and far-reaching. They included the collective affirmation that "all patients with active tuberculosis, regardless of drug susceptibility patterns, have a right to treatment"; that "resistance to antituberculous agents is an urgent problem demanding prompt attention"; and that "the current situation calls for a focused and concerted effort which, together with the global implementation of DOTS, can bring the eradication of tuberculosis finally within our grasp." The participants agreed that "in some settings DOTS alone is clearly insufficient," but that a "DOTS-plus approach to multidrug resistant tuberculosis would be most likely to succeed where DOTS was already established or being established."[34]

Following this meeting, a decision was made to create a WHO Working Group on DOTS-Plus for MDR-TB, one of whose primary charges was to develop guidelines for DOTS-Plus pilot projects based upon a consensus of its scientific panel. A codified "WHO Model List of Essential [Second-Line] Drugs" to manage MDR-TB was drawn up and, with the active participation of MSF, a so-called Green Light Committee selected from members of the Working Group was appointed to review and approve applications according to the guidelines. The projects approved were to be given the advantages of being able to purchase second-line anti-TB drugs at prices negotiated by this committee, and of receiving technical support from it.[35]

Partly overlapping in time and in content with WHO's response to MDR-TB was the publication at the end of 1999 of *The Global Impact of Drug-Resistant Tuberculosis*, a lengthy report by Harvard Medical School and Partners in Health, commissioned and funded by the Open Society Institute. One of its notable features was the amount of attention that it paid to the incidence of MDR-TB in Russia. The report was widely circulated in Russian medical and political milieux and covered heavily in the Russian press. Encouraged by the interest that it had sparked, the Open Society Institute made another grant to Partners in Health, along with the WHO and UNAIDS Stop TB Partnership Task Force on TB and Human Rights, to enable it to move forward with developing the plan for tuberculosis control outlined in the report.[36]

The Open Society Institute focused its largesse on tackling TB in Russian prisons, providing grants totaling $13 million (over four times the $3 million that MSF spent during its seven years in Kemerovo). Alexander Davidovich Goldfarb (generally known as Alex Goldfarb), a microbiologist born in Moscow, who had earned his PhD at the Weizmann Institute in Rehovot, Israel, and done postdoctoral research at the Max Planck Institute for Biochemistry in Munich, was appointed its project director, working under the auspices of the Public Health Research Institute (PHRI), of which he was a member.[37]

Goldfarb, in some ways a rather enigmatic man, with a complex personal, political, and professional history, had emigrated from the Soviet Union to the United States in 1975 and settled permanently in New York in 1982, becoming a naturalized American citizen. His scientific career in the United States—first at Columbia University, and then at PHRI—was bound up with his role as an activist, particularly on behalf of prominent Russian dissidents. The PHRI/Open Society Institute–funded project in Russia was centered on furthering the control and treatment of TB—especially MDR-TB—in Russian prisons and in civilian settings surrounding them, particularly in the Tomsk region of Siberia. As its director, Goldfarb oversaw activities that included building a TB-relevant infrastructure in that context, training laboratory and medical personnel, and providing appropriate first- and second-line drugs. He also sought support for the program from influential TB experts in the Russian medical community and powerful figures in the Ministry of Health and the Ministry of Justice. Once the program in Tomsk was set up, PHRI invited Partners in Health to act as consultants to it, and subsequently to manage it. Over the course of 2001–2002, PHRI transferred the entire Tomsk program to Partners in Health, which assumed primary responsibility for clinical care.

In the midst of this chain of events, the existence of MDR-TB in the penal colonies throughout the Kemerovo region became ominously apparent.

Grappling with MDR-TB in Kemerovo

As early as September 1996, laboratory studies showed that the conversion rate from "smear positivity" to "smear negativity" of prisoners with tuberculosis in Colony 33 who had been treated intensively with the DOTS regimen was worrisomely low. Alarm about the low cure rate was raised to a new pitch following a visit made to the project in March 1998 by Drs. Francine Matthys, director of the Medical Department of MSF Belgium in Brussels, and Michael E. Kimerling, MSF Belgium's medical advisor to the Colony 33 Prison Tuberculosis Program, and also one of the chief investigators at the Gorgas Tuberculosis Initiative at the University of Alabama in Birmingham, where he was a faculty member in the Department of Medicine.[38]

"[I]t is now clear," Matthys and Kimerling wrote in the conclusion of their report, "that MDRTB is *the* [authors' emphasis] major threat to TB control in the colonies. Its prevention must become the primary goal and focus of any future MSF program. A failure to do so will only lead to a colony of chronic patients with incurable tuberculosis. Given the resistance patterns found and an overall cure rate of only 46%, it also implies that the currently used Category II regimen [of retreatment with DOTS] is not adequate."[39] They strongly urged the project to move from the "curative" orientation limited to Colony 33 to a broader public-health outlook aimed at breaking the transmission of MDR-TB and preventing its spread within the larger Kemerovo penal system.

In 2000, Kimerling extended this analysis of the crisis in Colony 33 further. Despite the greater "management success" achieved through "a comprehensive reorganization of prison diagnostic and treatment systems," he wrote, "a plateau in the treatment failure [had] emerged that approach[ed] MDR rates reported in two patient cohorts."[40] He attributed this to the dual epidemics in the prison:

> Once drug-resistant strains become established and represent a significant . . . proportion of cases, and these cases are either not cured or do not die (as in Colony 33), then primary transmission of resistant strains becomes a second mechanism directly impacting the MDR-TB epidemic. The latter mechanism ultimately becomes independent of the initial process that created the MDR strains, forming a unique epidemiology of disease that requires a new control strategy. This appears to be happening in Colony 33.[41]

In addition, Kimerling pointed to evidence that suggested the epidemics were not only associated with imprisonment, but that a "civilian drug resistance epidemic [was] developing in parallel to that in prisons." Therefore he strongly recommended what he called a "Russian paradigm" for tuberculosis control that would "move in a direction of coordination and collaboration between civilian and prison services, at least on a regional level."[42]

Obstacles to the Control of MDR-TB

MSF and Dr. Vezhnina recognized the seriousness of the MDR-TB problem. But many factors converged to slow and, in the end, deter the implementation of a DOTS-Plus regimen in Colony 33, and throughout the Kemerovo penitentiary system and civilian region.

To begin with, both MSF and Dr. Vezhnina believed that for a number of reasons it would be unwise to start a DOTS-Plus treatment program immediately, without first making more progress with problems contributing to the epidemic—including the overcrowding, inadequate nutrition, and poor communication between the penitentiary system and the civil sector into which the prisoners were eventually released. Because the DOTS-Plus regimen was a lengthy one (extending over a period of up to two years, in contrast with the six-to-eight-month DOTS protocol), the communication gap between the prison colonies and the civil sector seemed especially problematic. It increased the possibility that during the course of that extended time period, prisoners' treatment with DOTS-Plus second-line drugs might be prematurely interrupted by their being released from prison, whether because their term of incarceration had ended or because they were transferred to another colony. Dr. Vezhnina and MSF greatly feared that such prisoners would develop resistance to the second-line DOTS-Plus as well as to the first-line DOTS drugs—the dreaded condition known as XDR-TB—that would also be disseminated to the civilian population. Its likelihood was increased by the prospect that in June 2000, in honor of the fifty-fifth anniversary of the victory of the Soviet Union over Nazi Germany, and linked to the recent election of Vladimir Putin as president of the Russian Federation, some ten thousand prisoners were being amnestied.

Before a DOTS-Plus program was launched, MSF and Dr. Vezhnina agreed, it had to be ascertained how these second-line drugs of internationally accepted quality could be obtained, and how their cost, which was more than one hundred times greater than that of DOTS first-line drugs, could be covered. They were aware that the Green Light Committee had made arrangements with both proprietary and generic drug firms to provide lower-priced, second-line TB drugs to certified DOTS-Plus pilot projects, and that this was a potential means of their gaining affordable access to them. However, they realized that they were as yet unequipped to meet all the laboratory, clinical, and organizational conditions required by a rigorous MDR-TB program. They were also concerned by the mismatch between the WHO recommendations on dosage and treatment regimen for MDR-TB patients, and the pharmacological and treatment regulations accepted by the Russian Ministry of Health. Indeed, in 2001, when MSF Belgium received approval from the Green Light Committee to begin treatment of a hundred and fifty MDR-TB patients in Kemerovo, and submitted its application to the Russian Ministry of Health, the WHO protocol was turned down because it relied on drugs that had not yet been registered in Russia.

In the meantime, during 2000 to 2002, with active input from Kimerling, short, two-week courses on TB control were organized at the University of Alabama for several key Russian physicians in Colony 33 and some health-care managers and administrators from the civilian sector. Dr. Andrei Slavuckij, an MSF physician, who later became the medical coordinator of the MSF tuberculosis program in that region, spent 1998–2000 at the University of Alabama studying for a master's degree in its School of Public Health, with Kimerling as his major teacher. In 2001, in a joint Gorgas Institute and MSF initiative, a Center of Excellence (COE) was created in the Kemerovo region to serve as a catalyst for the revision and improvement of TB control there.

Throughout the entire period during which MSF was searching for a response to the MDR-TB outbreak, its relations with a number of the Russian physicians who were caring for prisoner-patients, and with the local members of GUIN, the main Directorate of Corrections of the Ministry of Internal Affairs that supervised the prisons, were growing more strained. During 2000, the tensions between GUIN and MSF escalated and became more political. The conflict ended in the firing of Dr. Vezhnina from her position as assistant head of GUIN's Medical Division in the Kemerovo region. Her close collaboration with MSF had made her vulnerable to being viewed as "working for MSF rather than for the Russian authorities." In addition, the stand that she took, along with MSF, against accepting a prospective, large World Bank loan for a TB control program in Russia, shook GUIN's confidence in her.

MSF's main objection to the loan stemmed from the fact that the proposal associated with it called for establishing a "cluster system" of regional penal colonies, within which all MDR-TB prisoner-patients would be transported from wherever they were incarcerated in Russia to specified colonies in the oblasts of Tomsk, Nizhny Novgorod, and Kemerovo. In MSF's and Dr. Vezhnina's shared view, this risked increasing the logistical problems endemic to treating MDR-TB in a prison setting, because it entailed moving large numbers of highly contagious inmates across the country and made the interruption of their treatment more likely. They also questioned it from a human rights point of view, since it would alter the usual arrangements of imprisoning inmates in their home regions, where their families could easily visit them. At a crucial May 2000 meeting concerning negotiations with the World Bank, Dr. Vezhnina gave voice to her strong objections to the terms of the loan. Rather than doing good, she said, it would worsen the situation. The most important thing was to develop an efficient system of TB control in order not to create resistance; and it was dangerous to take up the treatment of drug-resistant TB when the blueprint for dealing effectively with the ordinary form of it had not yet been established. She did not want her children to have to pay for an enormous loan that was likely to aggravate the epidemiological situation in the penal system by creating a "bacteriological monster" of "super-resistance" to the tuberculosis bacillus. In turn, MSF sent a protest letter to the World Bank, not only expressing their objections to the proposal, but also requesting that Colony 33 be taken out of the project.

In this charged atmosphere, two commissions from the Moscow office of GUIN made several visits in July and August 2000 to the MSF TB project in Kemerovo. The GUIN representatives were highly critical of MSF. They accused it and Dr. Vezhnina of disrespecting Russian law by not following the guidelines of the Ministry of Health in their treatment of TB patients, and of contributing to the occurrence of MDR-TB through their treatment regimens. The GUIN visitors raised concern over the patients who were *not* being treated because consensus on the MDR-TB treatment regimen had not been reached, and also because MSF was cleaving so tightly to WHO recommendations to give priority to patients who were smear-positive, putting them on DOTS as soon as they had been identified, and including no more than twenty percent of those who were smear-negative in the total patient load. This kind of public-health-oriented triage, which entailed an aggregate process of patient selection and deselection, ran counter to the traditional approach of Russian physicians, who inclusively and individually treated all patients.

Following these GUIN visits, Dr. Vezhnina was dismissed from her position. This action was officially explained as an "early retirement." Dr. Vezhnina's position was eliminated, and in its place another comparable one was created with the title of Main Specialist in TB in the Medical Department of GUIN of the Kemerovo Region, to which a conservative phthisiatrist committed to long-standing traditions of Russian medicine and clinical care was appointed.

In addition, GUIN issued a warning to Dr. Oleg Sheyanenko, a Russian physician who had been trained by MSF and Dr. Vezhnina to be the DOTS coordinator of MSF's TB program, who was a leading proponent of DOTS-Plus in Colony 33.

Paul Farmer's Criticism of MSF

Paul Farmer now weighed in against MSF. In response to an article in the *International Journal of Tuberculosis and Lung Disease* by Michael Kimerling, Hans Kluge, Natalia Vezhnina et al.,[43] Farmer published an editorial in the same issue of that journal that bluntly criticized the way in which the "Russian prison medics and . . . the expatriate medical staff of Médecins Sans Frontières" were dealing with drug-resistant tuberculosis in Colony 33 and other prisons. The "bad news from the Siberia . . . story here," he wrote, was "one of decreasing treatment efficacy in the face of a burgeoning epidemic." A striking "clinical failure" had occurred both in spite of and as a consequence of the "managerial success" in carrying out and enforcing a "strict DOTS protocol" in that setting. "[D]rugs used in conventional DOTS regimens cannot cure MDR-TB," he declared. What were called for were "new strategies." While "DOTS must remain the cornerstone of effective TB control throughout the world," DOTS-Plus was called for if MDR-TB was to be controlled.[44]

Kimerling and his coauthors did not respond with acrimony to Farmer's stinging rebuke. However, they felt that Farmer had not taken into account the obstacles that MSF had to overcome in Kemerovo before it could go forward with implementing this treatment regimen. In addition, having come into the Russian penal system in 1996, in the wake of a TB epidemic partially attributable to unsystematic patterns of treatment, the MSF physicians and Dr. Vezhnina were conditioned to be wary of launching a patient on a treatment course before they knew that it would not be interrupted.

In the exchanges that we (Fox and Shevchenko) had with him, Paul Farmer attributed the shortcomings of the MSF program to the fact that "they used the wrong drugs, gave the prisoners the wrong treatment." This was partly because it was more cost-effective than DOTS-Plus, he claimed. In his view, the medical consequences had been tragic, resulting in numerous deaths among the prisoners. He also expressed both perplexity and dubiety about the degree to which MSF "blamed" the difficulties they faced on "the intransigence" of the Russian government. "[Th]e prison system is federal, not oblast-specific," he pointed out. "We were . . . working with the very same authorities" in the Tomsk region. "If they . . . were so intransigent," he asked, "then why were we able to introduce dot-plus [*sic*] in Tomsk? . . . [W]e worked with the same people and they supported our project fully."[45]

Why were the authorities willing to adopt the DOTS-Plus approach in Tomsk, but not in the Kemerovo region? The involvement of Alex Goldfarb as a go-between in Tomsk seems to have been a contributing factor. He played "a major role," Farmer said. "[T]hough the collaboration wasn't perfectly smooth at first, he did come around to support proper therapy and helped us to point out that it was not right to deny prisoners access to that therapy on the grounds that it 'wasn't cost-effective.'" As director of the $13 million Soros/Public Health Research Institute (PHRI) tuberculosis project in Russia, Goldfarb had funds at his disposal that greatly exceeded those of MSF, and the authority to make decisions about how they were distributed. As a former citizen of the Soviet Union who had championed dissidents in the USSR and post-Soviet Russia, he also knew how to deal with Russian apparatchiki. He appears to have been able to arrange for the Tomsk project to be accorded a singular status as a Russian pilot project, supported by all relevant regional authorities, which was not centrally controlled on a national level, but was backed by the "right people" on that level.

The deepest sources of Paul Farmer's critique of MSF, however, were philosophical—rooted in his worldview and most militant values. Farmer is committed to a human-rights-based, doctor-patient-centered conception of effective medical care of high quality that he believes every person is individually and morally entitled to receive. This includes prisoners, the poor, and those who are afflicted, marginalized, or disenfranchised in other ways. For him, "the best way to protect the rights" of prisoners with MDR-TB is to "cure them of their disease"—a disease that at this medical-historical juncture he regards as "completely curable." "And the best way to protect the rights of other prisoners, and those who take care of them is to prevent transmission by treating the sick"[46]—ideally in a way that "maintain[s] the chance for the doctor to act as a doctor, proceeding as if there were only one patient in the world."[47]

Farmer is not unmindful of the relationship among social, political, and economic factors, the illnesses to which people are prone, and the medical care they receive. He makes frequent reference to what he terms the "structural violence"[48] to which the inequality and injustice embedded in the social order subjects persons—including the role they play in the susceptibility of the imprisoned to a disease like tuberculosis and their lack of quality care. He also recognizes the importance of a public-health perspective, which extends the doctor-patient relationship and medical care to the health of whole populations. But with regard to a disease like tuberculosis, he contends, for which efficacious medical therapy now exists, placing too much emphasis on such "structural" transformations that lie outside the orbit and competence of physicians and medicine, and waiting for them to come to pass, is not justifiable, nor is evaluating the worth of health expenditures on the basis of their cost-effectiveness.[49]

Criticisms from Inside MSF

Criticisms of MSF Belgium's operations in Siberia also came from inside of MSF itself. In their retrospective concluding report on the MSF Belgium TB project, Dominque Lafontaine and Andrei Slavuckij attributed some of the difficulties the program had encountered to MSF's excessive tendency to engage in analysis and decision-making done "internally" or "entirely by MSF." MSF had involved "only a restricted number" of people on the Russian medical staff of Colony 33 and in GUIN, and "sometimes deliberately ignored key persons who had much more power but were not convinced" about MSF's espousal of DOTS and DOTS-Plus.[50]

The strongest internal criticisms emanated from MSF France, however. For several years MSF Belgium had hoped that MSF France would become a participant in the Siberian TB project. MSF Belgium and MSF France would each have had their own heads of mission in the field; but there would have been a single, joint medical coordinator for the two missions, who, because of MSF Belgium's long history in Russia, would be affiliated with the Belgian section. MSF France did not find the decision-making authority that this triangular structure accorded to MSF Belgium acceptable. Another source of strain between the two sections concerned their conceptions of the division of labor between them with respect to the prison and the civilian aspects of the TB program. MSF Belgium proposed MSF France taking major responsibility for the program's civil society services—including the follow-up of released prisoners—while it continued to concentrate on patients inside the prison colonies. MSF France, which was only minimally interested in working outside the prisons, considered this an unsatisfactory arrangement.

There were also fundamental differences in the medical-philosophical orientations of MSF Belgium and MSF France—which had some similarities to Paul Farmer's perspective on medical humanitarian action. Dr. Vinciane Sizaire (who was then affiliated with MSF Belgium, had previously worked for MSF France, MSF Luxembourg, and MSF Holland, and was serving as the regional advisor for all of the MSF TB programs in the Russian Federation) described the differences in the outlooks of MSF Belgium and MSF France to Olga Shevchenko.[51] MSF Belgium has "more of a public-health approach," she said, whereas MSF France "wants to be really close to the patient." MSF France would treat a dying MDR-TB patient regardless of its larger project paradigm and plans. It had done so in the Nagorno-Karabakh Republic,[52] for example, where the population was so small that MSF staff knew each patient personally, "eye to eye." Sizaire was a consultant to that project, and when she returned from Nagorno-Karabakh, "reasoning as an MSF Belgium person," she advised MSF France that it was fine for them to treat particular MDR-TB patients on an individual basis. However, due consideration should also be given to providing "technical support" for the establishment of DOTS and DOTS-Plus programs in that setting. MSF France took exception to the notion of "technical support," she said, implying that it was antithetic to their paramount commitment to MSF's principle of "proximity" to patients. When Sizaire met with Francine Matthys, the-then director of MSF Belgium's medical department, and Francis Varain, a long-time leader of MSF's TB working group, they suggested that she delete the term "technical support" from her recommendations, because it would not please that section's operations department.

An explosive confrontation occurred between representatives of MSF Belgium and MSF France in the latter's Paris office. It concerned Michael Kimerling, the medical advisor to the program associated with MSF Belgium. As recounted to us by Kimerling, at this hostility-pervaded meeting, members of MSF France's operations department expressed unwillingness to work in partnership with him, because he was an American physician, affiliated with an American research institution (the Gorgas Tuberculosis Initiative at the University of Alabama) receiving funding from the U.S. Agency for International Development (USAID), which they called "dirty money."[53] A more implicit component in this encounter was the French operations desk's view of Kimerling as a proponent and expediter of the kind of public-health approach that they regarded as the antithesis of the one-on-one, doctor-patient-centered treatment that they considered to be the quintessence of medical humanitarian interventions. Unsurprisingly, what transpired at this meeting played a capital role in Kimerling's decision to end his relationship as an adviser to the program. His departure constituted a significant loss for the program's capacity to systematically collect and evaluate data important for making informed decisions about its tuberculosis control actions.[54]

The Rift with the Russian Authorities

Meanwhile, following the dismissal of Dr. Vezhnina and her replacement by a conservative physician, the relationship of MSF Belgium's TB project to local Russian authorities worsened.

Previously, MSF Belgium's greatest difficulties had arisen with federal officials; it had been easier to handle the pragmatic issues raised by regional officials. However, although the specialist who replaced Vezhnina had agreed to be listed as a coauthor of several of the papers published by members of MSF in collaboration with Michael Kimerling and the Gorgas Institute, she shared the hostile opinions about MSF, DOTS, and Vezhnina of General Alexander Kononets, the medical head of the federal Prison Administration, GUIN. Furthermore, the head doctor of the hospital in Colony 33, who had previously been Vezhnina's assistant, now did everything possible to manifest his loyalty to the policies and combative attitude to MSF of the new main TB specialist, Dr. Starchenkova. MSF was ejected from the office that it had occupied in Colony 33 on the grounds that it was needed for the extension of the pharmacy, and Starchenkova built a special room in which she treated TB prisoner-patients with the salt air and natural crystal salts of an alternative medicine system known as speleotherapy. She also defiantly responded to MSF's "inaction" with regard to MDR-TB by starting a small group of such patients on what she called a "therapy of despair," which consisted of a cocktail of several available first- and second-line drugs, complemented with some folk and traditional remedies such as pine-oil inhalations, controlled breathing exercises, and products that abounded in vitamins C and E.

The breaking point in the relations between MSF and the GUIN authorities occurred on March 24, 2003, when a high-ranking medical professor from the Central Russian Institute of Tuberculosis of the Russian Academy of Medical Sciences visited Colony 33. Given the Institute's status as a progressive medical establishment friendly to WHO protocols, the MSF volunteers had hoped that this visit would lend credibility to their opposition to the erratic MDR-TB treatment regimens advocated by the new Main Specialist. Instead, to their bewilderment and indignation, the visiting dignitary "massacred the WHO regimen," encouraging the gathered personnel to use available second-line drugs intermittently, for periods of time much shorter than those recommended by WHO, and to switch them without regard to the internationally accepted protocol.

In response, Dr. Andrei Slavuckij, MSF's medical coordinator, openly questioned the treatment strategy approved by a GUIN consultant—saying that it contradicted the international treatment standards recommended by WHO and risked creating an extremely drug-resistant form of TB (XDR-TB). On the same day, after an emergency meeting in their office, Slavuckij and Dominque Lafontaine, the project coordinator, wrote a letter to Kemerovo GUIN in which they announced that they were putting the MSF project on standby until further notice.[55]

Grave consequences followed. MSF's access to the colony was revoked. Dr. Oleg Sheyanenko who, under the auspices of MSF, had received special training in administering DOT-Plus treatment, was dismissed by GUIN for "disciplinary reasons." He was accused of being responsible for the death of an MDR-TB patient in Colony 33; although some second-line TB drugs were available in the colony, his failure to treat this patient with those on hand, GUIN charged, constituted criminal negligence. To his MSF colleagues, Sheyanenko was unjustly "disgraced" because he had taken a firm position defending MSF's approach to DOTS-Plus.

In conversation with us, Slavuckij attributed his principled position to what he described as a "Go to the Square" mentality, which he associated with an historic event known as the "demonstration of the seven." On August 21, 1968, the USSR sent Warsaw Pact troops and tanks to Czechoslovakia to crush the "Prague Spring" reforms that Alexander Dubček, the first secretary of the Communist Party of Czechoslovakia, had set into motion. On August 25, rallying around the cry "Go to the Square," seven Russian dissidents gathered in Moscow's Red Square to protest the invasion. They were quickly arrested, and they paid for what Slavuckij called their "five minutes of freedom and action," with many years in prison. What their cry meant to him, he said, was: Come to a conclusion. Take a stand against a totalitarian system, for the freedom to choose according to conscience, and in support of competence.[56] He had brought this outlook with him when he first began to work with MSF in Angola in 1991,[57] and he felt it was in keeping with the "spirit" of the movement:

There have been political struggles in MSF [he averred], and also struggles over principles, finances, and human resources. There is much that is not written down in the MSF Charter. But the spirit of MSF, I feel in myself. After ten years I have concluded that you can do what you believe in this organization, but you have to argue for it, and prove it.[58]

Although Slavuckij was particularly outspoken, his passionate forthrightness was compatible with MSF's precepts of self-examination, self-criticism, and accountability, and with its culture of debate. However, he was increasingly viewed by the national and regional Russian authorities as a primary source of their problems with MSF.

MSF Belgium Calls a Halt

In a letter dated September 9, 2003, signed by Dr. Tine Dusauchoit, in her capacity as director-general of MSF Belgium, MSF Belgium formally conveyed to relevant Russian officials its decision to terminate its involvement in TB control in the Kemerovo Region at the end of the year 2003. "Taking this decision has been very difficult," she wrote:

It . . . brings us sadness, because of all the consequences it will have for the patients, our staff in the region and for our Russian colleagues that we leave on their own to tackle this deadly disease. However, in the given circumstances and for the reasons outlined . . . , my organization has no other choice than to stop its commitment. . . .

[O]ur organization cannot and will not be involved in [a] treatment strategy we strongly disagree with. Not because of the fact of this disagreement, but because we cannot be involved in a treatment strategy that does not cure patients.

Dusauchoit outlined the sequence of events that had led to this. "[O]ur doctors have been faced with an important number of patients suffering from drug resistant TB, which cannot be cured with the first-line TB drugs we provided," she recounted. In 2002, together with the regional authorities in Kemerovo, MSF had therefore come up with a comprehensive plan for the treatment of such patients based on WHO DOTS-Plus recommendations. This was submitted to WHO's Green Light Committee, which approved MSF's starting to use second-line drugs, initially to treat one hundred and fifty prisoners.

However, when the proposal was submitted to the Russian Ministry of Health, it rejected it (in spring 2003).

> We were informed that the treatment schemes proposed in the project were in contradiction with the regulation of the Russian Pharmaceutical Committee. We were advised to review the project document, which we did with support of leading and recognized authorities in the field of TB treatment. This new project did not change in essence the treatment schemes that are in conformity with WHO recommendations. It received a written approval by the CTRI [the Central Tuberculosis Research Institute], linked through agreement with the GUIN, and of the Novosibirsk TB Institute, responsible to monitor the TB activities in Kemorovo region. In June of this year the GUIN again submitted the project for approval by the MoH [Ministry of Health]. In September, the MoH rejected the project for the second time. The reasons given referred to Russian legislation that prohibits extended use of certain 2nd line anti-tuberculosis drugs.[59]

In effect, this meant that the DOTS-Plus pilot project was classified as "experimental," and therefore forbidden under national law within the penal system. "In order to comply with the existing legislation," MSF was being asked to "implement a treatment strategy for drug resistant TB that [was] in complete contradiction with the one proposed by WHO, which must be followed if we want to provide adequate care to patients," Dusauchoit concluded.

Thus, "[a]fter years of efforts, we are back at square one," Nicolas Cantau, MSF Belgium's head of mission in the Russian Federation, declared: "We are forced to quit, as the only alternative would be to provide incomplete, inadequate treatment to the patients. We have no options left, but given the scale of the problem with TB in Siberia and our investment over seven years in trying to tackle it with the Russian authorities, our decision to leave feels like a very painful defeat."[60]

In October 2003, the Russian deputy minister of justice, Yuri Kalinin, was asked at a press conference on reform of the Russian penitentiary system to comment on "the recent scandal" connected with the cessation of the collaboration of MSF in the Kemerovo penal institutions. In a press release titled "MSF could not find common language with the penitentiary system of RF," emanating from the REGNUM News Agency (a federal Russian news service), Kalinin responded that the "causes for the conflict," in his opinion, were that MSF had tried to use "drugs with limited shelf lives," which were "not registered by the Ministry of Health," on Russian TB prisoners; that they had imposed "requirements for prisoners' living conditions that conflicted with Russian legislation"; and that "they thought . . . we are [still] somewhere in 1994, when we needed any kind of assistance." Kalinin "stressed" that "a quite well established system" of treating "socially significant diseases" existed "nowadays" in the Russian Federation's penitentiary system—including their treatment in "polyresistant forms." Notwithstanding his criticisms of MSF, he said that "we are very thankful to [them] for the assistance provided," and that he was confident that the issues between the Ministry of Justice and MSF would eventually be resolved.[61]

Recriminations

That there was little remaining hope of a resolution became dramatically apparent at the meetings of the High Level Working Group and of the Russian and International Partners on Financial Mobilization for Tuberculosis Control, chaired by Deputy Minister of Health and Social Development Dr. R. A. Khalfin, that were convened consecutively at the Russian Ministry of Health in Moscow on November 20 and November 21, 2003. Andrei Slavuckij and Oleg Sheyanenko took notes throughout the proceedings, recording verbatim passages from the most acrimonious exchanges concerning MSF Belgium.[62]

In response to some of the allegations made by Dr. Natalia Antonova, head of the Division for the Organization of Medical Care of Infectious Diseases in the Russian Ministry of Health, in her presentation on "The MDR-TB Problem and the Ways to Solve It," Slavuckij rose to say that "[t]aking the MSF project in the Kemerovo region as an example, I would like to [take note of] a striking difference between the approach of WHO recommendations and the regulations of the Ministry of Health":

> Because of it MSF was forced to stop its activities on TB control in the Kemerovo region. . . . MSF . . . tried to follow WHO recommendations, but the project prepared on these grounds . . . was rejected by the Ministry of Health. We have to remember that second-line drugs are . . . [being] sent to the regions and are already in use in accordance with Ministry of Health regulations.

As a consequence, Slavuckij implied, "the process of super-resistance development [was] going on everywhere" in Russia.

To this, Antonova angrily retorted: "You, MSF Belgium, love to raise a scandal when everything is finished in hope that [nobody will] be able to respond to you":

> When you organized a press conference dedicated to the end of your project, you never invited us, fearing that there [would] be someone to respond to you.[63] I would divide this problem in two parts—political and clinical. For the clinical part I will let Professor Sokolova respond to you. . . . [T]he political part of it is that you left because you got ready to leave anyway, because you did not have enough money for MDR-TB treatment. And you never carried out the TB control in that region; for that there is a specialized anti-TB service present there. . . . [O]ur clinicians have solved this problem and now Professor Sokolova will tell you about it.

Dr. G. B. Sokolova, a member of the Pharmacological Committee of the Ministry of Health, and a close colleague of the Russian Chief Phthisiatrist, Dr. Mikhail Perelman, then gave a long talk in which she stated that Russian physicians had been trained to treat TB and drug-resistant TB in an "overall" and "individualized" way. Grave consequences could ensue from treating them otherwise. Particularly serious were the side effects of long-term treatment with second-line drugs integral to the DOTS-Plus regimen, which could "turn patients into invalids." Her statement was challenged by Dr. Richard Zaleskis, regional advisor for Tuberculosis Control in the WHO Regional Office for Europe in Copenhagen, who contended that recently published scientific evidence had demonstrated the benefit of long-term treatment with second-line drugs, and that this was no longer a matter of debate.

Slavuckij took the floor next, reacting with indignation to the remarks that Natalia Antonova had made about MSF. "I do not know how it is possible to say the help brought by MSF is nothing, or something insignificant in TB control activities in the Kemerovo region," he exclaimed:

> During seven years of our involvement MSF directly invested in the Kemerovo TB program more than U.S.$3.5 million. How can one suggest that MSF planned "anyway" to withdraw from its involvement, [when one takes] into consideration [the] significant investment in the reference laboratory that since 2000 is ready for DOTS-Plus, [and] all the second-line drugs [that] with difficulties . . . finally arrived and were available since May of this year. Financial argument is simply not true. Our DOTS-Plus protocol, approved by the Green Light Committee of WHO, was simply repeatedly rejected by the Ministry of Health referring to experiments

on prisoners. The problem is there—[the] non-agreement of WHO and the Ministry of Health on the treatment of drug-resistance.

At the end of the first meeting day, Mr. Smirnov, representing GUIN, made a presentation listed on the program as "Information about the MSF Project in the Penitentiary System of the Kemerovo Region."[64] Its title notwithstanding, it consisted mainly of a recitation of GUIN's achievements in the struggle with TB. The only mention of MSF was a perfunctory expression of gratitude for its help, accompanied by the assertion that TB treatment methods remained strictly the prerogative of the Ministry of Health. This triggered another outraged response from Slavuckij. "According to the title of your presentation," he declared, "[you were supposed] to give information about the MSF project in the Kemorovo penal system; but we did not hear anything concrete on the MSF project itself":

> MSF not only invested [a] considerable financial amount, but [the MSF project] is . . . the [main] efficient system of TB detection, diagnosis, and treatment created, with clear diagnostic algorithms and treatment protocols. [I]t is twelve laboratories in peripheral colonies, also [a] bacteriological laboratory in Colony 33 that has no analogues in the whole of Siberia, . . . a series of continuous trainings [sic] that should be mentioned as well, and [much] more. . . .
>
> MSF is not a sponsor. MSF is a humanitarian-implementing NGO. Simple people in Belgium confer [sic] their offerings to MSF, for this organization, in the best possible way . . . [to give] help to the Siberian people in need. I am not a Belgian, and I know that Russian people are famous for their hospitality. . . . I would not expect that there [would be] such a hostile attitude—not one word of gratitude, transmitted or published, to [the] Belgian people.

"We are grateful for the experiment in Kemerovo," Smirnov responded, "and we regret the ceasing of the joint work." (It was notable that he persisted in referring to MSF's action as "experimental.")

Toward the close of the meetings, General Kononets (the medical head of the federal GUIN) asked for "the opportunity to clarify the situation with regard to MSF Belgium," because, he said, "there are differences in interpretation." He went on:

> Some time ago, when we had difficulties with the supply of anti-TB drugs, MSF helped very much in the Kemerovo region, not only with the drugs, but in setting

up the network of laboratories, with additional food for patients, and so on. However, when the necessity to treat MDR-TB patients arose, I was waiting a long time for MSF to start the DOTS-Plus project; but they never got permission to import drugs, as part of these drugs were not registered in Russia. After waiting for half a year, I supplied the region with second-line drugs that we had obtained by that time. And then the problems started. MSF protested against the way we used these drugs and finally they closed their project because of the disagreement with the Ministry of Health. That is it, as simple as it is.

Slavuckij once more tried to set the record straight about "the sad story" of MSF's withdrawal from the TB control program in Kemerovo. In his view, it "should be studied as a case-study":

This is the story of how good people in Belgium conferred their means [*sic*] to MSF, wishing to help many suffering people in Kemerovo; how MSF, armed with the best, worldwide renowned, and recommended by WHO treatment methods, . . . with the best quality drugs (though obtained with a lot of difficulties) had difficulty in bringing this help to patients, [and] thus was prevented [from doing] good.

He ended with an exhortation:

All of us have to be honest with ourselves. . . . We have to open our eyes and look at what is going on now. In many regions of Russia the treatment using second-line drugs is going on without clear guidelines, without necessary conditions created. Already now the future unbearable problem of extensively drug-resistant TB [has been] created. Urgent measures have to be taken to address this problem today. Once again we urge all of you to seriously think about this—about the non-agreement in treatment approach between the Ministry of Health and WHO, because [the] more this agreement is delayed, [the] more it contributes to the growth of super-resistance. All of us bear responsibility.

The meeting was closed by its chairman, Deputy Minister of Health Dr. Khalfin, with a parable-like story, drawn from his childhood:

A boy and a girl were busy drawing. The boy asked the girl to give him a green-colored pencil. The girl refused to give it to him. After a while, however, she decided to give him the green pencil. But the boy did not need it anymore, because he had filled in the leaves of the tree he was drawing with his black-colored pencil.

The moral that he drew from this tale—"It is necessary to *give* in such a way that the recipient will want to *take* it"—was received by the assemblage with approving laughter and applause. For many of them "the boy" in the story represented the Russian physicians, and governmental health and penitentiary authorities who were involved in the treatment and control of tuberculosis, and "the girl" represented MSF Belgium.[65]

Glimpses of the Aftermath

"I was in Moscow, and worked with MSF on the capitalization [*sic*] of MSF projects [*sic*] that took place in the Kemerovo region," Dr. Natalia Vezhnina wrote in an e-mail message to us (Fox and Shevchenko) on November 11, 2003:

> We discussed articles to be published in medical [journals] and in the mass media in order to inform the community about the situation in Russia, about the impending catastrophe of [the] increase [in the] number of cases with pan-resistance. MSF and other international organizations shouldn't bear responsibility for the things that are going on . . . because treatment protocols suggested by them [according to] WHO standards were not supported by the Ministry of Health of the Russian Federation.[66]

While in Moscow, she continued, she was offered a position with the AIDS Foundation East-West (AFEW). AFEW is an international, nongovernmental humanitarian public-health organization, whose stated "mission is to make a major contribution to the reduction of HIV/AIDS in the Newly Independent States of the former Soviet Union."[67] Founded in the Netherlands in 2001 by four MSF Holland staff members who had been involved since 1996 in dealing with the rapidly growing epidemic of HIV/AIDS in the Russian Federation, Ukraine, and Mongolia, it characterized itself as "rooted in the traditions and activities of MSF Holland,"[68] and as a "bridge between East and West"[69] in tackling the challenges of preventing and treating HIV/AIDS in a context where its epidemic had had a "late start," but was becoming "the fastest growing [one] in history."[70] The job with AFEW that Dr. Vezhnina was invited to fill, she explained, was that of a coordinator in a project concerned with the protection of inmates' health in prisons of Central Asia (in Kazakhstan, Uzbekistan, Tajikistan, and Kyrgyzstan). Among the inducements for her to accept this position, she said, was the fact that Nicolas Cantau, former head of the MSF Belgium mission in Russia, was now running AFEW's projects in Almaty (formerly known as Alma-Ata), Kazakhstan.[71] "I think that today I will finally give an official consent" to take this position, she wrote, though "it is very hard and painful for me," because "the work will be connected with HIV/AIDS education," and this means that "I will step aside from TB. . . . My main dream is to continue work on TB."[72]

In the same e-mail, Vezhnina expressed great regret and shame about what had become of Michael Kimerling's efforts through the Gorgas TB Initiative and the University of Alabama to create the possibility for TB control in the prisons and the civil society of the Kemerovo region, and to "disseminate modern world [scientific and medical] knowledge and experience." The Center of Excellence project that he had created to coordinate these activities was "very effective," she commented, but it had had "no continuation in the area of practical activity." And now, she reported, almost before it had begun, Kimerling's project was about to be shut down due to many of the same factors that had closed MSF Belgium's TB program.[73]

We learned from Vezhnina that there had been a "great staff turnover" in Colony 33.[74] Most of her collaborators had left MSF Belgium when the TB project was dissolved. MSF had treated the national Russian personnel very well. Several had found positions working for AFEW. Some of the younger women and men had gone to Moscow to look for jobs in commercial companies. Dr. Oleg Sheyanenko had been engaged in a succession of MSF Belgium and MSF Switzerland TB-relevant missions in Kyrgyzstan and Ukraine. And Andrei Slavuckij had become deputy medical director for operations in the Geneva office of MSF Switzerland.

Although Vezhnina continued to think that it would be wonderful if MSF could one day return to the Kemerovo region, where they had "laboriously created . . . a system of detection, diagnosis, and treatment of TB," and begin DOTS-Plus at this "site which ha[d] such a long history," this did not seem possible to her. The "state structures . . . did not want anyone meddling in their business," she said, and for MSF, it was "hard to step into the same river twice." She continued to insist that there were no grounds for the disagreements over DOTS-Plus between MSF, the Ministry of Health, and WHO. "Quite simply, MSF was too active," she declared. "[T]hey did not keep silent and were not yes-men. . . . Because . . . they did not only treat, but also witness. Because they did not rush to please every time some establishment figure . . .

wanted to dictate to them how to run their organization. . . . [They] did not yield and simply wanted to do good honest work." Although geographically dispersed, the members of the MSF Belgium staff who had participated in the Kemerovo tuberculosis program continued to feel connected, interpersonally and emotionally, by the moral as well as the medical meaning of their work, and by what their shared commitment had "put them through": in Vezhnina's words, "the blow . . . we sustained in Kemerovo that left scars, probably for the rest of our lives." They were delighted when they had occasion to meet professionally. At the Thirty-Fifth World Conference of the International Union Against Tuberculosis and Lung Disease, held in Paris on October 28–November 1, 2004, for example, Vezhnina, Michael Kimerling, and Hans Kluge (who had served as a medical coordinator for the MSF-TB project)[75] were happily reunited. Kluge and Kimerling chaired a session on TB in prisons at which Vezhnina presented a paper on the dual epidemic of TB and HIV/AIDS in the prisons of the Central Asian Republics.[76] The large audience included General Alexander Kononets, the head of GUIN's medical section, who, at the end of the session, to Vezhnina's great surprise, effusively told her how proud they all were of her, and of how she was moving ahead.

As the paper Vezhnina delivered indicated, her passionate interest in TB was unabated. A postcard that she sent from Paris to the Russian physician who was now serving as head doctor in Colony 33 conveyed that in giving this paper, her "heart and soul . . . were with my doctors at Colony 33, [to whom] I am deeply grateful for their work."

Some Patterns

The patterns observable in MSF Belgium's tuberculosis program in the Russian Federation's penitentiary system have recurred in other MSF humanitarian projects. Notwithstanding its commitment to politically independent action, MSF has often had to struggle with local and national political authorities. The internal disagreements that developed around issues connected with the authority structure, the division of labor, the sponsorship, and the outlook of the TB control program in the Kemerovo region were not unique occurrences within MSF's "culture of debate." And MSF Belgium's "witnessing" in reaction to the Russian Ministry of Health's refusal to endorse DOTS-Plus treatment for prisoners with MDR-TB expressed a foundational principle that MSF has exercised in many other contexts.

There were, however, some aspects of the patterning of these phenomena in Russia that distinguished it from other MSF projects. To begin with, MSF Belgium was enmeshed in an extraordinarily complex skein of social systems. It involved relating to and functioning within a penitentiary system that was just emerging from the Gulag era—a prison system organized as a hierarchical military entity, and that functioned under the aegis of three national ministries, within a newly postsocialist state, in which political power was becoming more centralized. MSF also had to handle relationships with several international organizations (principally the World Health Organization and the World Bank), an institute in an American University (the Gorgas TB Initiative at the University of Alabama, and its funding by USAID), the Public Health Research Institute (PHRI) when it was located in New York City,[77] and the power-wielding representative of a U.S.-based NGO, the Soros Foundation/Open Society Institute. In addition, MSF Belgium was confronted with contentious questions—which were as cultural, philosophical, ethical, and ideological as they were biomedical—about the optimal treatment of tuberculosis in its various forms. These were issues and differences arising from the juxtaposition of a one-on-one, care-centered doctor-patient perspective, an individual human rights emphasis, and a public-health outlook, on the one hand, and the ensemble of traditional attitudes and practices staunchly upheld by Russian TB "phthisiatrist" specialists, on the other.

MSF Belgium's reasons for terminating its project in Siberia differed markedly, too, from the circumstances under which MSF has usually made this kind of decision. Generally, such closures occur when the security conditions in a field situation are too perilous for the staff to continue its work in that locale, or when an MSF mission can be competently carried on by local personnel under other than MSF auspices. Furthermore, in contrast to the finality of MSF Belgium's departure from the Kemerovo region, MSF staff have often returned to the scene they had left, and resumed their work there. Finally, another unusual feature was that even after exiting from Siberia, MSF Belgium continued to engage authorities there in debate about the reasons that had driven its members from the field, and to exhort the Russians to take urgent action to address the spread of MDR-TB and XDR-TB—action for which MSF still felt some responsibility.

A Retrospective Testimony

Looking back at his experiences with the MSF Belgium TB project in the Siberian prisons of the Russian Federation unleashed what Andrei Slavuckij described as "an explosion of emotion" within him:

> The enormity of the endeavor and works performed by MSF guys! . . . Nurses, doctors, lab technicians, logisticians, administrators, drivers! . . . [N]ot only expats . . . but also national staff. [T]hey were really devoted, enthusiastic, motivated!! It was a huge collective effort . . . mental, psychological, professional, spiritual, physical. Temperatures minus 30–40 [degrees Centigrade], sometimes down to minus 50!!! Covering huge territory, to the remote colonies, deeply in snow, bringing hope and such awaited aid. This effort should not be underestimated. . . .
>
> Among 10,500 patients treated for TB, nearly 7,000 were treated successfully! This is a spectacular result that everyone has a tendency to forget, concentrating uniquely—though rightfully—on the fact that we never started MDR!! **Seven thousand people** were successfully treated. Can this be considered simply "a failure"? . . .
>
> [W]e were proud of what we were doing, not because of vanity . . . but because every day we have seen, we were witnesses to, incredible scenes of human suffering and miraculous effects resulting from our efforts, and feelings of devastation when it did not work. Devastation! THIS gave to all of us additional forces; this was the subject of feverish debates, disputes, sleepless nights spent in discussing how to do better, whether it was in Mariinsk, in a Russian *izba* [log cabin] 800 meters from Colony 33 where the team lodged, in Kemerovo, Novokuznetsk, or Moscow headquarters. . . .
>
> All of us have LIVED this project as . . . the most important [thing] that happened in our lives.[78]

Remembering the Past and Envisioning the Future

Doctors Without Borders / Médecins Sans Frontières celebrated its fortieth anniversary and held the first meeting of its newly created International General Assembly on December 16–18, 2011, in Saint-Denis, a commune in the suburbs of Paris, at a conference center called L'Usine (The Factory).

Throughout the nineteenth and twentieth centuries, until the 1970s, Saint-Denis was one of the most heavily industrialized communities in France. It declined economically after that; its factories closed; unemployment became widespread; and its immigrant population grew.[1] It is also the locale of the Royal Cathedral Basilica of Saint-Denis, named after the first bishop of Paris, a patron saint of France, and a model for numerous Gothic cathedrals, particularly in northern France and England.[2] The other notable physical landmark of Saint-Denis is a secular one, and of recent vintage: the Stade-de-France, a modern stadium where the 1998 World Cup football (soccer) finals were held, and a structure that is viewed as a harbinger of Saint-Denis's recovery.

L'Usine is located near the Stade-de-France. Built in 1862, it was a central factory of the pharmaceutical company founded by Émile-Justin Menier in 1816, which prepared and sold medicinal powders, and used chocolate to coat the bitter-tasting pills it produced. Over time it developed into the Menier Chocolate Company, the largest chocolate maker in France, and one of the leading chocolate manufacturers in the world—statuses that it maintained until the end of World War I.[3]

It was coincidental that the locale of this meeting was contextually related to a factory that once manufactured medical drugs, and to the habitat of an immigrant population—which are both foci of MSF's concerns and action. However, it was not accidental that its venue was in Paris, France, and that MSF France hosted the meeting. For, as MSF's international president Unni Karunakara stated at the opening of the meeting, "[I]t was here in Paris . . . forty years ago, [that] the band of volunteers . . . started our sans-frontières movement."

Three hundred members of MSF attended, including two representatives from each of MSF's nineteen sections,[4] and also from the four new MSF "entities"—MSF Brazil, MSF East Africa, MSF Latin America, and MSF South Africa—that were applying to the Assembly to become full-fledged members of MSF International. Parts of the proceedings were live-streamed, so that wherever they were located in the world, MSFers could view and hear and ask questions in real time, or tune in later to the sessions, discussions, and debates that had already taken place. I attended the entire meeting as an invited guest. "It is a great pleasure for me to invite you to MSF's first International General Assembly," MSF's International President Karunakara had written to me:

> This assembly coincides with our 40th anniversary and will mark the conclusion of a two-year reform process and the implementation of a new, more inclusive governance set-up. The event is a key moment in the life of our movement. . . . [It] will be both an opportunity for reflection on forty years of medical humanitarian action and a discussion about the future, examining our ambitions and ongoing commitment to medical action.[5]

Commingled in the agenda of the meeting and its opening atmosphere were festive sentiments of reunion and comradeship; an ebullient commitment to MSF as a movement; a collective sense of appreciation for what MSF had accomplished; a self-questioning awareness of its shortcomings and limits, and of old and new challenges that it faced in the field; and an emerging vision of MSF's future as pragmatic as it was utopian. Permeating the meeting were positive expectations about how the reform of MSF's international governance, through the establishment of an International General Assembly and an International Board, might make the organization's inner and outer functioning more global, in spirit and fact, and more responsive to change.

The Meaning of the MSF T-Shirt

Most attendees were dressed casually—many in blue jeans and T-shirts. I saw fewer wearers of MSF T-shirts than at other MSF gatherings I have attended, but a book of photographs available for purchase paid tribute to their symbolic importance.[6] This album-like volume was conceived, assembled, and edited by Rip Hopkins, a professional photographer, who had worked with MSF for five years, doing photojournalism reports and making documentary films about field missions in South Sudan, Bosnia, Liberia, Uganda, Ingushetia, East Timor, and elsewhere. In that capacity, he wrote, he was "proud to wear the Médecins Sans Frontières T-shirt," but he "did not feel that [he] deserved it. . . . I was not equal to this symbol, this sign."[7]

The book consists of a series of full-page portraits of sixty persons posed in MSF T-shirts in a way that evoked how they imagined an MSF volunteer in the field might live. Hopkins asked them to provide a citation for the photo expressing their commitment to freely doing something for others to "keep them from falling," without expecting anything in return. The subjects of the photos included actors and actresses, musicians, writers, journalists, scientists, mathematicians, athletes, theatrical directors, a dancer, a circus performer, a financial advisor, and a cook. Interspersed among these photos were those of thirteen members of MSF in their roles of physician, nurse, pharmacist, logistician, laboratory assistant, head of mission, and administrator.[8]

In his introduction, Hopkins speaks to the meaning of this "white cotton garment with a red and black logo":

> In the field, no need of papers, nor to explain one's self, the MSF T-shirt suffices. It justifies the presence of its wearer, with little importance attached to who is inside it. It can be put on in order to pass check-points, to infiltrate a camp of refugees, to escape imprisonment. . . .
>
> This white cotton garment with a red and black logo is more than a symbol. One shares it, it protects us from the sun, the heat, the cold and from being looked at, it hides our nudity and our own identity. It gives a status, a family, a reason for being, a direction. It is also a torch, a sponge, a filter, a strap, a sack, a bucket, a hat. Everything depends on the circumstances.

Anybody can be an MSF volunteer. But it is not easy. It involves work, sweat, reflection and suffering. Even well-known persons must be willing to undergo a little pain in order to deserve to wear this T-shirt.[9]

Four New Associations

After the welcoming and opening remarks delivered by the president of MSF France (Marie-Pierre Allié) and Unni Karunakara, representatives of MSF Brazil, MSF East Africa, MSF Latin America, and MSF South Africa delivered oral and video presentations about their origins, geographical scope, membership, funding, activities, links to other MSF sections, associations and operational centers, and their "messages" and "added value" to the MSF "movement." A flurry of procedural discussions then occurred before a vote was taken on the resolution to the effect that: "The International General Assembly approves the [four] associations . . . as institutional members of MSF International." Each of the associations was unanimously approved. The outcome of the voting was received with enthusiastic applause, expressing the general sentiment that the ratification of these associations went far toward making MSF a "truly international and global association," adapting to the "changing world."

Partly because the status that the new associations had just attained seemed to me to be rather vague, I had some doubts concerning how much influence they would have with regard to fundamental organization- and movement-wide issues. Each of the four new associations would have two elected representatives to the International General Assembly (IGA). Nevertheless, they would be heavily outnumbered by the nineteen sections of MSF, whose directors, it seemed to me, would retain the dominant decision-making powers.

I had occasion to think about these matters again when, on the third day of the meeting, at the so-called "Vision Feedback" session, a member of the East Africa Association raised challengingly pertinent questions about the "in-between status" of the new associations, and the "nebulous space" that they occupied. "How are they going to be integrated into the movement?" she asked in a ringing voice.

The President's and Treasurer's Reports

Most of the rest of the first day's session was centered on the overview reports given by Unni Karunakara and by MSF's treasurer, Martin Aked, on the activities in which MSF had been engaged during the previous year (2010) and their financial concomitants.

Before turning to the contents of his report, Karunakara mentioned two colleagues, Montserrat Serra and Blanca Thiebaut, who had been abducted in Dadaab, Kenya, on October 13, 2011, while providing humanitarian assistance there to Somali refugees. As he spoke of them, their computerized photos appeared on the conference room screen. We are thinking of them and their families, Karunakara said, and doing everything we can to bring about their safe release. Silence descended momentarily on the previously animated assemblage.[10]

Karunakara began his president's report on MSF's activities by characterizing the past year as a period marked by natural disasters—most notably, a 7.0 magnitude earthquake in Haiti, and catastrophic floods in five provinces of Pakistan. MSF had mobilized its largest-ever emergency response to the catastrophe in Haiti, he reported, including helping contain the subsequent cholera epidemic. In Pakistan, in addition to basic needs for medical care, MSF's interventions had centered around water and sanitation, and the treatment of children suffering from severe acute malnutrition.

Karunakara detailed MSF's response to the 2011 Tohoku earthquake in Japan, the most powerful (9.0 in magnitude) ever to have hit the country, and the destructive tsunami waves that it had triggered. MSF Japan had worked in coordination with the Japanese Disaster Medical Assistance Team, assessing relief needs, identifying pockets of people not yet reached by the national aid effort, and setting up temporary mobile clinics to treat them. MSF Japan also organized a team of psychologists to help survivors of the earthquake and tsunami cope with the emotional impact of the disaster.[11]

Karunakara next turned to some of the places where MSF was engaged in medical action in the midst of war and civil violence. Prominent among them were Afghanistan, the Central African Republic, the Democratic Republic of Congo, Somalia, and Sudan. "MSF has returned to Afghanistan," he said matter-of-factly. At the end of August 2004, in the wake of the targeted killing of five of its staff members in Badghis province, and after working in Afghanistan since 1980, MSF had closed its medical projects there, handing most of them over to local groups, other international NGOs, or to the Afghan Ministry of Health. Only after negotiating with all warring parties had MSF started working again in Afghanistan, in a district hospital in East Kabul and a provincial hospital in Lashkargah.

He moved on to identify outbreaks of infectious diseases to which MSF had responded. They included epidemics of measles in Malawi, Chad, the Democratic Republic of Congo, Nigeria, South Africa, Swaziland, Yemen, and Zimbabwe, where MSF helped vaccinate millions of children; cholera in Papua, New Guinea, as well as in Haiti; and polio in both the Democratic Republic of Congo and the Republic of Congo, where MSF conducted widespread vaccination campaigns.

Applause greeted Karunakara's announcement of a breakthrough in dealing with HIV/AIDS. New evidence revealed that providing antireroviral treatment earlier in the course of the disease, before the virus seriously undermines a patient's immune system, could prevent opportunistic infections—notably TB—and reduce its transmission to sexual partners. Still, he pointed out, funding for HIV/AIDS was in danger of seriously declining; because of the economic recession in donor countries, the Global Fund to Fight AIDS, Tuberculosis and Malaria was canceling its Round 11 subsidy.

MSF had also been reaching out, Karunkara said, to "invisible populations": to migrants being held in detention centers under inhumane conditions in Greece and in South Africa, for example, where strong xenophobic prejudices festered.

We need to collect more qualitative and quantitative data, Karunkara stated, in order to better evaluate how we are doing in all these spheres of action.

Concluding his report, Karunakara called attention to a list of members of MSF who had died in action, which was posted outside the conference rooms. And he paid tribute to the founders of MSF, several of whom were present at the meeting. "Although [w]e have since become more professional, more international, and gained recognition in large parts of the world," he declared, "the core values [that they] first developed in 1971 continue to drive and inspire us."

In his treasurer's report, Martin Aked indicated that MSF's income had increased from 278 million euros in 2009 to 813 million euros in 2010, due mainly to the donations received in the wake of the Haiti and Pakistan emergencies. These donations had come from more than five million individuals and private institutions, and constituted ninety-one percent of MSF's total income. MSF's expenditures in 2010 had amounted to 813 million euros, an increase of 196 million euros over 2009. MSF's activities had increased thirty-two percent over the year. Eighty-two percent of those funds (666 million euros) had been allocated to MSF's "social mission" (work in the field), and five percent (forty-three million euros) to management and administration office expenses. The largest allocations of funds (102 million euros) had gone to the work in Haiti, in the Democratic Republic of Congo (54 million euros), and in Sudan (39 million euros).

A question-and-answer session followed these reports, led by a panel comprised of the members of the former International Council.[12] One comment evoked applause from everyone present: "We are speaking out less and less about political things," someone exclaimed, "and we take too much time to do so!" At the end of this session, one of my MSF acquaintances humorously remarked to me that its "conclusion" was "inevitable" for MSF—namely, that "we could have done more, and we could have done better."

Before exiting from the first day's meeting, I paused to look at the poster on which the names of the members of MSF who had been killed in the field were displayed. Where they had died and the dates of their deaths were listed next to their names. I did not count the total number of names on the list, but they filled three long columns. Later, in an essay published by the president of MSF France, I read that between 2004 and 2008 alone, as many as "nine members of Médecins Sans Frontières were killed in the course of their missions in Afghanistan, Central African Republic and Somalia."[13]

An Independent Humanitarian Actor?

"MSF: An Independent Humanitarian Actor?" was the title of one of the more spirited sessions of the meeting, a "panel debate" on the afternoon of its second day. It grew out of MSF's two-year-long period of reflection on the conditions under which its members operate. Those in-house discussions had focused on the tensions between MSF's medical action and its human rights witnessing. Prior to the meeting, a volume of essays that grew out of these discussions had been published in French and in English, focusing on case studies of MSF's humanitarian interventions in Sri Lanka, Ethiopia, Yemen, Afghanistan, Pakistan, Somalia, the Gaza Strip, Myanmar, Nigeria, India, South Africa, and France.[14] The Paris panel debate explored the themes highlighted in the book—whether MSF was speaking out less and compromising its independent humanitarian principles more than it had in the past; and to what extent, and in what ways, it should be willing to do so, in response to the suffering and needs of the populations it tries to assist. Weighing in on these questions were two invited guests whose opinion of its witnessing action MSF considered to be of great importance: Reed Brody, legal counsel and spokesperson in Brussels for Human Rights Watch (a leading international nongovernmental organization dedicated to defending and protecting human rights), and Yves Daccord, director-general of the International Committee of the Red Cross.

Brody's comments were predominantly admiring and reassuring. Your capacity for self-observation and self-criticism is remarkable, he told the assembled group. I have done missions where I have relied on MSF to get information that I needed. And when MSF speaks out, he attested, you have a great impact—frequently greater than that of Human Rights Watch—because you are so close to people in crisis.

Yves Daccord of the International Red Cross Committee (ICRC) was more frankly critical of MSF. The ICRC did not doubt that MSF was strongly independent with regard to "access, acceptance, and relevance," he said. MSF and the ICRC had been the only humanitarian organizations present in Afghanistan, Libya, and Somalia. Both took the "risk of proximity." Perhaps MSF was more honest than the ICRC about the "forced negotiations" that this could entail. But in its witnessing, its modus operandi, and in their relationship, MSF was now more conservative than the ICRC. "[I]ncreasingly you act and don't communicate; or you communicate and don't act," Daccord declared, evoking applause from the audience.

MSF was good at communication, Daccord affirmed. That was apparent in its fund-raising. Nevertheless, MSF was not as effective in its field-based communication with local and regional audiences, as it was in its international communication. It was still launching messages from Europe, rather than choosing decentralized communication hubs. The world was changing, and what constituted testimony had changed with it, which posed a challenge for both organizations. People now had cell phones. There was the Worldwide Web. It was not necessary to give "testimony for the people" in the same way as in the past. That could be patronizing. The role of the MSF and ICRC was now to be "independent validators."

Put communication back into action and into negotiations, Daccord concluded. You are on the ground rendering medical services. So are we. Please play with us, he urged. That will make a difference. The audience strongly applauded his exhortation, which was supported by the panelists' comments that followed. Christopher Stokes, general director of MSF's Operational Center in Brussels, was the most articulate among them. He agreed with Daccord that MSF had too much of a tendency to approach the relationship between action and communication as a "zero-sum game"—meaning that it opted either to stay in the field and not communicate, or to leave the field and communicate—and that in certain ways local communication was becoming more important than international communication. MSF's operations had improved, but its communications had not. MSF had too many layers, Stokes said, and too many players; and it tended to see communications as likelier to hinder its operations than facilitate them.

In the corridors of the meeting after this session was over, members spoke of Daccord's "straight, gloves-off" commentary as "historic" and "excellent." I was struck, as I always am, by the place that criticism, along with self-criticism, occupies in MSF's sense of identity and distinctive culture. Praise from Daccord, I mused, would not have been as appreciated or considered as authentic by the MSF assembly as his critical assessment of how they negotiated, witnessed, and communicated.

Forty Years of MSF—A Tale in Four Acts

The emotional high point of the meeting came at the end of its second day, in a session on MSF's forty years of history, billed as "a tale in four acts."[15] The oral presentations made were interspersed with photographs of international events that had occurred during each of those periods (including armed conflicts, natural catastrophes, epidemics, and famines to which MSF had responded), and of MSF members at work in the field. These images were accompanied by music popular at the time. Partly in order to avoid "glorifying" MSF by "recall[ing] past experiences as a kind of exhilarating, heroic, idealized self-history,"[16] the presenters were told not to be too "serious," but rather to relate "amusing anecdotes" drawn from their personal MSF memories.

The 1970s Physician-Founders

Even though they did their best to follow these instructions, the group that represented the first decade of MSF's history—the 1970s—profoundly moved the audience, because it was composed of three of the thirteen "French doctors" who had founded MSF: Xavier Emmanueli, Pascal Greletty-Bosviel, and Max Récamier. ("It was quite emotional just to *see* them," an MSFer commented to me.)

As these three men, who were now in their seventies, described MSF's first act, the camaraderie and the humanitarian passion of their youth were still apparent. They recounted details of the legendary story about how "it all began in Biafra." "With the whole gang, we were all there working for the International and the French Red Cross in the midst of Nigeria's 1967–1970 civil war, helping the population of the Biafran region that had seceded from the Nigerian central government." When they observed what they perceived as the "genocidal" intentions of the Nigerian government in blocking the distribution of food to Biafrans, they reacted against the Red Cross policy of " neutrality" and its reserve about protesting such a violation of human rights. This impelled them to create a new association combining medical humanitarian and human rights witnessing action.[17] At first it was called the Organisation pour la lutte contre le génocide au Biafra (Organization for the Fight Against Genocide in Biafra). One year later, it was renamed the Groupe d'intervention médicale et chururgicale en urgence (GIMCU—Emergency Medical and Surgical Intervention Group). The formation of this group, Emmanuelli pointed out, coincided with an early stage of the development of the field of emergency medicine.

During this same period, a cyclone hit East Pakistan,[18] leaving severe flooding and some 500,000 victims in its wake. This was the "second episode that caused us to get together again," Emmanuelli, Grelety-Bosviel, and Récamier continued. Along with some of his colleagues, Raymond Borel, who was then the editor of *Tonus*—"the medical journal that every physician in France received at that time"—founded an aid organization called Secours Médical Français (SMF—French Medical Relief), under whose aegis some French physicians went to East Pakistan to assist the distressed population. The members of GIMCU and of SMF decided that it made sense for them to merge their two groups into one association. But before they did so a name for it had to be chosen. Call it what you will, Borel said, but it must have *médecins* in its name.

The idea of "frontiers" emerged, not only with regard to geography, but also in reference to groups who were "isolated" by society, like women and homosexuals. It had some relationship as well to the willingness of these physicians to "leave their homes, go far, and incur danger."

The "anagram MSF" evolved from SMF—the acronym for Sécours Médical Français—and Médecins Sans Frontières became the agreed-upon name. At the beginning, they said, "we made our team available to other groups that did not have medical training. We added a medical touch to what other [humanitarian] organizations were doing." Among "the slogans that we used to launch the idea of MSF" were: "Finding ourselves going toward others"; "We dare to go where others do not go"; and "Two billion people in their waiting room."[19]

"We all had this humanitarian streak in us," they declared. We could not let two million deaths happen in Biafra, among them children who were starving and dying. "We were also boy scouts who disregarded orders" and insisted on our "independence from government. We focused on getting out of government claws."

The three men took turns describing how, lubricated by Scotch whiskey, they argued about "burning issues" until four in the morning—including the issue of *témoignage*—"bearing witness"—and whether or not they had the right, and beyond that the duty, to contravene Red Cross policy by speaking out about human rights abuses they saw in the field.

Talking about the intensity of their youthful arguments and "flying debates" led them to recount—with some regret in their voices—the bitter 1979 dispute within MSF that resulted in an irremediable internal split: the exodus of a group of members, led by Bernard Kouchner, from MSF, and their creation in 1980 of another medical humanitarian organization—Médecins du Monde (Doctors of the World). Precipitating the split was the "boat for Vietnam" project initiated by a group of illustrious French intellectuals, which was vigorously supported by Kouchner, the first president of MSF and the most famous of its founder-physicians. The project involved chartering a ship to help evacuate Vietnamese refugees who were fleeing the ravages of the war taking place between North and South Vietnam. The plan entailed fitting it out like a hospital ship, the participation of physicians to deliver medical care to the Vietnamese "boat people," and the presence of journalists to publicize the violation of human rights under the Vietnamese Communist regime. Inside MSF there was a confrontation between persons who belonged to two "different schools of thought": on the one hand, stood those who were more "technician/mission-oriented" and, on the other, those, led by Kouchner, who were "more media-driven." "We were young. We were passionate," Grelety-Bosviel and Recamier exclaimed. "We were brothers. We came from the same family. We came from the same culture. But we could not get over this divide." In retrospect, they intimated, "Kouchner's boat" might have had its "advantages." It showed a "symbolic presence," and even if it generated conflict within MSF, it was a "model" that was "taken up" later by other organizations. Emmanuelli did not join them in expressing these sentiments. (I knew that as vice president of

MSF during the "boat for Vietnam" episode, Emmanueli's confrontation with Kouchner had been especially bitter, and had included publishing a severely critical article about Kouchner and his relationship to the boat project).[20]

The physician-founders ended their presentation with an emotional affirmation: "We had a vocation," they said. "People can dream when they are young men and women who are willing to leave their homes, stand up for their dreams, and die for them." They paused here to refer to the list of members of MSF who had died in the field, posted on a wall in the meeting.

"We were privileged to give birth to a legend of which we are a part," they concluded. There was a moment of silence, and then the entire audience rose to give them a standing ovation that went on and on.

The 1980s

The chief spokespersons for the 1980s were Rony Brauman, an early member of MSF, president of MSF France from 1982 to 1994, and Philippe Laurent, a founder of MSF Belgium in 1980, and its first director. Brauman started by paying tribute to "the grandfathers" of MSF, and proceeded to tell an anecdote about the first time he met Xavier Emmanuelli. As a long-haired young "leftist," Brauman had arrived at the office of MSF in Paris with the desire to be sent into the field on a mission—even to a place where "the bullets were flying." But Emmanuelli refused him an assignment, and for a while after that, Brauman "did not want to have anything to do with MSF." However, he continued, he returned to the MSF office several years later—"with shorter hair." Emmanuelli did not recognize him, and this time he was sent on a mission.

Philippe Laurent took up the narration from there to describe the beginnings of MSF Belgium, the first section of MSF established after the founding of the organization in France. It was started by a group of Belgian physicians, he related, who wanted to utilize their training in tropical medicine at the Institute of Tropical Medicine in Antwerp in a place where it was needed. ("That's what we were driven to do.") They had difficulty in finding an organization that would send them into the field until they made contact with MSF in 1989. Laurent reminisced about meeting with members of MSF in their "crummy" Paris office. Notwithstanding the physical surroundings, he said, "there was chemistry" in that meeting. . . . When we went through the door, it felt like home. . . . This is what we were looking for." Several of them joined members of MSF on a field mission, and "the experience that we had was great." "Why don't we do it in Belgium?" they enthusiastically asked upon their return. But when they proposed the idea of creating a branch of MSF in Belgium, "the French said, 'No.'" We can't find enough doctors for MSF in France, they declared. It is even more doubtful that you could do so in Belgium.

At this juncture, Brauman and Laurent exchanged recollections of MSF France's opposition to the idea of an MSF Belgium, or to the creation of any other sections of MSF. "We were not happy about MSF Belgium," Brauman frankly admitted. "They started criticizing us," he continued. "I was absolutely convinced that there was a horrible Belgian plot to dominate us," he jokingly added.

A founding member of the Spanish section of MSF joined the discussion to say they had had a comparable experience with MSF France. In Spain, as in Belgium, young people with "dreams and courage" comparable to those of MSF's French physician-founders, were "driven by the idea" of creating an MSF Spain. MSF France did not think that this was a good idea because, in their view, it would strengthen MSF Belgium's "notion of the autonomy of sections." Nevertheless, he stated with satisfaction, in spite of these "internal conflicts, MSF Spain happened anyway."

The 1980s had been "benchmarked" by "fights" (*bagarres*) between the sections that were successively created (Belgium and Switzerland in 1980, Holland in 1984, and Luxembourg and Spain in 1986). There was general agreement that such episodes were now behind us.

Disagreement erupted when someone (identified by Rony Brauman as "Jacques") rose to say that what was "a failure" was that "we have never been able to work out in the field how to 'de-nationalize' MSF"—for example, to demonstrate that when MSF France is in the field in a former colony, like the Côte d'Ivoire, it has nothing to do with France. "The attachment of sections to home countries is a mistake," he declared. Brauman immediately retorted:

> I am going to reactivate an MSF tradition [by saying that] I don't agree with what Jacques said. I'm not for nationalism, but you cannot erase reality. We are doctors with passports, who intervene to act in the world. Everyone comes with a country, a region. Despite our beautiful name, I don't think that a world "without borders" is [likely] to be a happy utopia.

"I will end here in order not to prolong the dispute," Brauman said with good humor, closing the 1980s panel.

The 1990s and the 2000s

The panel on the 1990s highlighted the awarding of the Nobel Prize for Peace to MSF in 1999. Because of MSF's conception of participatory democracy, and the tensions that existed between its sections, it took three months to write the acceptance speech, the panel revealed, and its final draft had not been ready until the very day of the ceremony.[21]

One of the panelists ventured that there was a sense in which the 1990s had been "all about [MSF's] inner tensions." That decade had seen many new MSF sections,[22] but there had been resistance to them in virtually every instance. What was more, he said, although personnel from different sections had collaborated when they were in the field together—for example, during the 1990s when MSF France, Belgium, and Holland had jointly responded to a catastrophic flood in the People's Republic of China—upon their return from the field, it "all started up again," with MSF France emphasizing the importance of supporting field hospitals, MSF Belgium, the importance of witnessing via the media, and MSF Holland, the further development and increased use of kits of medical supplies that could be stored easily in a central warehouse and quickly transported into the field.

The discussion of the 1990s ended on a positive note, with remarks typical of MSF:

Without disputes, there would be no innovation.
One of the strengths of our association is that we are willing to discuss
    our mistakes and our failures with one another.
We should be proud that everything works much better on the
    international level now. But, of course, we should continue to be
    critical.

Reflection on MSF's fourth decade, the 2000s, was relatively brief. It included a critical and self-ridiculing reference to the dominance of "expatriate," largely western European MSF staff over "national" staff who live in the countries where MSF is in the field—even though "nationals" occupy a large majority of MSF field positions, and do a great deal of the work.[23] A comic imaginary incident was recounted that depicted "expatriates" being observed by "nationals." The "expatriates" are portrayed absorbed in nonfunctional activities, such as "rearranging offices" with successive MSF groups as they arrive on the scene. "In the corridors," the amused "nationals" watching them decide to "forgive the expats," because they were "trying to find something to do, and there was *nothing* for them to do." This scenario evoked the heartiest laughter of the day.[24]

Day Three: Election of Members to the New International Board

The third and final day of the meeting began with a short question-and-answer session about the election of the new International Board members, scheduled for that morning. Thirteen members of MSF had previously presented themselves as candidates. Their profiles, CV's, application letters, and photographs had been made available throughout MSF on its website. (It is noteworthy that with the exception of one from the United States and one from New Zealand, all the candidates were western Europeans—Austrian, British, Dutch, French, German, and Norwegian; and only two of them were women.) Six members were to be elected to the board, for staggered terms of three-and-a-half, two-and-a-half, and one-and-a-half years—which would bring its total membership to twelve persons. The voting instructions stated that out of these six, "two at least shall be medical, to meet the quota of [having] two-thirds [of the board] members with medical backgrounds."[25]

At the end of the morning, while the scheduled "Vision Feedback" sessions were in progress, MSF members turned in their ballots for the International Board candidates. At the end of the morning, the names of the six who had been elected to the board were announced to the assembly—rank-ordered by the votes each had received. Number one was Morten Rostrup, a Norwegian physician, who was currently working part-time at the Oslo University Hospital in emergency and intensive care. He joined MSF in 1996, became the founding president of MSF Norway in that same year, subsequently served as international vice president of MSF, and in 2000 was elected MSF's international president for a four-year term. During his fifteen-year-long affiliation with MSF, he had been on many field missions in Africa, the Americas, Asia, Europe, and the Middle East—some of which were long-term in nature, and others, short-term emergency undertakings.

Ranked sixth among those elected to the Board was the only woman elected to the new board, Clair Mills, a New Zealand physician, currently working as a public-health doctor in the far north of her country and teaching and doing research on health inequalities at the University of Auckland. After previous stints as a field doctor and a medical coordinator for MSF in southern Sudan, western Congo, Somalia, and Sri Lanka, and subsequently with the World Health Organization and with Save the Children, she returned to MSF to take up the position of medical director of its operations center in Amsterdam for four years (2004–2008). At the end of 2010, she joined a short-term MSF mission in Papua, New Guinea, to combat a cholera outbreak.

In rank-order, the other four persons who were elected to the International Board were: number two, Darin Portnoy, a U.S. physician; number three, Colin McIlreavy, an Irish engineer; number four, Michalis Fotiadis, a Greek logistician; and number five, Jean-Marie Kindermans, a French-Belgian physician. Like Morten Rostrup and Clair Miles, they all had in common many years of association with MSF—fourteen, thirteen, seventeen, and thirty years, respectively—and wide-ranging field experience on multiple MSF missions in an array of world areas. In a number of cases, they had returned to MSF after an interlude of working with other humanitarian agencies—among them, the European Association for Development and Health, Human Rights Watch, and the GOAL development organization in Sudan, Kenya, and Tanzania, as well as Save the Children, and the World Health Organization—bringing value-added experience gained in those contexts to MSF. Within MSF, all the newly elected International Board members had held numerous positions of responsibility—including as project and medical coordinators, heads of missions, medical directors, presidents of MSF sections, members of the boards of multiple sections, and in international posts that included president and vice president of the International Council, secretary-general of the International Office, International Association coordinator, and the organization's so-called flying coordinator in the Middle East, eastern Europe, Central America, and Africa. In addition, several of them had been key participants in MSF's processes of internal reform.[26]

Afterward

Eleven days after the meeting, MSF issued the following press release:

Mogadishu/Nairobi/Brussels, December 29, 2011

It is with great sadness that Médecins Sans Frontières (MSF) confirms that two staff members were killed this morning as a result of a shooting in the organization's compound in Mogadishu [Somalia]. . . .

The victims are Belgian and Indonesian nationals. Philippe Havet, a 53-year-old from Belgium, was an experienced emergency coordinator who had been working with MSF since 2000 in many countries, including Angola, the Democratic Republic of Congo, Indonesia, Lebanon, Sierra Leone, South Africa, and Somalia. Andrias Karel Keiluhu, better known as "Kace," was a 44-year-old medical doctor who had worked with MSF in his native Indonesia, as well as in Ethiopia, Thailand, and Somalia. . . . Philippe and Kace were in Mogadishu working with the MSF teams to provide emergency medical assistance to displaced persons and residents of the city.

We are deeply shocked by this tragic event and we will greatly miss Philippe and Kace. We extend our heartfelt sympathy and condolences to their families and friends.

MSF has been working in Somalia continuously since 1991 and currently operates 13 projects in the country, including medical activities related to the ongoing emergency, vaccination campaigns, as well as nutrition interventions. MSF also assists Somali refugees in camps in Dadaab, Kenya, and Dolo Ado, Ethiopia.[27]

On January 19, 2012, another MSF press release was published, this time announcing that MSF "sees itself forced to end all activities" in the Hodan district of Mogadishu, the Somali capital, "including the closure of two separate 120-bed medical facilities for the treatment of malnutrition, measles and cholera." "The closure of activities in this district halves the assistance MSF is providing in Mogadishu," the article went on to say. However, "for now, MSF projects will continue to provide medical care in the other districts of the capital as well as in 10 locations in the rest of Somalia." Christopher Stokes, general director of MSF Belgium, was quoted as saying, "It is hard to close health services in a location where the presence of our medical teams is genuinely lifesaving every day, but the brutal assassination of our colleagues in Hodan makes it impossible for us to continue working in the district of Mogadishu."[28] The press release ended with an appeal for the release of the two MSF staff members kidnapped while caring for Somali refugees in Kenya, about whom Unni Karunakara had expressed concern in his opening remarks to MSF's Paris meeting.

Closing Reflections

Attending this both backward-looking and forward-looking meeting constituted my last interlude of field research inside MSF. As someone who has been
observing MSF for many years, what struck me most about it was the extent to
which the issues around which it was oriented were ones with which MSF has
grappled throughout its history. Predominant among them: collective struggles to continue to be a humanitarian movement that realizes its foundational
moral principles through its "in-the-field" medical and witnessing action,
and its efforts to embody its "sans frontières"/"without borders" worldview
more fully by becoming more internally as well as externally international
and transnational. In the name of achieving these goals—particularly that
of transcending the persistent national "borders" between its sections and
its operational centers—the 2011 Paris meeting inaugurated reforms in MSF's
governance structure intended to further this process. In the light of MSF's
ideal conception of itself as a nonbureaucratic "association" of persons with
a common purpose, in which equality and participatory democracy prevail,
and "institutionalization" is held in check, there is an element of paradox in
MSF's recurrent recourse to elaborating its organizational structures. A number
of participants were aware of how such an investment in the reform of MSF's
structure might be inconsistent with its self-image as a "movement" rather
than "just an organization." In this connection, sporadic complaints were
voiced about how many "layers" and "bureaucratic hurdles" already existed
in MSF, and how complicated and hard to comprehend its structures were.

Within this overarching framework, the meeting centered on an array of
issues that MSF has repeatedly confronted and vigorously debated over the
years. These included questions regarding MSF's medical and witnessing action, their relationship to each other, their place in the movement's history
and ethos, and what their optimal attributes ought to be. On the one hand,
there was consensus about the paramountcy of MSF's medical action, while
on the other, there was agreement that it should neither eclipse nor subvert its
human rights witnessing. Great concern was expressed over any diminution
of MSF's "speaking out" in revelatory protest about the suffering and abuses
to which the people they were assisting were subject. This restraint was attributed in part to the reluctance of MSF personnel to jeopardize conditions
negotiated with the countries where they had missions, which enabled them
to be present and deliver medical care in a way that was in keeping with their

scientific and clinical standards, and with the moral principles enunciated in MSF's Charter.

In turn, these aspects of the discussions at the Paris meeting opened onto the consideration of another set of questions with which MSF has been constantly preoccupied: What kinds of "compromises" ought and ought not to be made to stay in the field? When, in the face of what conditions, should MSF exit from an area or country where it is embedded and engaged in committed work? And although MSF's Charter states that MSF workers should be "aware of the risks and dangers of the missions they undertake," when do these become so great that an organizational decision to leave the field is both necessary and justified? As I prepared to leave the meeting, I wondered how many more anniversaries MSF would celebrate, and how the global problems it has addressed would change over time. The medical and moral issues MSF has faced throughout its history are intrinsic to humanitarian action, and transcending national "borders" takes generations to achieve. So it seems likely that as long as MSF exists, it will be dealing with the questions around which the 2011 Paris meeting was structured.

What about MSF's determination to continually rekindle its spirit as a movement and avoid overinstitutionalization? Max Weber provided social scientists with a classical set of concepts that delineate the progressive routinization and structuration a charismatic movement can be expected to undergo as it evolves into a stable, enduring organization.[29] But Weber's paradigm can't predict how long MSF the organization can preserve the ethos of MSF the movement.

As I walked out of the conference center, I paused to look again at the many names of MSF members who had been killed in the field. In keeping with MSF's "anti-heroic heroism," its members would not want me to dwell on those deaths. Nor would they want me to exaggerate how I felt as I took leave of them, or to magnify what accompanying them through my research has meant to me.

Acknowledgments

At its inception, my sociological quest to know and understand Doctors Without Borders / Médecins Sans Frontières (MSF), out of which this book grew, was given intellectual and moral impetus by three inspiring individuals: Willy De Craemer, Jonathan Mann, and Ernest Drucker. Albeit in differing ways, each of them had been involved in firsthand humanitarian action to which he was strongly committed, while remaining keenly aware of the dilemmas it posed, its limitations and imperfections, and the unintended harm it could cause.

Willy De Craemer, a fellow sociologist and a Jesuit priest, was the one with whom I had the closest professional and personal relationship. In a missionary capacity, he had been a teacher and the director of a center for sociological research in Congo/Zaïre, where he initiated me into the social and cultural worlds of Africa south of the Sahara, and of the Catholic Church–affiliated personnel who worked there.[1]

Jonathan Mann was a physician, renowned for having uncovered the existence of an epidemic of HIV/AIDS in sub-Saharan Africa (from a base in Zaïre), for his international battle (as first director of WHO's AIDS program) against the pandemic it became, and as a leading figure in linking AIDS and global health with social problems and human rights issues. He was also a founder of the American branch of Doctors of the World (the humanitarian organization that resulted from a schism in Doctors Without Borders).[2] We became acquainted through these links, our respective publications, and our Harvard connections. (After his term with WHO he returned to the Harvard School of

---

1. I have written extensively about Willy De Craemer's background, professional career, my relationship to him, and my years of research and teaching in Congo/Zaïre (now the Democratic Republic of Congo) in my autobiography, Renée C. Fox, *In the Field: A Sociologist's Journey* (New Brunswick, NJ: Transaction Publishers, 2010).

2. For more details about this schism and the foundation of Médecins du Monde / Doctors of the World, see chap. 2 of this book.

Public Health, where he was director of the International AIDS Center, and of the Bagnoud Center for Health and Human Rights.)

For twenty-five years, the psychologist Ernest Drucker was director of Public Health and Policy Research at the Albert Einstein College of Medicine's Montefiore Medical Center in New York City. Throughout his career his policy- and human-rights-oriented research, conducted in Africa as well as the United States, has centered on drug addiction, the reduction of drug-related harm, and the relationship between drugs, crime, HIV/AIDS, and "mass incarceration" (which he regards as an epidemiological, plaguelike phenomenon.)[3] In the first phase of my research when I was considering making a comparative study of Doctors Without Borders and Doctors of the World, it was Drucker, at that time a member of the board of Doctors of the World, USA, who arranged for me to become a participant observer in its New York City office.

Willy De Craemer died from complications of Parkinson's Disease in 2005. Jonathan Mann perished in 1998 in a Swissair crash, en route to Geneva to participate in global strategy sessions on HIV/AIDS, sponsored by WHO and the UN. Ernest Drucker, an emeritus professor, is still involved in humanitarian action and advocacy. I shall always be thankful to each of them for encouraging and aiding me to undertake a study of MSF, and for infusing it with added meaning through their example.

I am profoundly grateful to the members of MSF for the unreserved access they gave me to their lived experiences within their organization/movement—including to their questions and disputes about the humanitarian action in which they are ardently engaged. They are likely to say there was nothing exceptional about what they willingly shared with me—that it was in keeping with MSF's culture, its commitment to transparency and critical self-examination, and its conviction that "ideas matter for action." Nevertheless, I hope this book will demonstrate to readers how remarkable, and in many ways admirable, these attributes of MSF's culture are, as well as how vital to the research I was able to conduct.

I am especially grateful to members of MSF who have been important teachers, exemplars, providers of key information and documents, and sources of

3. I was introduced to Ernest Drucker by Robert Klitzman, who is presently a professor of clinical psychiatry at the College of Physicians and Surgeons, and in the Mailman School of Public Health at Columbia University, and director of the Master of Science in Bioethics Program in Columbia's School of Continuing Education. Klitzman has extensively studied and written about ethical, social, and psychological issues in medicine and psychiatry.

emotional and moral support. They include Eric Goemaere, James Orbinski, Jean-Marie Kindermans, Alex Parisel, Jean-Hervé Bradol, Ulrike von Pilar, Unni Karunakara, Nicolas de Torrente, Revka Papadopoulou, Sharon Ekambaram, Hedwige Jeanmart, Alexei Nikiforov, Andrei Slavuckij, Kenneth Tong, Stephanie Short, Fiona Terry, Rony Brauman and, through the medium of his brilliant cartoons, Samuel Hanryon ("Brax"). The parts that some of these persons have played in MSF are chronicled in the body of the book.

In addition, along with other MSFers, some of these individuals performed crucial roles in reading, commenting on, and when necessary correcting, the contents of the book's chapters. All of its chapters underwent this kind of scrutiny and review by the principal persons who appear in or are relevant to them.

In a number of ways writing this book has been a collective process. Throughout its course, I have not only been surrounded by members of MSF, but by a bevy of friends and colleagues, and also some of my former students, who were indefatigably interested in the book, and in how it was progressing. Among them were Peggy Anderson, Isabelle Baszanger, the late Robert Bellah, Evelyn and Solomon Benatar, Harold Bershady, Judith Brown, Pamela Bump, Nicholas Christakis, Anne Fadiman, Tovia and William Freedman, Gail and Allen Glicksman, Mark Gould, Jonathan Imber, Jan Jaeger, Carole Joffe, Robert Klitzman, Gail Kotel, Victor Lidz, Kenneth Ludmerer, Mary Ann Meyers, Keith Robinson, Olga Shevchenko, Neville Strumpf, Judith Swazey, Emiko Ohnuki-Tierney, Jan Vansina, Lydwine Verhaegen, Renée Waissman, and Yves Winkin.

Several persons in this local, national, and international entourage carried out tasks that were indispensable to the development and production of the book. Foremost among them was Olga Shevchenko, who coauthored the chapters that deal with MSF's missions in Russia, and who played a capital part in collecting and analyzing the field data on which they are based. Nicholas Christakis helped me to comprehend the cultural meaning of the existence of a section of MSF in Greece and to conduct interviews in Athens with members of its staff. He also enabled me to climb the hill to the Acropolis, from whose panoramic summit I contemplated the import of Greece's ancient history. Judith Swazey, my companion in much of the medical sociological research that I have conducted since we first met in 1967, made several journeys into the field with me: to MSF's "La Mancha" meeting in Luxembourg, to its fortieth anniversary meeting in Paris, and, once, to its HIV/AIDS program in Cape Town, South Africa. She brought the astute observations that she made in those settings, along with her usual combination of intelligence, candor, and kindness to her reading of the penultimate drafts of most of the book's chapters. In addition, her "wordsmithing" helped me to craft the book's title. And notwithstanding the arduousness of checking the book's references and bibliography, obtaining permissions for the inclusion of certain materials in it, proofreading its text, and constructing its index, Judith Watkins was enthusiastically insistent about taking on these assignments, to which she unrelentingly applied her consummate skills as an information specialist.

Dr. Natalia Nikolayevna Vezhnina does not fit neatly into any of the foregoing groups of persons to whom I am indebted; but in common with them, she made an essential contribution to the book. She is a Russian physician who is a central figure in the chapter on MSF's tuberculosis project in the prison colonies of Siberia. The detailed oral history of the project and of her relationship to it that she generously and courageously related to Olga Shevchenko and me was indispensable to writing that chapter.

This book had a master editor—Jack Beatty. He had been described to me by those who knew him as a highly "admired editor," who was very "smart," "talented," "well-informed," "sophisticated," and "deep." He brought all these qualities to bear on the editing of my book, along with personal warmth, gusto, and vigorous, forthright opinions about my writing that were also flexible and open-minded. I had been told that he had only one "imperfection": his notoriously "terrible handwriting." This proved to be true. But I did not have much trouble reading the valuable notes that he scrawled all over the pages of my manuscript.

I would be remiss if I failed to mention that my author-editor relationship with Jack Beatty was made possible by another outstanding editor—William Whitworth—whom Beatty considers his mentor, and on whose staff Beatty worked as a senior editor during Whitworth's distinguished tenure as editor-in-chief of the *Atlantic Monthly*.[4] Whitworth edited my autobiography. He was the first editor, and the only editor—other than copy editors—I ever had for the books I previously published.[5] He was not free to undertake the editing of this book, he told me when I consulted him about it; but he recommended

4. Whitworth, currently editor emeritus of the *Atlantic*, was its editor-in-chief from 1981 to 2001. Prior to that, beginning in 1966, he was a member of the staff of the *New Yorker*, first as a writer and then as associate editor.

5. On this experience, see Renée C. Fox, "'Dear Mr. Whitworth/Dear Professor Fox': Ode to an Editor and to Editing," *Society* 48, no. 2 (March–April 2011): 102–111.

a short list of alternative editors to me. At the top of that list was Jack Beatty, whom he contacted on my behalf, and with whom he said he would "put [me] in touch when the end of [my] book was in sight"—which he did. I am sure that having William Whitworth as my intermediary was a determining factor in Jack Beatty's assenting to become the editor of this book. And so it is to both of them that I express my appreciation for this good fortune.

The sorts of contributions that two other persons made to writing this book and readying it for publication should not be underestimated. Initially, I was overwhelmed by the volume of field data and documents about MSF that I had amassed during the years of my research. How to organize them in a way that would make it easier to find the material I needed at specific points in the writing process was a daunting challenge. It was Yizhar Gilady, a personal assistant, who helped me create a set of files that enabled me to do this, to consolidate the books in my library that had bearing on MSF in particular and humanitarian action more generally, and to locate the files and books together in a small room in my apartment designated for them. The results of his efforts were so impressive that I felt it entirely appropriate to affix a special sign to the door of that room reading: *Archives.*

Jeff Katz, an information technology (IT) specialist, did more than keep my computer in working order as I typed the pages of this book, communicated via e-mail with MSF informants and respondents, and searched on the Internet for additional data and to fact-check some of the data I already had. He also set up a system on my computer to file and safeguard the unfolding chapters of the manuscript and to store the photos and cartoons I had collected as potential illustrations for the book. He accompanied these tasks with supportive therapy for an anxiety-ridden, marginally competent computer user like myself, who has little understanding of how computers work. And at one crisis-ridden juncture he rescued me, psychologically as well as technically, from a computer crash that had imperiled the entire manuscript of the book.

Kenneth Ludmerer took the initiative of informing Jacqueline Wehmueller, executive editor at Johns Hopkins University Press, that this book was in an advanced stage of being written, and suggested to her that it might be of interest to the Press. She, in turn, contacted me, and with alacrity set the process in motion that eventuated in the book being accepted for publication by the Press. In a continuous, hands-on way, she accompanied the book and me throughout all the stages of its being reviewed and readied for publication— bringing to the manuscript meticulous, astute attention to detail, her literary craftsmanship and artistic sense of design, and, most important, her deep understanding of its wellsprings. Working with her, and with senior editorial assistant Sara Cleary, was one of the most gratifying publishing experiences I have ever had.

I am indebted to all these persons for whatever merits this book may possess. I hope that it will be judged to be a worthy portrayal of MSF, and of the medical humanitarian care and assistance that, in the words of its Charter, MSF provides to people "in distress, to victims of natural or manmade disasters and to victims of armed conflict . . . irrespective of race, religion, creed or political convictions."

NOTES

Unless otherwise stated, all translations from the French in the text and notes are by Renée C. Fox.

THE QUESTS: An Introduction

1. "History & Principles—Doctors Without Borders," www.doctorswithoutborders .org/aboutus/2012 (accessed 12/21/2012). Doctors Without Borders/Médecins Sans Frontières is usually referred to throughout this book by its acronym MSF or, where appropriate, by the abbreviated name of a section—e.g., MSF France; MSF USA, etc.

2. Over the course of the many years during which my study of MSF took place, the research was funded by relatively small grants from the Acadia Institute, the Social Sciences Research Fund associated with the Honorable Walter H. Annenberg Chair in the Social Sciences at the University of Pennsylvania, the Andrew W. Mellon Foundation, and the Nuffield Foundation (in the United Kingdom).

3. For a detailed narrative account of some of my research in Belgium, the Congo, and France, and what it involved ethnographically, see Renée C. Fox, *In the Belgian Château: The Spirit and Culture of a European Society in an Age of Change* (Chicago: Ivan R. Dee, 1994). See also Fox, *In the Field: A Sociologist's Journey* (New Brunswick, NJ: Transaction Publishers, 2011), 135–200.

4. See chaps. 7 and 8, which are based on this field research.

5. See Renée C. Fox, "Exploring the Moral and Spiritual Dimensions of Society and Medicine," in Carla M. Messikomer, Judith P. Swazey, and Allen Glicksman, eds., *Society and Medicine: Essays in Honor of Renée C. Fox* (New Brunswick, NJ: Transaction Books, 2003), 257–271, at 268; Fox, *In the Field*, 367.

6. Jonathan Sacks, *The Great Partnership: God, Science and the Search for Meaning* (London: Hodder & Stoughton, 2011), 237, 248. Chapter 12 of Rabbi Sacks's book reflects on "the problem of evil" and the questions of meaning it poses; the quoted words were not intended by Sacks to refer to MSF, but they nevertheless aptly and eloquently articulate key characteristics of its worldview.

7. In the early, exploratory phase of my research, my intention was to study MSF within a framework that would enable me to view it in relation to Doctors of the World (Médecins du Monde), another international medical humanitarian organization of French origin, which was established in 1980 as a consequence of a split within MSF between members of its founding and next generations (for a detailed account of the genesis, dynamics, and consequences of this split, see chap. 2). After doing a significant amount of participant observation in the New York office of Doctors of the World,

conducting face-to-face interviews with members of Médecins du Monde in Paris, and a field trip to visit the organization's program with homeless children in Saint Petersburg, Russia, I decided that even if I made Doctors of the World a comparative case secondary to MSF, I would be undertaking more than I could realistically handle. Nevertheless, the research that I did on Doctors of the World illuminated not only certain aspects of MSF's history but also some of its characteristics.

8. The anthropologist Clifford Geertz first applied the philosopher Gilbert Ryle's concept of "thick description" to what Geertz regarded as the defining characteristics of "doing ethnography"—to the kinds of cultural data that are gathered, and how they are inscribed, analyzed, and interpreted by social scientists conducting ethnographic research. See Clifford Geertz, "Thick Description: Toward an Interpretive Theory of Culture," in *The Interpretation of Cultures: Selected Essays by Clifford Geertz* (New York: Basic Books, 1973), 3–30.

9. See chaps. 4, 5, 10, and 11. In Greece, I was assisted in this field research by Nicholas Christakis, and in Russia, by Olga Shevchenko, both of whom are U.S.-based sociologists. Christakis (who is also a physician) has Greek origins, and Shevchenko, Russian ones. I had the privilege of teaching each of them when they were studying for their PhDs in sociology at the University of Pennsylvania.

10. This was the case, for example, with regard to my efforts to obtain charts or diagrams of MSF's evolving organizational structure and to identify and enter into communication with the webmaster for the "blogs from the field" that I analyze in chap. 1, and with the member of MSF who drew the cartoons at its "La Mancha" meeting that I describe in chap. 6. I finally did succeed in obtaining this information and making these contacts thanks to the help of Unni Karunakara, the international president of MSF, Hélène Ponpon, Karunakara's assistant in MSF's International Office in Geneva, the offices of MSF Holland in Amsterdam and MSF UK in London, and Kenneth M. Tong, manager of Online/International Media in MSF Canada's Toronto office.

11. "A Vision for MSF: Statement of Ambitions for 2012–2021" (MSF internal document, April 2012), 1, 3.

12. Within the theoretical framework of the eminent sociologist Max Weber, such organizational developments would be seen as concomitants of the process whereby "charisma" is stabilized and institutionalized into ongoing authority structures. According to Weber, if a social organization is to survive and continue to function, some form of "routinization" of its original charismatic authority must take place. In the case of MSF, this appears to have entailed some movement in the direction of the development of what Weber would have termed a more "rational-legal authority" structure. See Weber, "The Types of Authority and Imperative Coordination," pt. 3 of *Max Weber: The Theory of Social and Economic Organization*, trans. A. M. Henderson and Talcott Parsons (New York: Oxford University Press, 1947), 324–407.

13. "Vision for MSF," 1.

14. Craig Calhoun, "The Idea of Emergency: Humanitarianism and Global (Dis) Order," in Didier Fassin and Mariella Pandolfi, eds., *Contemporary States of Emergency: The Politics of Military and Humanitarian Intervention* (New York: Zone Books, 2010), 29–58, at 54–55.

15. The phrase "global and multicultural" comes from a speech delivered by the late president of the Czech Republic Václav Havel on the occasion of his receiving the

Liberty Medal at Independence Hall in Philadelphia on July 4, 1994. "Politicians are rightly worried by the problem of finding the key to insure the survival of a civilization that is global and multicultural," he said in the course of his speech. "The central political task of the final years of this century is the creation of a new model of coexistence among the various cultures, peoples, races and religious spheres, within a single interconnected civilization."

16. Antonio Donini, "Humanitarianism, Perceptions, Power," in Caroline Abu-Sada, ed., *In the Eyes of Others: How People in Crises Perceive Humanitarian Aid* (New York: MSF, Humanitarian Outcomes, and the NYU Center on International Cooperation, 2012), 183–192, at 191, www.doctorswithoutborders.org/publications/book/perceptions/?id= 5945&cat=perceptions.

17. "Every night when I go to bed, I worry about how I'll fulfill all the promises I've made. And every morning when I wake up, I think I haven't made enough promises," the physician and anthropologist Paul Farmer says of the medical humanitarian work in which he is engaged in association with Partners in Health, an organization he cofounded (https://donate.pih.org/page/contribute/donate).

18. For very thoughtful and richly documented analyses of these dilemmas of humanitarian action, see, e.g., Fiona Terry, *Condemned to Repeat? The Paradox of Humanitarian Action* (Ithaca, NY: Cornell University Press, 2002), and David Kennedy, *The Dark Sides of Virtue: Reassessing International Humanitarianism* (Princeton, NJ: Princeton University Press, 2004).

19. James Orbinski, *An Imperfect Offering: Humanitarian Action in the Twenty-First Century* (Toronto: Doubleday Canada, 2008).

20. "MSF's primary mandate is to bring emergency medical assistance to populations in need. To reach those who need our help the most, we often work in conflict and postconflict regions. Each region involves different risks according to the context in which our humanitarian intervention takes place. . . . Field workers must abide by security rules and procedures throughout their mission. There is a clear chain of responsibility regarding security management" (www.msf.org.uk/working-overseas-safety-and-security).

21. Kenny Gluck, "Of Measles, Stalin and Other Risks—Reflections on Our Principles, Témoignage, and Security," in *My Sweet La Mancha: Invited and Voluntary Contributions* (internal MSF document, published in 2005, "within the framework of the La Mancha process launched in 2005," which was "not meant for diffusion or use outside of MSF").

22. In MSF parlance, "national" staff members are indigenous to the countries where MSF projects are located and "expatriate" staff are involved in projects located outside their countries of residence.

23. Samuel Hanryon, a member of the Communications Department of MSF France, drew this cartoon, using the nom de plume Brax.

24. The lyrics of the song "The Impossible Dream" were written by Joe Darion. The composer of the music for it was Mitch Leigh.

CHAPTER ONE: Voices from the Field

1. Prinitha Pillay, "A South African Doctor in Darfur," May 5, 2008, MSF field blog entry "I'm struggling to close the chapter," http://blogs.msf.org/Prinitha.

2. Kenneth Tong, e-mail to the author, September 19, 2012. Tong said he based his opinion that "prohibiting things never works" on what "we know . . . from alcohol

prohibition," "promoting safer sex practices," and "harm reduction programs for responsible drug use."

3. Ibid. The primary language in which these blogs are written and recorded is English, but translations of them into other languages, including French, Dutch, German, Russian, Spanish, and Swedish, are also available online. I am indebted to Kenneth Tong, with whom I conducted telephone interviews on June 15 and on September 7, 2012, for providing me with the information about the history of the development of the MSF field blogs in this chapter, and for printed spreadsheet data that he sent me on the bloggers' countries of origin, the "mission countries" from which they wrote their blogs, and the status roles they occupied in the field.

4. Kenneth Tong, e-mail to the author, September 4, 2012.

5. South America is strikingly absent from this list.

6. Trish Newport, "Brown bread revolutionary: Community outreach and nutrition," January 16, 2011, MSF field blog entry "Right to be here," http://blogs.msf.org/trishn/2011/01/16. Bashir and Zara were children suffering from severe malnutrition in the midst of a widespread malnutrition crisis that was occurring in Niger at the time that this blog was written. Trish Newport, who wrote this blog, was a community outreach nurse who was supervising the nutritional survey of the region that MSF was making.

7. Nazanin Meshkat, "Off the beaten path . . . PNG (Papua New Guinea)," October 1, 2007, MSF field blog entry "Writer's Fork," http://blogs.msf.org/NazaninM/2007/10/01.

8. Lauralee Morris, "Lauralee in Lankien," May 25, 2008, MSF field blog entry "Blogging as Insurance Against 'New Fridge Syndrome,'" http://blogs.msf.org/LauraleeM/2008/05/25.

9. Chantelle Assenheimer, "Honeymoon in Chad," November 30, 2010, MSF field blog entry "Dear Diary," November 30, 2010. http://blogs.msf.org/honeymooninchad/2010/11/30.

10. James Maskalyk, "Suddenly . . . Sudan," August 4, 2007, MSF field blog entry "an end," http://blogs.msf.org/jamesm/2007/08/an-end.

11. Steven Cohen, "Farchana Nights," July 14, 2008, MSF field blog entry "In a Gentle Way," http://blogs.msf.org/StevenC/2008/07/14.

12. Meshkat, "Off the beaten path . . . PNG," October 4, 2007, MSF field blog entry "a latte and a martini," http://blogs.msf.org/NazaninM/2007/10/04/4.

13. Edith Fortier, "Vakaga Sky," July 20 and November 14, 2008, MSF field blog entries "Adrenaline" and "Why do I do this work?" http://blogs.msf.org/EdithF.

14. Raghu Venugopal, "Awakening in CAR [Central African Republic]," September 11, 2009, MSF field blog entry "Perhaps, one of the best jobs in the world," http://blogs.msf.org/raghuv/2009/09/11.

15. This testimony by Zakariah Mwatia, a Kenyan community health nurse who served as the project coordinator of MSF's mission in Epworth, Zimbabwe, was elicited in an interview conducted by Paul Foreman, a long-time member of MSF, who has filled many roles in the organization, and who worked with Mwatia in Zambia. "So what is it that makes you spend so much time away from home—what is it about MSF that you like so much?" Foreman asked Mwatia. Paul Foreman, "Positive Thinking: Blogging from Zimbabwe," December 12, 2011, MSF field blog entry "Zak," http://blogs.msf.org/paulf/2011/12/12.

16. Joe Starke, "Medicine at the frontier," September 8, 2009, MSF field blog entry "The grinding burden of chronic disease," http://blogs.msf.org/jstarke/page/2.

17. Cohen, "Farchana Nights," June 11 and 19, 2008, MSF field blog entries "The Women of Farchana Refugee Camp" and "Where is the outrage?" http://blogs.msf.org/StevenC/2008/06/19/41/ and http://blogs.msf.org/StevenC/2008/06/32.

18. Jess Cosby, "Jess in Zim," May 18, 2010, MSF field blog entry "This world is crazy, mixed up," http://blogs.msf.org/jessc/2010/05/18.

19. Cohen, "Farchana Nights," April 28, 2008, MSF field blog entry "Fruit in a Bowel" [*sic*], http://blogs.msf.org/StevenC/2008/04/28/18.

20. Maeve Lalore, "TB in Uzbekistan—continued," February 26, 2011, MSF field blog entry "The Highs and Lows," http://blogs.msf.org/maevel/2011/02/26.

21. Grant Assenheimer, "Pré Avis in the Congo," February 22, 2010, MSF field blog entry "Molaw," http://blogs.msf.org/drcdubie/2010/02/22/molaw.

22. Pillay, "South African Doctor in Darfur," January 17, 2008, MSF field blog entry "Gorgeous apple-cheeked Waly," http://blogs.msf.org/Prinitha/2008/01/17.

23. Edith Fortier, "Vakaga Sky," September 23, 2008, MSF field blog entry subtitled "This little girl," http://blogs.msf.org/2008/09/23.

24. This phrase was capitalized by the blogger.

25. Pillay, "South African Doctor in Darfur," February 12, 2008, MSF field blog entry "I grieve for the little one," http://blogs.msf.org/Prinitha/2008/02/12.

26. This phrase is quoted from the MSF Charter.

27. Cohen, "Farchana Nights," "Fruit in a Bowel."

28. Elisabeth Canisius, "Smiles after starvation: Critical care malnutrition in Zinder, Niger," November 14, 2011, MSF field blog entry "Gradual recovery and slow change in season," http://blogs.msf.org/elisabethc/2011/11/14.

29. Emmett Kearney, "My New Friend ROSS," November 22, 2011, MSF field blog entry "Friendliness, smiling faces and fist-bumps in Raja," http://blogs.msf.org/emmettk/2011/11/14.

30. Edith Fortier, "Vakaga Sky," August 3, 2008, MSF field blog entry "Falling in Love," http://blogs.msf.org/EdithF/2008/08/03.

31. Kartik Chandaria, "TB doc in Tajikistan," December 22, 2011, MSF field blog entry "Mystical men and Christmas in Dushanbe," http://blogs.msf.org/kartikc/2011/12/22.

32. Chandaria, "TB doc in Tajikistan," November 15, 2011, MSF field blog entry "Weather and language lessons," http://blogs.msf.org/kartikc/2011/11/15.

33. Douglas Postels, "RUNDRC," August 20, 2009, MSF field blog entry "Gifts," http://blogs.msf.org/douglasp/2009/08/20/gifts.

34. Cosby, "Jess in Zim," July 13, 2008, MSF field blog entry "One foot in front of the other," http://blogs.msf.org/jessc/2010/07/13.

35. Cohen, "Farchana Nights," January 29, 2008, MSF field blog entry "The Farchana Sky," http://blogs.msf.org/StevenC/2008/01/29.

36. Kevin Barlow, "Dear Darfur," February 14, 2008, MSF field blog entry "The Sea of Sticks and Plastic," http://blogs.msf.org/KevinB/2008/02/14.

37. Starke," Medicine at the frontier," December 22, 2009, MSF field blog entry "Closing snapshots of life and work in NWFP," http://blogs.msf.org/jstarke/2009/12/22.

38. Pillay, "South African Doctor in Darfur," "I'm struggling to close this chapter"; Fortier, "Vakaga Sky," "Falling in Love."

39. The blogger is referring here to the Canadian health care system.

40. Grant Assenheimer, "Pré Avis in the Congo," June 8, 2010, MSF field blog entry "Hard Goodbyes," http://blogs.msf.org/drcdubie/2010/06/08.

41. This passage was extracted from a blog entry reproduced in James Maskalyk, *Six Months in Sudan: A Young Doctor in a War-Torn Village* (New York: Spiegel & Grau, 2009), 300.

42. These are packets of "Plumpy Nut," a ready-to-eat nutrition supplement for children suffering from severe malnutrition.

43. Abeyei is a north-south border town in the south of Northern Sudan, where this blogger spent a six-month-long MSF mission.

44. Maskalyk, *Six Months in Sudan,* 281–282.

45. Grant Assenheimer, "Pré Avis in the Congo," June 2, 2010, and June 21, 2010, MSF field blog entries "Thanks for the chickens" and "Pré Avis," http://blogs.msf.org/drcdubie.

46. Cohen, "Farchana Nights," "In a Gentle Way."

47. Sandy Althomsons, "TB in Uzbekistan," August 10, 2010, MSF field blog entry "Good bye and good luck," http://blogs.msf.org/sandya/2010/08/10.

48. Joe Starke, "Medicine at the frontier," December 22, 2009, MSF blog entry "Closing snapshots of life and work in NWFP," http://blogs.msf.org/2009/12/22.

49. Elina Pelekanou, "Thoughts from the Palestinian Territories," September 5 and September 15, 2008, MSF field blog entries "Days go by . . . " and "Belongings," http//blogs.msf.org/ElinaP.

50. Cohen, "Farchana Nights," "In a Gentle Way."

51. Starke, "Medicine at the frontier," December 28, 2009, MSF field blog entry "On saying goodbye," http://blogs.msf.org/jstarke/2009/12/28.

52. Maskalyk, "Suddenly . . . Sudan," "an end."

53. Starke, "Medicine at the frontier," "On saying goodbye."

54. Shauna Sturgeon, "Shauna in DRC," April 10, 2008, MSF field blog entry "Home now…orsomethingcalledhomeanyway,"http://blogs.msf.org/ShaunaS/2008/04/10/47.

55. Ibid.

56. Maskalyk, *Six Months in Sudan,* 3–4.

57. Ed Rackley, "MSF Changed My Life," in *Un regard dans le rétroviseur de l'année 2000* (MSF internal publication, September 2000), 57.

CHAPTER TWO: Origins, Schisms, Crises

1. Tony Judt, *Past Imperfect: French Intellectuals, 1944–1956* (New York: New York University Press, 2011), 1.

2. Stanley Hoffmann, "Raymond Aron (1905–1983)," *New York Review of Books,* December 8, 1983, www.nybooks.com/articles/archives/1983/dec/08/raymond-aron.

3. Between 1956 and 1962, eighteen French colonies in Africa gained independence: Tunisia (1956), Morocco (1956), Guinea (1958), Cameroon (1960), Senegal (1960), Togo (1960), Mali (1960), Madagascar (1960), Benin (1960), Niger (1960), Burkina Faso (1960), Ivory Coast (1960), Chad (1960), Central African Republic (1960), (French) Congo (1960), Gabon (1960), Mauritania (1960), and Algeria (1962). Most traumatic of all for France was the Algerian War that took place between France and Algerian independence movements from 1954 to 1962, which resulted in Algeria's independence.

4. The journalists were associated with *Tonus*, a French medical journal.

5. Xavier Emmanuelli, *Les Prédateurs de l'Action Humanitaire* (Paris: Flammarion, 1990), 16.

6. Xavier Emmanuelli, *Au Vent du Monde* (Paris: Flammarion, 1999), 18.

7. In a challenging paper, Rony Brauman has questioned whether what was deemed "genocide in Biafra" actually took place, or was intended. See "Dangerous Liaisons: Bearing Witness and Political Propaganda. Biafra and Cambodia—the Founding Myths of Médecins Sans Frontières" (CRASH [Centre de Réflexion sur l'Action et les Savoirs Humanitaires], 2006), www.msf-crash.org/drive/877a-rb-2006dangerous-liaisons-%28fr-p.14%29.pdf.

8. "Why Doesn't the ICRC Denounce Unacceptable Behavior More Often?" Question 15 in Bernard Obserson, Nathalie Floras, et al., *ICRC: Answers to Your Questions* (Geneva: ICRC, Public Information Division, 1995), 34.

The text states that the ICRC "does not remain silent about violations of humanitarian law," but uses "confidential approaches, oral and written, to those responsible, and sends reports and recommendations to the parties in the conflict." If these confidential approaches "prove ineffective, the ICRC may break its self-imposed rule of discretion, but only if certain criteria—which are in the public domain—are met" (34).

9. http://association.msf.org/sites/files/documents/Principles%20Chantilly%20EN.pdf.

10. These Paris-based intellectuals included Raymond Aron, André Glucksman, Bernard-Henri Lévy, Claude Mauriac, Edgar Morin, Jean-François Revel, and Jean-Paul Sartre.

11. In connection with their sense of mission to rescue the Vietnamese refugees, it should be noted that France had been involved, religiously, politically, and economically, with Vietnam since the seventeenth century. Vietnam was a part of French Indochina, France's colony, from 1885 to 1954, when at the end of the First Indochina War, it won its independence.

12. Malhuret became president of MSF in 1978.

13. In addition, in a more diffuse way, Brauman's influence within MSF France had become considerable. It is not surprising that he succeeded Malhuret as president in 1982, or that he held this office for twelve years (until 1994).

14. This article was published in the December 4, 1978, issue of *Le Quotidien du médecin*. Emmanuelli titled it "Un bateau pour Saint-Germain des-Prés," making sarcastic reference to the association of the "Boat-for-Vietnam" project with the Paris *arrondisement* of Saint-German-des-Prés (the 16th) on the Left Bank of the Seine, a haunt of post–World War II existentialists—notably of Jean-Paul Sartre, Simone de Beauvoir, and their entourage.

15. Rony Brauman, *Penser dans l'urgence: Parcours critique d'un humanitaire. Entretiens avec Catherine Portevin* (Paris: Seuil, 2006), 79. Xavier Emmanuelli and Raymond Borel were the only ones of the founding group who stayed with MSF.

16. Since 1988, Bernard Kouchner has been secretary of state in the [French] Cabinet for Humanitarian Action (1988); French minister of health (1992–1993); a member of the European Parliament (1993–1997); minister of health again (1997); UN special representative in Kosovo (1999–2001); and French minister of foreign and European affairs (2007–2010).

17. Brauman, *Penser dans l'urgence*, 112.

18. Tribunal de Première Instance de Bruxelles, *Audience publique des référés du 15 juillet 1985*, 5.

19. Brauman, *Penser dans l'urgence*.

20. Tribunal de Première Instance de Bruxelles, *Audience publique*, 5. See Rony Brauman, ed., *Le Tiers-mondisme en question: Actes du colloque de Liberté sans frontières en juillet 1985* (Paris: Olivier Orban, 1986).

21. The MSF Charter was issued in 1971, at the time of MSF's founding.

22. Tribunal de Première Instance de Bruxelles, *Audience publique*, 6.

23. Ibid., 7–8. At the end of the official document containing her decision and the legal grounds for it, the vice president of the Tribunal signed herself simply as "Halsberghe."

24. P. H., "Guerre franco-belge chez Médecins Sans Frontières," *Libération*, July 10, 1985.

25. Max Weber, "The Sociology of Charismatic Authority," chap. 9 in *From Max Weber: Essays in Sociology*, trans. from Weber's *Wirtschaft und Gesellschaft*, pt. 3, chap. 9, by H. H. Gerth and C. Wright Mills (New York: Oxford University Press, 1946), 245–252; Talcott Parsons, *Max Weber: The Theory of Social and Economic Organization*, trans. A. M. Henderson and Talcott Parsons, ed. Parsons (New York: Oxford University Press, 1947), 64–77, and chap. 3, "The Types of Authority and Imperative Coordination," esp. 358–373.

26. The document in my files that contains this provisional statute is not headed by a title, dated, or signed. However, it is attached to a communication and an editorial dated January 20, 1985, which were sent together to the members of MSF Belgium by its director, Philippe Laurent, and that contain the section's strong objections to Liberté Sans Frontières. It is notable that notwithstanding its "sans frontières"/"without borders" appellation, at this stage in its history and development, MSF's conception of "internationalizing" was confined strictly to becoming more European.

27. Judt, *Past Imperfect*, 282.

28. Claude Liauzu, "Le tiersmondisme des intellectuals en accusation," *Vingtième Siècle* 12, no. 12 (October–December 1986): 73–80, at 73, 74, and 75, doi: 10.3406/xxs.1986.www .persee.fr/web/revues/home/prescript/article/xxs_0294–1759_1986_num_12_1_1515.

29. See Stany Grelet and Mathieu Potte-Bonneville, "qu'est-ce-qu'on fait là?" (interview with Rony Brauman), *Vacarme* 04/05 (1997) 1–7, at 1–2, www.vacarme.org/article 1174.html. Like Brauman, Claude Malhuret, the co-organizer of the colloquium, had also made a transition from the political Left to the political Right. In 1986, he had been a militant member of the Parti Socialiste Unifié (PSU), a small radical party that dissolved itself a few years later, and the founder and director of one of the Sorbonne University sections of the student syndicate, Union nationale des Étudiants en France. Brauman referred to Malhuret as his "accomplice" in this era.

30. Grelet and Potte-Bonneville, "qu'est-ce-qu'on fait là?" 2. With regard to his complex ideological and political orientation, his conviction that the ideals of the Enlightenment and the Rights of Man were crucial to the human condition, and his excoriation of intellectuals for overlooking the repression and tyranny of Communist regimes, Brauman felt strongly identified with the thought and writing of the renowned French sociologist, historian, philosopher, and journalist Raymond Aron, whose works he greatly

admired and studied, and to whom he attributed the "theoretical support" that he needed for his own "militant humanitarian liberal democratic anticommunist" outlook.

31. Brauman, *Penser dans l'urgence*, 107.

32. Grelet and Potte-Bonneville, "qu'est-ce-qu'on fait là?" 2; Brauman, *Penser dans l'urgence*, 108.

33. Rony Brauman, personal communication to the author, August 21, 2011.

34. Brauman, *Penser dans l'urgence*, 117.

35. Ibid., 109–110, 117.

36. These ideas are expressed in an anonymous, undated, seven-page photocopied typescript in my files, on whose first page the letterhead and the icon of the "Fondation Liberté Sans Frontières Pour l'Information sur les Droits de l'Homme et le Développement" are printed.

37. Brauman, *Penser dans l'urgence*, 131.

38. Fiona Terry, *Condemned to Repeat? The Paradox of Humanitarian Action* (Ithaca, NY: Cornell University Press, 2002), 48–49. Terry has spent more than twenty years involved in humanitarian relief operations in different parts of the world. From 2000 to 2003, she worked as a research director in MSF France's Paris office. She holds a PhD in international relations and political science from the Australian National University.

39. Ibid.

40. Ibid.

41. MSF Belgium, which was present in a different area of Ethiopia in 1994 than MSF France, disagreed publicly with the stance that the latter had taken, because of the role it played in MSF France's enforced withdrawal from Ethiopia, and its consequent inability to render further assistance to the Ethiopian population. MSF Holland also took exception to MSF France's decision.

42. Grelet and Potte-Bonneville, "qu'est-ce-qu'on fait là?" "Rony Brauman s'est trompé sur la vraie nature du communisme," 3.

43. Ibid.

44. Rony Brauman, personal communication to the author, August 21, 2011. Two members of MSF Belgium told me that after Liberté Sans Frontières expired, Brauman quietly expressed some after-the-fact regrets about having created it and deemed this to have been a "mistake." However, this is not a sentiment to which he gave voice in the several conversations that I had with him. The closest that he came to saying this was in the form of a passing remark that he made to the effect that he should have realized how "political" Liberté Sans Frontières was.

45. Brauman, *Penser dans l'urgence*, 115.

46. Mitterand's first term as president of France was during the years 1981 to 1988, and his second term ran from 1988 to 1995.

47. Claude Malhuret became more politically conservative over time. By 1986, when he was appointed secretary of state for human rights in Prime Minister Jacques Chirac's government, he had left MSF. In 1989, he was elected mayor of Vichy, an office that he held until 2001. Rony Brauman continues to be associated with MSF France. Working out of its Paris office, he is a director of its Centre de Réflexion sur l'Action et les Savoirs Humanitaires (CRASH). As described in its mission statement, CRASH was created by MSF in 1999. "Its objective is to encourage debate and critical reflection on the humanitarian practices of the association. CRASH carries out in-depth studies and analyses of

MSF activities. This work is based on the framework and the experience of the association." The mission statement continues: "In no way, however, do these texts lay down the 'MSF party line,' nor do they seek to defend the idea of 'true humanitarianism.' On the contrary, the objective is to contribute to the debate on the challenges, constraints, and limits—as well as the subsequent dilemmas—of humanitarian action. Any criticisms, remarks or suggestions are most welcome."

48. Personal communication to the author from a long-standing member of MSF, May 24, 2006.

49. Terry, *Condemned to Repeat?* 2 and 245.

CHAPTER THREE: "Nobel or Rebel?"

1. James Orbinski, *An Imperfect Offering: Humanitarian Action in the Twenty-First Century* (Toronto: Doubleday Canada, 2008), 334.

2. Ibid.

3. "MSF Japan Members Celebrate Nobel Prize," *Daily Yomiuri*, October 17, 1999, 2.

4. Patrick Wieland, "Don't Give Up the Fight," MSF *Nobel Peace Prize Journal* (produced on the occasion of receiving the Nobel Peace Prize in 1999), 15.

5. Jean Guy, ibid.

6. Alex Parisel, "The Day After the Night Before," ibid., 7.

7. Albert Camus, *L'Homme Révolté*, trans. Anthony Bower as *The Rebel: An Essay on Man in Revolt* (New York: Vintage Books, 1991), 13, 16, 22, 302–303, 305.

8. The debate took place in a mixture of French and English. The excerpts from it here were all taken from a transcript entitled "Nobel ou rebelle, a Nobel without a cause?"

9. Wieland, "Don't Give Up the Fight."

10. Philippe Biberson and Rony Brauman, "'The Right of Intervention'—A Deceptive Catch-Phrase," *Nobel Peace Prize Journal*, 7.

11. Parisel, "Day After."

12. The nineteen MSF sections were created in the following order: France (1971), Belgium and Switzerland (1980), Holland (1984), Luxembourg and Spain (1986), the United States and Greece, (1990), Canada and Italy (1991), Japan (1992), Sweden, Denmark, Germany, and the United Kingdom (1993), Australia, Austria, and Hong Kong (1994), Norway (1995).

13. James Orbinski, "Where to From Here?" (internal MSF document, November 24, 2000).

14. Parisel, "Day After."

15. It was not until January 1997 that MSF established an international council. Before that no entity existed within it that facilitated communication and coordination among its sections.

16. James Orbinski served as president of the International Council from 1998 to 2001. He had worked with MSF since 1992—including in the setting of Baidoa, Somalia, in 1992–1993, during a time of civil war and famine; in Kigali, Rwanda, in the midst of the 1994 genocide there; and in Goma, Zaïre (now the Democratic Republic of Congo), while it was undergoing a Rwandan refugee crisis.

17. The International Office of MSF was located in Brussels at this time. It is currently in Geneva.

18. My account of this MSF France board meeting, and all the passages that I quote from it, are taken from the November 19, 1999, transcript (*procès-verbal*) of the meeting.

19. For an extensive, firsthand account of MSF's TB project in Russia, see chap. 11 of this book.

20. Orbinski, *Imperfect Offering*, 334.

21. Ibid., 338.

22. The five operational sections of MSF at this time were MSF Belgium, MSF France, MSF Holland, MSF Spain, and MSF Switzerland.

23. The partner sections (known as "delegate offices" until 1997) were Australia, Austria, Canada, Denmark, Germany, Greece, Hong Kong, Italy, Japan, Luxembourg, Norway, Sweden, the United Kingdom, and the United States.

24. Orbinski, *Imperfect Offering*, 338–339.

25. I believe I first heard the term "informal hierarchy" from Jean-Marie Kindermans in the course of a personal conversation about my continuing perplexity regarding how decisions are made in the "everyone is equal," "anti-institutionalization" context of MSF. Kindermans (born in France), a physician, whose special fields are public health and tropical medicine, is also a qualified engineer. He first became associated with MSF in 1982 and has worked in Thailand, Chad, Afghanistan, Lebanon, Vietnam, and Central America. Among the positions that he has held in MSF are those of director of MSF Belgium, member of MSF Belgium's board of directors, member of MSF's International Council, and secretary-general of MSF.

26. December 10, the anniversary of Albert Nobel's death, is the day that the Nobel Peace Prize is traditionally awarded.

27. This so-called Second Chechen Campaign was initiated in 1999. The First Chechen Campaign launched by Russian troops in an attempt to stop Chechnya from seceding from the Russian Federation had taken place in 1994 to 1996. Officially, the conflict between Chechnya and Russia ended in 2000, but insurgent activity continued.

28. The murals on the walls of the Central Hall were painted by Henrik Sørensen between 1938 and 1950.

29. Orbinski, *Imperfect Offering*, 339.

30. The acceptance speech was thirty-five minutes long. The passages that I have excerpted from it and quoted above are not presented in the order in which they appear in the speech. For a complete, verbatim transcript, see "The Nobel Prize Acceptance Speech," December 10, 1999, www.doctorswithoutborders.org/publications/article .cfm?id=708.

CHAPTER FOUR: MSF Greece Ostracized

1. Minutes of the meeting of the International Council of MSF, Brussels, September 9, 1994.

2. Ibid.

3. The letter, originally written in French, is reproduced in *L'Odyssée de Médecins Sans Frontières–Grèce* (*The Odyssey of MSF–Greece*), a 1997 MSF "memorandum" printed in both French and English versions, Annex 7, 43.

4. Ibid., 27–28.

5. Ibid., Annex 8, 44.

6. Ibid., Annex 9, 45.

7. See http://en.wikipedia.org/wiki/Srebrenica_massacre. The Srebrenica massacre (which became known as the Srebrenica genocide) entailed the killing of more than eight thousand Bosniaks (Bosnian Muslims), mainly men and boys, in and around Srebrenica (a small town and municipality in the east of Bosnia and Herzegovina) by units of the Army of Republika Srpska (also referred to as the Bosnian Serb army), and members from a paramilitary group from Serbia known as the Scorpions.

8. "Movement" is written with a capital "M" in Orbinski's communication.

9. *"Memorandum présenté par Médecins Sans Frontières–Grèce: MSF victime du conflit du Kosovo"* (memorandum presented by Médecins Sans Frontiers–Greece: MSF Victim of the Kosovo Conflict), Brussels, January 26, 2000, 4.

10. Ibid., 8–9.

11. Ibid., 14.

12. Nicholas Christakis subsequently became professor of medicine and of sociology at Harvard. On July 1, 2013, he moved to Yale to become the Sol Goldman Family Professor of Social and Natural Science.

13. Our relationship began when Christakis was studying for his PhD in sociology at the University of Pennsylvania, where I was his one of his teachers, his faculty advisor, and the director of his dissertation.

14. For an account of this split, see chap. 2.

CHAPTER FIVE: The Return of MSF Greece

1. The two persons who had carried out the fact-finding mission to MSF Greece were Laure Delcros and Kostas Moschochoritis. They made an oral presentation to the International Council meeting based on their written report about the mission. My account of the report and the presentation, and of what transpired at the International Council meeting, is based on "IC [International Council] Meeting Minutes, Barcelona, November 22–24, 2002."

2. Among the sections of MSF that the "invited guests" at this meeting represented were MSF France, MSF Holland, MSF Switzerland, MSF Germany, MSF UK, and MSF Sweden.

3. The quoted words and the account of what transpired at this Extraordinary General Assembly centered on the "Kosovo debate" that follows are taken from "Report on Kosovo Debate—XGA MSF GR, 13th January 2007," which, in effect, constitutes detailed minutes of the meeting.

4. These countries included Portugal, Spain, Italy, and Ireland.

5. By late 2010, the unemployment rate in Greece had reached eighteen percent, rising to thirty-five percent for young persons between the ages of fifteen and twenty-nine. Rachel Donadio, "With Work Scarce in Athens, Greeks Go Back to the Land," *New York Times*, December 9, 2012, A1 and A7.

6. This paragraph is based on three documents, from which the quoted passages were drawn: "MSF–GR Annual Plan 2011: Executive Summary"; "MSF–GR Annual Plan 2012: Executive Summary"; and "MSF Greece: Medical-Operational Support Unit (SOMA)."

7. "MSF Malaria Intervention in Greece: Executive Summary," Athens, December 1, 2011.

8. In the longer run, what was contemplated was the possibility of integrating these malaria interventions into the entrance points and detention centers for refugees and immigrants located in Evros, Greece. See ibid.

9. Reveka Papadopoulou, personal communication to the author, February 14, 2012.

10. Reveka Papadopoulou, personal communication to the author, September 19, 2011, from which all the quotations in this paragraph are drawn.

11. Michaël Neuman, interview with Reveka Papdopoulou, "En Grèce, des bidonvilles sont dans une situation comparable à celle de terrains plus traditionnels de MSF," *Libération*, March 12, 2012, http://humanitaire.blogs.liberation.fr/msf/page/3.

12. Reveka Papadopoulou, personal communication to the author, February 14, 2012.

CHAPTER SIX: La Mancha

Epigraph. "The Impossible Dream (The Quest)" is sung by Don Quixote all the way through the musical *Man of La Mancha*. Copyright 1965. Words by Joe Darion. Music by Mitch Leigh. Andrew Scott Music, Helena Music Company, ASCAP. Permission for use of lyrics from "The Impossible Dream" has been granted by Alan S. Honig.

1. Rowan Gillies, "Why La Mancha?" in *My Sweet La Mancha* (internal MSF publication, December 2005), 10–15, at 10.

2. Rowan Gillies, "From Here to the La Mancha Agreement," *La Mancha Gazette* (internal MSF newsletter), May 2006, 1–2, at 1.

3. "What Is the La Mancha Process?" (internal MSF document).

4. "Brax" is Samuel Hanryon, a member of the Communications Department of MSF France.

5. I was present as an observer at the La Mancha meeting, by permission of the president of the International Council, Rowan Gillies, and with the assent of MSF members who knew me. In an e-mail sent after the meeting, Gillies wrote me: "Thank you very much for coming to the La Mancha conference. I think it was ideal for us to have a semi-outside person there, but one who understands the peculiarities and particularities of MSF."

6. This is a consequence of two developments: as a result of MSF's expansion and greater internationalization, most of its sections are no longer headquartered in French-speaking countries; and at this historical juncture, English has succeeded French as the global language.

7. There were only a few incidental exceptions to this pattern that I observed, when several French and Belgian attendees who had been members of MSF for many years referred jokingly to their affiliation with Marxism or Maoism in their youth.

8. The phrase "nonideological, apolitical ideology" is my own coinage.

9. Personal communication from an MSF member, May 24, 2006.

10. The tale, which originated in India, has been widely diffused, and exists in many different versions.

11. Marie Buissonière, "La Mancha, here we come!" *La Mancha Gazette* (internal MSF newsletter), May 2006, 2–3.

12. At this time, seventy-eight percent of MSF's financial resources came from more than three million private donors.

13. Sudan, the Democratic Republic of Congo, and Angola were the sites of the three biggest MSF interventions in 2004, collectively entailing more than thirty-four percent of its operational expenses.

14. Buissonnière, "La Mancha, here we come!"

15. Ulrike von Pilar, "Sharing Knowledge! The La Mancha Training Centre," *La Mancha Gazette* (internal MSF newsletter), May 2006, 12. The self-accusations of being "colonialist" that were voiced at the conference probably had some connection with MSF's complex institutional and personal relationships with the history of colonialism in Africa. Belgian, French, and British members of MSF, for example, are members of societies that were once colonial powers in Africa, and some of them have relatives who went to Africa as missionaries, physicians, government administrators, or commercial agents during the colonial era. For these reasons, they may be especially inclined to feel strongly identified with Africa and Africans, on the one hand, and highly condemnatory of colonial ways of thinking, feeling, and behaving, on the other.

16. Vincent Janssens, "If the Glove Doesn't Fit, Shrink the Hand?" in *My Sweet La Mancha*, 181–182, at 181. I have retained the author's unconventional style.

17. "Movement" is often written with a capital "M" in MSF documents.

18. James Orbinski, "MSF: Where to From Here?" (internal MSF document), November 24, 2000, 1–6, at 1 and 3.

19. "Final—La Mancha Agreement—June 25, 2006, Athens."

20. Erwin van't Land, "At Our Core, a Resounding Non!" in *My Sweet La Mancha*, 186–187, at 186.

21. Ibid., 187.

22. Gillies, "Why La Mancha?" 13.

23. Report from the June 1989 MSF France board of directors meeting, cited in Jean-Hervé Bradol and Elizabeth Szumlin, "AIDS: A New Pandemic Leading to New Medical and Political Practices," in Jean-Hervé Bradol and Claudine Vidal, eds., *Medical Innovations in Humanitarian Situations* (New York: MSF USA, 2011), 178–199, at 181. For more details of these earlier MSF debates about the pros and cons of MSF becoming involved with HIV/AIDS, see chap. 7.

24. MSF inaugurated the International Campaign for Access to Essential Medicines in 1999, with its Nobel Peace Prize money. See chap. 3.

25. Quoted in Eric Goemaere, "HIV/AIDS Programs' Impact on Our Operational Principles—A Subtle Balance Between Political Involvement and Medical Responsibility," in *My Sweet La Mancha*, 214–219, at 214.

26. This program was established in the township of Khayelitsha, Cape Town, South Africa where, in greatly expanded form, it still exists. For a detailed account of its history, development, and operation, based in part on my firsthand field observations, see chaps. 7 and 8.

27. Goemaere, "HIV/AIDS Programs' Impact," 215.

28. Ibid., 216.

29. Kenny Gluck, "Measles, Stalin, and Other Risks—Reflections on Our Principles, Témoignage, and Security," in *My Sweet La Mancha*, 150–155, at 150.

30. The other MSF staff member who was abducted in this area was Arjan Erkel, who at the time headed MSF Switzerland's mission in Dagestan. In August 2002, he was kidnapped by gunmen, who kept him in captivity until April 2004. Furthermore, as many

as six members of the International Red Cross working in the area were murdered. As a result of these events, MSF reevaluated the role it would play in the Northern Caucasus. A reluctant decision was made to withdraw both all Russian and expatriate staff from the area and carry out whatever humanitarian activities were undertaken through a "remote control system of intervention," conducted by Chechens and Ingushetians, who were ethnic natives in the region.

31. Pierre Salignon, "From Taking Risks to Putting Lives in Danger?" in *My Sweet La Mancha*, 285–287, at 285.

32. Ibid.

33. Colin L. Powell, "Remarks to the National Foreign Policy Conference for Leaders of Non-Governmental Organizations, State Department, Washington DC, October 26, 2001," cited and quoted in Rony Brauman and Pierre Salignon, "IDEAS & OPINIONS FROM MSF: Iraq: in Search of a 'Humanitarian Crisis,'" April 16, 2004 (e-mail to the author).

34. Quotation from MSF's 1996 "Chantilly Agreement."

35. It is possible that what influenced Brax to use French rather than English for these cartoons is that a number of French humanitarian organizations figured prominently in a consortium of NGOS that were particularly outspoken in questioning the necessity of going to war in Iraq. They included La Croix-Rouge Française, Action Contre la Faim, Médecins du Monde, Première Urgence, and Solidarité et Enfants du Monde. Cited in Brauman and Salignon, "IDEAS & OPINIONS."

36. These General Assembly meetings took place during May 2006.

37. Key sentences were printed in bold type.

38. E-mail communication from a member of MSF to the author, May 2, 2006.

39. E-mail communication from a member of MSF to the author, May 22, 2006.

CHAPTER SEVEN: Struggling with HIV/AIDS

Epigraphs. Treating 1 Million by 2005: Making It Happen. The WHO Strategy, the WHO and UNAIDS Global Initiative to Provide Anti-Retroviral Therapy to 3 Million People in Developing Countries by the End of 2005 (Geneva: World Health Organization, 2003), 3–4; Peter Piot, *No Time to Lose: A Life in Pursuit of Deadly Viruses* (New York: Norton, 2012), x; Albert Camus, *The Plague*, trans. Stuart Gilbert (New York: Knopf, 1950), 35, 278.

1. As many as twenty-five new infectious diseases had emerged since the founding of MSF in 1971; and among the old infectious diseases that had reemerged, multi-drug-resistant forms of tuberculosis, malaria, and measles were some of the most serious.

2. Helen Epstein and Lincoln Chen, "Can AIDS Be Stopped?" *New York Review of Books* 49, no. 4 (March 14, 2002): 29–31. See Helen Epstein, *The Invisible Cure: Africa, the West, and the Fight Against AIDS* (New York: Farrar, Straus & Giroux, 2007).

3. Alex Parisel, personal communication to the author, January 10, 2002.

4. The HIV retrovirus was identified as the biological cause of AIDS in 1983–1984; anti-retroviral drugs to treat AIDS were introduced in 1987.

5. In 2001, MSF Belgium's board held a debate on "MSF and AIDS." Prior to, and in preparation for this, they sought the "opinions, attitudes and wishes" of its members on a number of AIDS-relevant questions. Among the documents circulated to members in this connection was one on "AIDS treatment for MSF employees. A kick-off for discussion." The text quoted above was written in response to this document by the head of the MSF Belgium mission in Rwanda, who sent it to the Brussels office by e-mail on May

14, 2001. In order to maintain confidentiality, he changed the names of the persons who he cited in it.

6. Gorick Ooms, "AIDS: Mega-Atomic Time Bomb" (MSF Belgium document, September 2000, 19–21, circulated internally as part of a collection of articles and reports issued in connection with the section's stocktaking at the end of the year 2000).

7. Eric Goemaere is a physician trained in economics, tropical medicine, public health, and epidemiology. He was the executive director of MSF Belgium from 1994 to 1999. Alex Parisel has an undergraduate university degree in business and management, and a graduate degree in the management of health institutions. He succeeded Goemaere as executive director of the section. Gorik Ooms is a human rights lawyer, with a PhD in medical sciences. He served as executive director of MSF Belgium from 2004 to 2008.

8. For a brief account of the nature of MSF's Campaign for Access to Essential Medicines, see chap. 3. Eric Goemaere was in charge of the portfolio for access to second-line drugs for multi-drug-resistant forms of tuberculosis.

Bernard Pécoul, a French physician, joined MSF France in 1983. He spent five years working on field projects in Latin America, Asia, and Africa. After his return to France in the late 1990s, he co-founded Epicentre, MSF's center for epidemiological research, in Paris and led its research and training until he was named executive director of MSF France, in which position he served for seven years. At the end of that term, in 1998, he assumed the role of executive director of MSF's Campaign for Access to Essential Medicines. Subsequently, in 2003, he became a founder and the executive director of the Drugs for Neglected Diseases Initiatives (DNDi), located in Geneva—a position that he still holds.

9. In calling Goemaere a member of the "1968 generation," Parisel was alluding to the student uprisings that took place on European university campuses during that period, and to the fact that when he was a student at the Université Catholique de Louvain in Belgium, Goemaere had seriously studied Marx's *Das Kapital* and considered himself to be a Trotskyite in his political outlook. He was also impressed and influenced by radically oriented students from Latin America who were enrolled at Louvain at the time—including disciples of Ernesto "Che" Guevara who were enrolled with him in a macro-economics course.

10. MSF was active in South Africa throughout the 1980s, until 1993, in assisting refugees from Mozambique.

11. At the time, the prevention-of-mother-to-child transmission (PMTCT) regimen consisted of giving AZT to pregnant women in the thirty-sixth week of their pregnancy, and during labor, following a pilot protocol (ACTG 076), which had been tested in Thailand. The results of this trial, published in 1998, had shown that administering AZT in this way reduced vertical transmission from mother to child by fifty percent.

12. "Coloured" in South Africa refers to persons of "mixed" ancestry, including black-white, black-Asian, white-Asian, and black-Coloured descendants.

13. The quotations in this paragraph come from an interview that I conducted with Eric Goemaere in Cape Town on September 25, 2002.

14. When Hermann Reuter began his medical education, Namibia (then South West Africa) was a South African mandated territory. He completed his medical studies in 1991, one year after Namibia gained its independence.

15. Interview with Hermann Reuter, September 17, 2002.

16. Eric Goemaere, interview, September 25, 2002. Goemaere attributed the nurses' failure to recognize how many of the patients they were seeing were infected with HIV partly to the fact that at this time, "hardly anyone was tested for HIV." "I recorded that only 450 HIV tests had been done in 1998 for the whole township," he told me.

17. Eric Goemaere to Renée Fox, September 29, 2011.

18. Toby Kasper, David Coetzee, Françoise Louise, Andrew Boulle, and Katherine Hilderbrand, "Demystifying Antiretroviral Therapy in Resource Poor Settings," *Essential Drugs Monitor* 32 (2003): 20–21; Quarraisha Abdool Karim, "HIV Treatment in South Africa: Overcoming Impediments to Getting Started," *Lancet* 363, no. 9418 (April 24, 2004), www.thelancet.com/journals/lancet/article/PIIS0140-6736%2804%2916055-8/fulltext.

19. Marleen Boelaert, *Consultancy Report: MSF Khayelitsha Project, South Africa* (Antwerp: Department of Public Health, Institute of Tropical Medicine, June 2002), 1.

20. All the quotations from Eric Goemaere in this paragraph are drawn from a personal communication to the author on February 1, 2005.

21. The Khayelitsha group has conducted and published a great deal of medical, epidemiological, public health, and primary-care-relevant research on its endeavors—much of it in collaboration with members of University of Cape Town's School of Public Health and Family Medicine. A major figure in this research is Katherine Hilderbrand, who is a research associate at HIV/TB Services of Khayelitsha and in the Centre for Infectious Disease Epidemiology and Research in the University of Cape Town's School of Public Health. She is also Eric Goemaere's wife.

22. These patients included 159 adults and 18 children under fourteen years of age. The mean age of the adults on HAART was thirty-two (ranging from fourteen to fifty-four), and sixty-nine percent of them were women. According to a joint "preliminary report" issued by MSF and the School of Public Health and Family Medicine of the University of Cape Town, there were more women on HAART than men "because more women [made] use of public facilities." Médecins Sans Frontières (MSF), and School of Public Health and Family Medicine, University of Cape Town, "Providing Antiretroviral Therapy at Primary Health Care Clinics in Resource Poor Settings: Preliminary Report, May 2001–May 2002," 5.

23. In 2002, Zackie Achmat, along with two other members of TAC (Matthew Damane and Nomandla Yako), and Joyce Phekane of the Congress of South African Trade Unions (COSATU) made a trip to Brazil to observe the Brazilian government's AIDS program, and to see how it had been able to circumvent the international drug companies' protection of the patents on anti-retroviral drugs in order to make affordable generic versions of them. They brought back to South Africa generic antiretrovirals from the Brazilian pharmaceutical laboratory Farmanguinhos for use in the MSF Khayelitsha project. All three of the TAC members were living openly with HIV, and two of them (Damane and Yako) were receiving treatment in Khayelitsha. The main witnessing and advocacy goal of their trip was to show that if the South African government took the necessary action, anti-retroviral drugs could be provided at half the price that was being charged by the multinational drug companies in South Africa.

24. For an ethnographic account of this research, see Renée C. Fox, *In the Field: A Sociologist's Journey* (New Brunswick, NJ: Transaction Publishers, 2010), 123–300.

CHAPTER EIGHT: In Khayelitsha

1. With the exception of the two phrases in brackets and some slight modifications, this description of Khayelitsha is excerpted from Renée C. Fox, "Khayelitsha Journal," *Society*, May–June 2005 (Culture and Society section): 70–76 (at 71–72).
2. Although this story is not factually true, there is a real sense in which it was true "in spirit." Because of the efforts of the Danish government and thousands of Danes from wide-ranging backgrounds, when the Nazis ordered the arrest and deportation of Danish Jews in October 1943, many of them had been hidden and sheltered by Danish citizens, and some 7,000 had been helped to escape in boats to Sweden, with which the Danish government had secretly negotiated an agreement to receive them. In the end, about 475 Danish Jews were deported to the Theresienstadt concentration camp (now in the Czech Republic), of whom twenty died en route, and fifty in the camp. See, e.g., "The Fate of the Jews of Denmark," www.holocaustresearchproject.org/nazioccupation/danish jews.html, and "The History of Jews in Denmark," www.jewishgen.org/scandinavia/ history.htm.
3. The nurses' epaulettes, which differed in color, indicated the various branches of nursing in which they were trained and registered.
4. This is a pseudonym.
5. Zidovudine (or AZT) and Nevirapine.
6. Women were given several options about how to feed their babies. At first the policy was to recommend formula feeding exclusively, in order to prevent the transmission of HIV to the baby through the mother's milk. Later, a "mixed feeding" option of breast and formula feeding was added, but as a less desirable alternative.
7. This, too, is a pseudonym.
8. She mentioned in passing that this desire on her part was partly connected with her membership in an Adventist Christian faith community.
9. Vuyiseka Dubula's account of how she became involved in HIV/AIDS issues, and a leading figure in the development of Ulwazi, was shared with me via a Skype-conducted personal interview with her on May 3, 2012.
10. Vuyiseka Dubula is now (in 2012) the secretary-general of TAC. Her work is still focused on HIV/AIDS, tuberculosis, and their interconnection, but her role has become more political, she said, more bureaucratic, and in certain ways "not as interesting" as her earlier activities in the context of Ulwazi.
11. This is taken from my field notes, and was published in Fox, "Khayelitsha Journal," 73–74, along with my overview account of the meeting.
12. In the afternoon, the group reconvened for a meeting that concentrated on instructing them how to teach others about HIV/AIDS—its symptoms, modes of transmission (especially through sexual relations), its prevention, and its treatment.
13. In 2011, Poole graduated as a medical doctor, and began specialty training in intensive care.
14. I had help from Colwyn Poole in translating the Xhosa.
15. A male TAC volunteer who sat next to me in the classroom kindly translated the Afrikaans for me, although I understood some of what was being said on my own, because Afrikaans is a Low Franconian, West Germanic language, derived from seventeenth-century Dutch, and from my years of research in Belgium, I am acquainted with West Flanders/Flemish Dutch.

16. "TAC Hands Over Submission to Operational Treatment Plan Task Team, Mass Rally in Gugulethu on Saturday," *TAC Newsletter*, September 23, 2003.

17. "Give Government Credit for Great Strides in Health Care," *Sunday Independent*, October 12, 2003, 8. This article contained an edited version of Graça Machel's speech.

18. For more detailed information about Dr. Hermann Reuter, see chap. 7.

19. "Open Letter to the South African Government From Médecins Sans Frontières," February 12, 2003, signed by Dr. Morten Rostrop, president, MSF International Council, and Dr. Eric Goemaere, head of mission, MSF South Africa.

20. At this time, the cost of treating a patient with antiretroviral drugs was approximately $8,000 a year. Given the magnitude of the epidemic of HIV/AIDS in South Africa, what it would have meant economically for the government to try to make this therapy available to all who needed it would have been economically staggering.

21. Katherine Hilderbrand, a research associate on the MSF Khayelitsha staff (for more on her, see chap. 7, n. 21), was the chief designer of the questionnaire, and it was she who invited me to meet with the group. My account of this meeting here coincides with the description of it in Fox, "Khayelitsha Journal," 72–73.

22. Ibid., 72. I identified these components of witchcraft from anthropological works about Central African societies and culture, and from my own firsthand knowledge of witchcraft in the Democratic Republic of Congo.

23. Willy De Craemer, Jan Vansina, and Renée C. Fox, "Religious Movements in Central Africa: A Theoretical Study," *Comparative Studies in Society and History* 18, no. 4 (October 1976): 458–475, at 461.

24. Contributing to the ability of the Khayelitsha program to increase its patient intake was the initiation of the national government plan for treatment and care of HIV/AIDS, which unlocked international funding, with the result that, beginning in July 2004, as much as eighty percent of Khayelitsha's antiretroviral drug supply was supported by the Global Fund to Fight AIDS, Tuberculosis, and Malaria. MSF also augmented its funding of the program. In addition, the majority of the staff began to be paid by the Western Cape Provincial Department of Health; and the sources of the high-quality, relatively low-cost generic forms of antiretroviral drug that it prescribed for patients had expanded from the Brazilian company from which they had originally been purchased to several Indian companies, along with Aspen Pharmacare of South Africa.

25. For a somewhat more detailed account of Khayelitsha's "patient selection" processes, and the ethical questions that they posed for the clinics' staff, see Renée C. Fox and Eric Goemaere, "They Call It 'Patient Selection' in Khayelitsha: The Experience of Médecins Sans Frontières–South Africa in Enrolling Patients to Receive Antiretroviral Treatment for HIV/AIDS," *Cambridge Quarterly of Healthcare Ethics* 16, no. 1 (Winter 2006): 302–312.

The difficulty that the Khayelitsha selection committees had in refusing treatment to patients reminded me of comparable problems that the Admissions and Policy Committee of the Artificial Kidney Center in Seattle, Washington, experienced during the 1960s when it was faced with the task of screening and selecting patients with end-stage renal diseases for chronic intermittent hemodialysis, in an era when a limited number of kidney machines and financial resources were available in the United States for this purpose. Like the Khayelitsha committees, the Seattle committee was disinclined to strictly apply the medical, psychological, and social patient selection criteria that it had developed. It was striking to observe, as the medical historian Judith Swazey and I did, how few of the selection/de-selection criteria that the Seattle committee was supposedly using ended up disqualifying a candidate for the procedure. The committee predominantly chose, rather than unchose, patients for dialysis. See Renée C. Fox and Judith P. Swazey, *The Courage to Fail: A Social View of Organ Transplantation and Dialysis* (Chicago: University of Chicago Press, 1974; 2nd, rev. ed. 1978, repr. with new introduction, New Brunswick, NJ: Transaction Books, 2002), esp. 226–265.

26. Although this is written in the first person, I was accompanied by my colleague Judith Swazey, and by a young woman physician, a Coloured South African general practitioner, who made regular visits to the hospice.

27. This constituted a major alteration in the "Directly Observed Therapy for the Treatment of Tuberculosis" regimen that the World Health Organization (WHO) had instituted and was recommending during the period in 1985 when I made my first field trip to Khayelitsha. At that time, the procedure for DOTS treatment that WHO advised involved having a trained health worker not only provide the prescribed TB drugs but also watch each patient swallow every dose.

28. South Africa has the highest incidence of rape in the world, only a fraction of which are reported. Studies conducted by the South Africa Medical Research Council, the World Health Organization, and the Community of Information, Empowerment and Transparency all confirm this extraordinarily high incidence.

29. This is a pseudonym.

30. The volume of clients seen by the rape clinic has continued to increase since my last field trip to Khayelitsha in 1995, and the clinic is now under the auspices of a local NGO.

31. www.boston.com/news/world/africa/articles/2011/06/04/s_africa_marks_milestone_in_aids_fight. Used with permission of The Associated Press Copyright © 2013. All rights reserved.

32. Statement by Eric Goemaere in *Khayelitsha 2001–2011* (Médecins Sans Frontières activity report, 2011), http://webdav.uct.ac.za/depts/epi/publications/documents/MSF_report_web_FINAL.pdf.

33. "Saying Goodbye to Lesotho's Highlands, Khayelitsha Heartland: Rachel Cohen, MSF Head of Mission, looks back at three years of making a difference," *MAMELA!* May 2009, 1–3, at 1. http://msf.org.za/Newsletter/MAMELA!/MAMELA_May09.html.

34. Personal communication to the author, March 29, 2009.

35. Peter Piot, *No Time To Lose: A Life in Pursuit of Deadly Viruses* (New York: Norton, 2012), 367.

36. According to an article in the *Lancet*, in 2007, SANAC endorsed a National Strategic Plan for HIV and AIDS and Sexually Transmitted Infections (2007–2011). "But a midterm review of implementation of the plan identified serious problems with SANAC. The review found that the high number and lack of definition of targets, weak coordination between different implementers, and between implementers and SANAC had seriously hampered reporting on national progress in the strategic plan." However, the article went on to say that with the very recent appointment of "widely respected" Dr. Fareed Abdullah as SANAC's new chief executive, who would lead the restructuring of the organization, there was now real promise that its Monitoring and Evaluation Unit would be "crucially strengthen[ed]" ("South Africa's AIDS Response: The Next 5 Years," *Lancet* 379, no. 9824 [April 14, 2012]: 1365). As recounted earlier in this chapter, in 1999,

Abdullah had initiated the program to prevent mother-to-child transmission of HIV/ AIDS in the Western Cape—long before it became legally obligatory for such treatment to be provided nationally. It was in this connection that he was one of the first persons to welcome Eric Goemaere to Khayelitsha.

37. Jon Cohen, "Reversal of Misfortunes," *Science* 339, no. 6122 (February 22, 2013): 898–903. The "alarming rise in coinfection with HIV and TB has been dubbed the HIV/ TB syndemic [the author of this article comments] because, for both biological and social reasons such as poverty, the two diseases have synergistic effects, with each making the other worse."

38. "Disappointment: The Ruling Party's 100th Anniversary Failed to Mask a Host of Worries," *Economist* 42, no. 8767 (January 14–20, 2012): 45.

39. "Breaking the Grip of Poverty and Inequality in South Africa, 2004–2014: Current Trends, Issues and Future Policy Options" (executive summary coordinated by J. P. Landman, with the assistance of Haroon Bhorat, Servaas van de Berg, and Carl van Aardt, December 2003), www.sarpn.org/documents/d0000649/P661-Povertyreport3b.pdf), 3, 5, and 7.

40. Lydia Polgreen, "Fatal Stampede in South Africa Points Up University Crisis," *New York Times*, January 11, 2012, A1 and A9, at A1).

41. Albert Camus, *The Plague*, trans. Stuart Gilbert (New York: Knopf, 1950).

42. Sophie Delaunay, "External Challenges: Working Group on Governance" (internal MSF document, May 2009), 2.

43. www.msf.org.za/download/file/fid/3706. This statement was issued by the Budget Expenditure Monitoring Forum (BEMF), a group of organizations concerned with HIV/AIDS funding in South Africa and the Southern African region. BEMF includes Section 27, the Treatment Action Campaign, Médecins Sans Frontières South Africa, the Centre for Economic Governance and AIDS in Africa, and the Free State Aids Coalition and World Vision. See www.tac.org.za/community/BEMF.

44. Eric Goemaere, personal communications to the author, November 30, 2011 and December 2, 2011. With regard to invoking the media, see, e.g., Alex Duval Smith, "World Aids Day: South Africa Pioneer Decries Cut in Global Funding: Eric Goemaere, a Médecins Sans Frontières Doctor Who Led Early Battle Against Aids in South Africa, Says Cut in Grants From Global Fund Threatens a Decade of Progress Against HIV in Africa," *Guardian*, December 1, 2011, www.theguardian.com/pioneer-eric-goemaer. In the e-mail that he sent to me on December 2, 2011, Goemaere (who by this time had become MSF South Africa's senior regional HIV/TB advisor) commented that, "unfortunately," in his view, this article (which was based on an extensive interview with him) was "too personal." Nevertheless, he added, "it says clearly what I believe might happen here."

45. See, e.g., Michel Sidibé, Peter Piot, and Mark Dybul, "AIDS Is Not Over," *Lancet* 380, no. 9859 (December 15, 2012–January 4, 2013): 2058–2059, www.thelancet.com/ journals/lancet/article/PIIS0140–6736%2812%2962088–1/fulltext:

Optimism and momentum [have] been building around the real possibility that an AIDS-free generation is imminent. Public enthusiasm is fuelled by news about the rapid scale-up of antiretroviral therapy evidence that HIV treatment can prevent new infections, and expanded coverage of programmes to prevent mother-to-child transmission of HIV. Yet the most recent estimates of HIV prevalence and incidence of AIDS-related mortality released by UNAIDS, together with data from the Global Burden of Diseases Study 2010 in *The Lancet,* make it clear that AIDS is not over. . . .

Looking at the most common causes of death globally, HIV/AIDS ranked sixth in 2004, and held the same position in 2010. The Global Burden of Disease study 2010 estimates 1.5 million AIDS-related deaths in 2010, whereas UNAIDS data show 1.8 . . . million AIDS-related deaths. Both estimates highlight a persistent, significant, and egregious burden of avoidable death. . . .

[D]espite substantial reductions in AIDS mortality rates in many countries, AIDS remains the leading cause of death in southern and eastern Africa. . . .

Thus, while much progress has been made in treatment and prevention, the persistent and substantial global burden associated with HIV and AIDS compels us to do more—and do better—to achieve the AIDS-free generation the world is waiting for.

CHAPTER NINE: A "Non-Western Entity" Is Born

1. For a detailed account and analysis of this meeting, see chap. 12 of this book.

2. See chap. 6 of this book.

3. ICB/ExDir Working Group New Entries, "Plan for MSF 'New Entities' and Related Considerations" (internal MSF document, June 2008, final version), 6.

4. Gorik Ooms, "Re: New MSF Entities in Brazil and South Africa" (internal MSF document, January 16, 2007), 1.

5. This refers to the fact that each MSF section has an association, which is composed mainly of persons working in the field, and persons who have returned from the field, and additionally, some persons working in MSF offices. Among these, one-third of the members are expected to be medical professionals. Each MSF section subscribes to the MSF Charter and its Chantilly text on MSF's identity and guiding principles. A general assembly is held annually by each section at which members of its board and the president of its board are elected. The board is not permitted to be "homogeneously national." The board presidents sit on the International Council (which, at the end of 2011, became the International General Assembly).

6. Ooms, "Re: New MSF Entities," 2.

7. Ibid., 4–5.

8. Eric Stobbaerts, with Erwin Van't Land, Sebastian Roy, and James Kliffen, "Feasibility Study: MSF Africa" (draft internal MSF document, March 2006), 7 and 105.

9. Gorick Ooms, e-mail to the OCB Board concerning "Creation of an MSF South Africa board (and perhaps an MSF Brazil advisory board")," January 27, 2007.

10. Subsequently, in 2007, after she felt that the new South African office had been successfully launched, and was "promoted" by MSF International to the status of a "delegate office," Ekambaram made a transition from general director to head of the Programs Unit—a post for which, in her opinion, she was suited by her attributes as an activist and organizer. She was succeeded as general director by Liz Thomson.

11. Sharon Ekambaram, personal communications to the author, January 28 and February 3, 2011.

12. http://aidsconsortium.org.za/About.htm#history.

13. Sharon Ekambaram, personal communication to the author, January 31, 2011.

14. Sharon Ekambaram, personal communication to the author, February 3, 2011.

15. Sharon Ekambaram, "MSF SA—Looking at Africa from an African Angle" (internal MSF SA document).

16. Sharon Ekambaram, personal communication to the author, February 1, 2012.

17. The exclamation mark is part of the newsletter's title.

18. These countries included the Central African Republic, the Democratic Republic of Congo, the Republic of Congo (Brazzaville), Somalia, and Zimbabwe.

19. "Xenophobic Violence: One Year on the Specter Still Lurks," *MAMELA!* May 2009, 1–2. http://msf.org.za/Newsletter/MAMELA!/MAMELA_May09.html. MSF Belgium also responded to these xenophobic attacks by sending a team of logisticians and medical personnel to assist with providing medical care and counseling for the foreign nationals living in makeshift shelters.

20. The name of the village in southern Sudan is Pagil. The town in the Democratic Republic of Congo—Masisi—is located in the country's North Kivu Province.

21. Stefan Schöne, "Pal Can Go Home Today," *MAMELA!* December 1, 2010, http://doctorswithoutborders.org/news/article.cfm?id+4824&cat=voice-from-the-field.

22. Josep Prior, "Pictures From Both Sides," *MAMELA!* November 20, 2008. http://msf.org.za/Newsletter/articles/From_The_Field/Josep_Pictures-011208.html. I have retained the punctuation used by the author of this article.

23. "Work With Us," *MAMELA!*

24. This paper, dated January–February 2010, was written for the MSF international conference on governance reform held in Barcelona on March 11–13, 2010, which was attended by Eric Goemaere and Hermann Reuter as delegates from MSF South Africa. The paper was endorsed by five MSF South Africa board members: Goemaere, an ex-officio member of the board; Reuter, then president of the board, and the focal point for drug-resistant TB management in a decentralized HIV/TB program in Swaziland, who was formerly the first South African staff member of the Khayelitsha program and subsequently the program coordinator who established the HIV/ARV program in rural clinics in the Eastern Cape; Elma de Vries, a member of the Family Medicine Department at the University of Cape Town and of the Rural Doctors Association of Southern Africa, and a former president of the MSF South Africa board; Prinitha Pillay, who received her medical education and training in Johannesburg at the University of the Witwatersrand, had worked with MSF since 2006, participating in medical missions in Lesotho, India, South Sudan, and Sierra Leone, and became president of MSF SA's Board following Hermann Reuter; and Haroon Salooje, a co-opted member of the board, who was head of community pediatrics at Witwatersrand University. For more details about Goemaere and Reuters, see chaps. 7 and 8 in this book.

25. The words "Migrant," "Black," "Muslim," "Civilian," "Armed Opposition," "Male," and "Citizen" were printed in boldface.

26. Foreigners arriving in South Africa from other African countries to the north usually did not speak any of the local African languages, and their "babble" sounded like *kwirikwirikwiri* to the local township inhabitants, who applied the onomatopoeic term *kwerikwere* (plural *amakwerekwere*) to them.

27. The data in this paragraph come from a "short profile" that MSF South Africa prepared as a candidate to become a new association, which it presented to MSF's International General Assembly in Paris on December 16, 2011. See chap. 12 in this book for a detailed account of this meeting.

28. Sharon Ekambaram, personal communication to the author, February 21, 2012. and April 14, 2012.

29. Sharon Ekambaram, personal communication to the author, February 21, 2012.

CHAPTER TEN: Reaching Out to the Homeless
and Street Children of Moscow

1. The course was based on Inkeles's scholarly work. See Alex Inkeles, *Public Opinion in Soviet Russia: A Study in Mass Persuasion* (Cambridge, MA: Harvard University Press, 1950); Inkeles and Raymond A. Bauer, *The Soviet Citizen: Daily Life in a Totalitarian Society* (Cambridge, MA: Harvard University Press, 1951); Alex Inkeles, *Social Change in Soviet Russia* (New York: Simon & Schuster, 1968).

2. The USSR (Union of Socialist Soviet Republics) was dissolved in 1991.

3. Olga Shevchenko's dissertation "Living on a Volcano: The Lived Experience of Social Change in Russia" was presented to the faculties of the University of Pennsylvania in partial fulfillment of the requirements for the degree of doctor of philosophy in 2002.

4. Olga Shevchenko, *Crisis and the Everyday in Postsocialist Moscow* (Indianapolis: University of Indiana Press, 2009), 8.

5. In June 2001, we also made a short trip to Saint Petersburg, where we met with several persons whom MSF staff members had recommended we see because of the significant roles they had played in MSF's homeless programs. We also spent some time there with personnel associated with the Paris and New York offices of Médecins du Monde / Doctors of the World, the organization that arose from the split in Médecins Sans Frontières in 1979–1980 between members of its founding generation. Between 1997 and 1999, MSF had run a medical and social assistance center for the homeless in Saint Petersburg, which closed after the city adopted an "Aid to Homeless Persons and Ex-Prisoners" program and opened a free medical center for them in the Botkin Hospital.

6. The First Chechen Campaign took place from 1994 to 1996, when Russian troops attempted to stop Chechnya from seceding from the Russian Federation. The Second Chechen Campaign was initiated in 1999 by an incursion of Russian troops into the area. In addition to continuing the fight to bring the breakaway Chechen Republic back under Russian rule, its stated objectives were to quell what were alleged to be bandits, criminals, separatist rebels, and terrorists in the region.

7. According to "The Trauma of Ongoing War in Chechnya," a report issued by MSF Holland in August 2004, more than fifty international humanitarian workers had been abducted in that region since 1995, and some of them [had] been murdered, including six members of the International Red Cross. During the period of our research in Russia, the two most publicized kidnappings of MSF personnel were those of Kenneth Gluck and Arjan Erkel. Gluck, a U.S. citizen associated with MSF Holland, was working as head of mission for the North Caucasus Project. He was abducted on January 9, 2001, while traveling in a humanitarian convoy near the village of Starye Atagi in Chechnya, and released on February 3, 2001. Erkel, a citizen of the Netherlands, was head of mission for MSF Switzerland's program in Dagestan when he was abducted in Makhachkala on August 12, 2002, by gunmen, who kept him in captivity until April 11, 2004.

8. In the course of our research, we also made a small "sub-study" of the relations between so-called national staff members of MSF (those who are indigenous to the

countries where MSF projects are located) and expatriate staff (those who are involved in projects outside their countries of residence). Our focus was on MSF's internal struggles to reconcile the distinctions that it made between these two categories of personnel, and its commitment to principles of universalism, egalitarianism, and equity. Our initial observations for this sub-study were made in the Moscow office of MSF Belgium. See Olga Shevchenko and Renée C. Fox, " 'Nationals' and 'Expatriates': Challenges of Fulfilling 'Sans Frontières' ('Without Borders') Ideals in International Humanitarian Action," *Health and Human Rights* 10, no. 1 (2008): 109–122.

9. Armenia declared its independence from the USSR on August 23, 1990.

10. Throughout the eighteenth and nineteenth centuries, and during the first years of the twentieth, an extensive network of charitable establishments and institutions existed in Russia, including places to live for the needy and hospitals for people without means. One of the most important of these was the Empress Maria Fyodorovna Department of Institutions, founded by and named for the wife of Emperor Paul I. In May 2000, a collection campaign was initiated in Saint Petersburg to erect a monument to the empress as part of what was called a "Russian charitable revival." The brochure issued in this connection mentions that plans to erect such a monument had already existed in 1911, but had been subverted by "historical events," and by the fact that "the word 'charity' was no longer in use."

11. Alexei Nikiforov, "Homelessness—Yesterday, Today and Tomorrow?" (unpublished MSF document).

12. "Special Report: Ten Years of Work With Moscow's Homeless," May 23, 2002, www.doctorswithoutborders.org/publications/article.cfm?id=1441.

13. Hedwige told us that throughout the stressful time that she and her colleagues had undergone, their solidarity remained strong. They talked to each other every day about what they were experiencing and feeling, and gave each other support. Upon their arrival in Moscow, MSF Belgium sent two persons from its Human Relations Department in Brussels to debrief them and provide them with psychological counseling. When they recounted what they had experienced in the field, Hedwige said, laughing, the human relations personnel were so stricken that "we had to console them," rather than the reverse.

14. Although we did not learn this from Alexei, Dr. Chazov was also celebrated because of the number of Russian and world leaders whose personal physician he had been, and because, in collaboration with the American cardiologist Dr. Bernard Lown, he cofounded International Physicians for the Prevention of Nuclear War. In 1985, IPPNW was awarded the Nobel Peace Prize, which Chazov and Lown received on behalf of the movement. Chazov "holds a Guinness Book world record for treating 19 leaders from 16 different countries," according to http://russiapedia.rt.com/prominent-russians/science-and-technology/evgeny-chazov.

15. *Bomji* is pronounced *bomzhi* in Russian.

16. The Center for Epidemiology and Sanitation was the first service in Moscow to recognize the needs of the homeless and to respond to them. In 1984, it gave homeless persons free access to three disinfection and sanitary stations, where those suffering from lice or scabies could receive treatment for these conditions and shower while their clothes were disinfected.

17. "Special Report: Ten Years of Work With Moscow's Homeless."

18. According to the social worker who we observed as she carried out consultations with a series of homeless persons in the MSF dispensary on June 1, 2000, and who we interviewed subsequently, the profession of social work had only existed for about five years in Russia at that time—since departments to train social workers had been created in state universities. She herself had previously been trained in electrical engineering and had worked in construction until she lost her job. She had gone to the employment agency to seek guidance regarding what to do next, and was offered training in social work as one alternative possibility. The state paid for her retraining. She became aware of the existence of MSF while she was studying to become a social worker through an article about it that she read in a magazine, went in search of them, and did an internship with them that included outstanding courses with psychologists. During her four years with MSF, she enthusiastically told us, she had experienced great satisfaction in her work because it enabled her to help people, and to inform them about their rights and how to claim them.

19. MSF received help from the Catholic relief agency Caritas, from religious Sisters belonging to Mother Teresa's Missionaries of Charity, from the Salvation Army, and from a few of the more progressive local Russian Orthodox churches in providing clothing and food for its homeless clients.

20. Jeanmart estimated that over the years, MSF sent more than one thousand letters to Moscow officials proposing that they open a municipal center for medical and social assistance to the homeless ("Special Report: Ten Years of Work with Moscow's Homeless").

21. Jeanmart had left MSF Belgium's Moscow office soon after this project was approved, primarily because she was expecting to give birth imminently to a second child; so at the time that Olga interviewed Alexei, he was working on it with another member of the MSF staff, project coordinator Gabriella Muretto, who had recently arrived in Moscow.

22. Interview with Jeanmart in "Special Report: Ten Years of Work With Moscow's Homeless."

23. Ibid.

24. Samusocial Moscow, which has French origins, is a "Russian non-commercial organization," associated with Samusocial International. Its Governing Board and Board of Trustees are "made up of both Russians and long-term expatriates, who are familiar both with the French approach and the local situation," and its members are "experts on issues concerning children, notably in the medical, psychological, legal, and financial sectors" (www.samu.ru/en/aboutus).

25. Mamar Merzouk, "End of Mission Report" (n.d.).

26. For example, MSF has been working in Sudan since 1979, in the Democratic Republic of Congo since 1981, in Russia since 1988, in Somalia since 1991, and in South Africa since 1999.

CHAPTER ELEVEN: Confronting TB in Siberian Prisons

1. MDR-TB is resistant at least to isoniazid and rifampin, the two most powerful, first-line anti-TB drugs. XDR-TB is also resistant to at least isoniazid and rifampin among the first-line anti-TB drugs, in addition to any drug in the fluoroquinolone group of

broad spectrum antibiotics, and to at least one of the three second-line, injectable anti-TB drugs.

2. Nicolas Cantau, "Aide Humanitaire en Russie: Médecins Sans Frontières Belgique" (internal MSF report), 35. Cantau headed the MSF Belgium mission in Russia from November 15, 1995, to January 8, 1998. He is now the Global Fund to Fight AIDS, Tuberculosis and Malaria's regional portfolio manager for Eastern Europe and Central Asia.

3. Margarita V. Shilova and Christopher Dye, "The Resurgence of Tuberculosis in Russia," *Philosophical Transactions of the Royal Society of London*, ser. B, 356 (2001): 1069–1075, at 1069 and 1074.

4. M. E. Kimerling, "The Russian Equation: An Evolving Paradigm in Tuberculosis Control," *International Journal of Tuberculosis and Lung Disease* 4, no. 12 (2000): S160–S167, at S160.

5. Paul Farmer, "Managerial Successes, Clinical Failures" (editorial), *International Journal of Tuberculosis and Lung Disease* 3, no. 5 (1999): 365–367, at 365.

6. Kimerling, "Russian Equation," S162.

7. Olga Shevchenko and Renée C. Fox, "'Nationals' and 'Expatriates': Challenges of Fulfilling 'Sans Frontières' ('Without Borders') Ideals in International Humanitarian Action," *Health and Human Rights* 10, no. 1 (2008): 109–122, at 118. "A TB patient cries twice—once when he is diagnosed, and once when he is cured," it was said of these patient entitlements in the Soviet era.

8. Yuri Ivanovich Kalinin, "The Russian Penal System: Past, Present and Future" (lecture at King's College, University of London, November 2002), 11, www.prisonstudies.org/info/downloads/website%20kalinin.pdf.

9. Deputy Justice Minister Yuri Ivanovich Kalinin, 1998 interview, shortened version (© Moscow Center for Prison Reform), www.prison.org/english/expkalin.htm.

10. Three of these institutions were pre-detention centers where persons were incarcerated while awaiting a trial and sentencing. The other twenty-three were so-called "general colonies."

11. Cantau, "Aide Humanitaire en Russie," 35–36.

12. In Russian medicine and medical schools, phthisiatry refers solely to tuberculosis and its concomitants. It is a specialty by itself, rather than being regarded as a branch of pulmonology.

13. Olga Shevchenko, interview with Dr. Natalia Nikolayevna Vezhnina, Moscow, June 7–8, 2003.

14. Dominique Lafontaine and Andrei Slavuckij, "MSF–Belgium TB Project in Siberian Region of Kemerovo, Russian Federation, 1996–2003: Conclusive Operational Report" (MSF internal report, May 2004), 5. Dr. Dominique Lafontaine served as the field coordinator of the MSF TB project in Siberia, and Dr. Andrei Slavuckij was its chief medical coordinator, beginning in 2000.

15. "Thieves in law" were the elite of the criminal world in Soviet times and were seen as the only legitimate enforcers of Russian criminals' code of honor both within and outside of prisons. See Federico Varese, *The Russian Mafia: Private Protection in a New Market Economy* (New York: Oxford University Press, 2001).

16. Olga Shevchenko, interview with Dr. Natalia Nikolayevna Vezhnina, Moscow, June 7–8, 2003.

17. What was envisaged in this regard included expanding the grounds for applying penalties and measures of restraint other than imprisonment or custody, and reducing the highest sentences for certain criminal offenses—particularly for petty ones.

18. Kalinin, 1998 interview (cited n. 9 above).

19. This was facilitated by the fact that the majority of the detainees came from the Kemerovo region of Siberia, where these pre-detention centers were located.

20. For a more detailed account of these attributes of the Russian penal system, and their implications for the incidence, treatment and spread of TB among its inmates, see Andrei Slavuckij, Vinciane Sizaire, Laura Lobera, Francine Matthys, and Michael E. Kimerling, "Decentralization of the DOTS Programme Within a Russian Penitentiary System: How to Ensure the Continuity of Tuberculosis Treatment in Pre-Trial Detention Centers," *European Journal of Public Health* 12, no. 2 (2002): 94–98.

21. These first-line anti-tuberculosis drugs were ethambutol, isoniazid, pyrazinamide, rifampicin, and streptomycin. In the standard short course, the drugs are given in a certain order of introduction, sequence of phases (a high-intensity phase followed by a continuation phase), for a differing number of months and of intermittent dosing. For example, isoniazid, rifampicin, ethambutol, and pyrazinamide are given daily for two months, followed by four months of isoniazid and rifampicin given three times a week.

22. Farmer, "Managerial Successes, Clinical Failures," 365.

23. Professor Mikhail Perelman, Chief Phthisiatrist of Russia and Academician of the Russian Academy of Medical Science, was one of the strongest, most prestigious, and influential proponents of the utilization of fluoroscopy for these purposes and for mass tuberculosis screening.

24. Kimerling, "Russian Equation," S162.

25. Farmer, "Managerial Successes, Clinical Failures," 367.

26. Although the "thief in law," also a TB patient, allowed his fellow inmates to take the DOTS drugs, he never agreed to do so himself. He died a few years later.

27. Lafontaine and Slavuckij, "MSF–Belgium TB Project," 12n16: "Protein biscuits were abandoned later due to logistical problems and difficulties [in assessing] the real intake." However, "nutritional input was made to the end of the program with regular survey of the nutritional status of the patients."

28. Kimerling, "Russian Equation," S613. Kimerling acknowledges that he received these data from the Colony 33 Statistics Unit via a personal communication from Slavuckij.

29. Shevchenko, interview with Vezhnina, July 7–8, 2003. The MSF physician who married the daughter of the Russian colony physician was Hans Kluge.

30. Kimerling, "Russian Equation," S163.

31. In July 2008, the name of the department was changed to the Department of Global Health and Social Medicine.

32. Paul Farmer, "Cruel and Unusual: Drug Resistant Tuberculosis as Punishment," in Haun Saussy, ed., *Partner to the Poor: A Paul Farmer Reader* (Berkeley: University of California Press, 2010), 206–219, at 218. This article was originally published in Vivien Stern, ed., *Sentenced to Die: The Problem of TB in Prisons in Eastern Europe and Central Asia* (London: International Centre for Prison Studies, King's College, 1999), 70–66.

33. Carole Mitnick, Jaime Bayona, Eda Palacios, et al., "Community-Based Therapy for Multidrug Resistant Tuberculosis in Lima, Peru," *New England Journal of Medicine* 348, no. 2 (January 20, 2004): 119–128.

34. The quoted passages about this meeting were all excerpted from Paul Farmer and Jim Yong Kim, "Community Based Approaches to the Control of Multidrug Resistant Tuberculosis: Introducing "Dots-Plus," *British Medical Journal* 317, no. 7159 (September 5, 1998): 671–674.

35. Scientific Panel of the Working Group on DOTS-Plus for MDR-TB, "Guidelines for Establishing DOTS-Plus Pilot Projects for the Management of Multidrug-Resistant Tuberculosis [MDR-TB]," ed. Rajesh Gupta and Thuridur Arnadottir (Geneva: World Health Organization, 2000).

36. *The Global Impact of Drug-Resistant Tuberculosis* (Boston: Program in Infectious Disease and Social Change, Dept. of Social Medicine, Harvard Medical School, 1999). The Stop TB Partnership Task Force on TB was established in 2010. The involvement of UNAIDS in this task force emanated from the relationship between HIV/AIDS and tuberculosis, and the mounting rate of HIV/TB co-infection that exists. TB is the commonest opportunistic infection and the primary cause of death among people with HIV/AIDS. In addition, people with latent TB are increasingly becoming infected with HIV, and many develop active TB because of the weakening of their immune systems by HIV.

37. PHRI, an independent, not-for-profit research organization, originally located in New York City, was founded in 1941 by Mayor Fiorello LaGuardia, primarily to study infectious diseases, and also applied immunology, nutrition, and physiology.

38. Kimerling had previously worked as a volunteer in several MSF field programs. He had been a member of MSF Holland and MSF Belgium missions in Cambodia in 1991–1993, and from June to December 1995, he had served as medical consultant for their malaria and tuberculosis control activities there.

39. Quoted in Lafontaine and Slavuckij, "MSF–Belgium TB Project," 19.

40. Kimerling, "Russian Equation," S163.

41. Ibid., S166.

42. Ibid., S167.

43. Michael Kimerling, Hans Kluge, Natalia Vezhnina, et al., "Inadequacy of the Current WHO Re-Treatment Regimen in a Central Siberian Prison: Treatment Failure and MDR-TB," *International Journal of Tuberculosis and Lung Disease* 3, no. 5 (May 1999): 451–453.

44. Farmer, "Managerial Successes, Clinical Failures," 365–367.

45. These quotations are excerpted from a series of e-mails between Olga Shevchenko, Renée Fox, and Paul Farmer on June 6, 2008.

46. Paul E. Farmer, "Rethinking Health and Human Rights: Time for a Paradigm Shift," in Saussy, ed., *Partner to the Poor*, 435–470, at 455.

47. Haun Saussy, "Introduction: The Right to Claim Rights," in Saussy, ed., *Partner to the Poor*, 1–24, at 15.

48. See, e.g., Saussy, ed., *Partner to the Poor*, 287–426.

49. Paul Farmer, "Social Medicine and the Challenge of Bio-Social Research," http://xserve02.mpiwg-berlin.mpg.de/ringberg/Talks/farmer/Farmer.html.

50. Lafontaine and Slavuckij, "MSF–Belgium TB Project," 14 and 22.

51. Interview by Olga Shevchenko with Vinciane Sizaire, Moscow, June 21, 2003.

52. Nagorno-Karabakh, a republic in the South Caucasus, borders Armenia to its west and Iran to its south. It is closely tied to the Republic of Armenia, uses the same currency, and has a predominantly Armenian Christian population. See www.nkrusa.org/country_profile/overview.shtml.

53. Renée Fox, telephone interview with Michael Kimerling, October 30, 2012. Kimerling's assessment of the causes underlying MSF France's objections to his involvement was not shared by Francis Varain, who was present at this meeting. "Working with Michael Kimerling was never seen as equivalent to accepting money from Gorgas or USAID," Varain claims. "Other priorities of MSF France at this time, in terms of TB, were involved" (personal communication to Fox, March 24, 2013).

54. At present (October 2012), Michael Kimerling is senior program officer in the Tuberculosis Program of the Bill and Melinda Gates Foundation in Seattle, Washington, and affiliate professor in the Department of Global Health in the Division of Infectious Diseases of the Department of Medicine in the School of Medicine of the University of Washington.

55. However, MSF continued to supply drugs and other necessary materials in order to avoid doing harm to the patients.

56. From an interview with Andrei Slavuckij, conducted by Renée Fox and Olga Shevchenko, June 19, 2001. The cry "Go to the Square" alluded to the Decembrist uprising in Imperial Russia on December 26, 1825, when Russian army officers led thousands of soldiers in a protest against Nicholas I's assumption of the throne.

57. Andrei Slavuckij first made contact with MSF in 1991 when he was working as an anesthesiologist with a Soviet organization that was rendering medical assistance in the interior of Angola where members of MSF were also present. Impressed by MSF's action and their "strong image," he joined their ranks as a member of MSF Belgium. During 1991–1994, he participated in a number of MSF missions in Bosnia, Rwanda, and Chechnya.

58. Fox and Shevchenko, interview with Slavuckij, June 19, 2001.

59. The second-line anti-TB drugs in question included olflaxacin, cycloserina, and capreomycin, which were available for Green Light Committee–approved programs at negotiated prices, as well as unregistered drugs such as amikacin and clofazimine.

60. "MSF Ends Tuberculosis Treatment in Kemerovo Region, Russia" (MSF press release, September 9, 2003).

61. "MSF could not find common language with penitentiary system of RF," the Russian nongovernmental REGNUM News Agency reported on October 21, 2003. MSF esteemed Kalinin and his reforms of the penal system. They interpreted his statement as a benevolent attempt to help foster a reconciliation between the hostile Ministry of Health and MSF.

62. Our account of some of the exchanges that took place at these meetings are drawn from the text of Slavuckij's and Sheyanenko's report.

63. The press conference to which Antonova was referring took place in Moscow on September 30, 2003, at the Press Development Institute. The chief presenters at the conference were Andrei Slavuckij, Nicolas Cantau, MSF's head of mission in Russia, and Mark Walsh, head of MSF's Press Office for its Cellular Information System. It was attended by numerous foreign as well as Russian correspondents (inter alia from the

BBC, Reuters, the Netherlands Press Association, Agence France-Presse, and *Le Monde*), representatives of several NGOs, and a delegate from the WHO Office of the Special Representative of the Director-General in the Russian Federation. See "Moscow Press Conference on Closure of the MSF Siberian TB Project" (internal MSF document).

64. According to the program, GUIN's chief TB specialist, Dr. Svetlana Sidorova, was to have made this presentation, but Smirnov, a new member of GUIN, spoke in her stead.

65. For Slavuckij, the meaning of this metaphor was both "precise" and grave, because he interpreted the black pencil as representing XDR-TB.

66. We (Renée Fox and Olga Shevchenko) maintained contact with Dr. Vezhnina after her dismissal from her position as assistant head of the Medical Division of GUIN in the Kemerovo region. In the fall of 2003, we invited her to act as a chronicler of the events that transpired in connection with, and in the aftermath of, the termination of MSF Belgium's TB program in Kemerovo, including follow-up news regarding the members of its staff and the Russian officials who were key figures in its history and its demise. She agreed to take on this role, principally because she thought that the story underlying what MSF Belgium had accomplished, the obstacles it had encountered, and the factors that had led to its closure ought to be documented, written up, analyzed as a case history, and eventually circulated. From mid-October 2003 through 2004, she sent us periodic communications, chiefly via e-mail, concerning what she knew about pertinent events taking place in and around Colony 33, and about the professional activities of its previous and present medical staff and relevant officials. She also provided us with a number of relevant documents.

67. AIDS Foundation East-West (AFEW), Annual Report, 2001–2002, 29.

68. Ibid., iv.

69. Ibid., v.

70. Ibid., 1.

71. Almaty, the former capital of Kazakhstan, is its largest city, and its major commercial and cultural center. Cantau and Slavuckij helped arrange for Vezhnina to be offered this position.

72. Subsequently, Dr. Vezhnina's "dream" was partially fulfilled. She was appointed to the position of advisor on HIV/TB and Penal System Projects with AFEW. In this capacity, she conducted training sessions on the mutually compounding effects of the HIV/AIDS and TB epidemics in the penal institutions of the Central Asian Republics. She has also piloted a number of projects relevant to co-infection with HIV/AIDS and TB that have been institutionalized and replicated throughout the system.

73. The plan had been for this training program to be funded by USAID through the Gorgas TB Initiative at the University of Alabama, and for its administrative and financial management to be provided by the Kemerovo Region Committee of the Russian Red Cross Society. Gorgas TB Initative, http://138.26.145.28/gorgas/Novokuznetsk.htm.

74. This information about what Dr. Vezhnina referred to as "the order of things in Colony 33" since the "dissolution" of MSF Belgium's TB project came to us via a long, undated communication that she sent to us in October 2004.

75. Hans Kluge, the Belgian physician who married the daughter of one of the Russian doctors in Colony 33, renewed his contract with the project three successive times.

76. Kazakhstan, Kyrgyzstan, Tajikistan, Turkmenistan, and Uzbekistan.

77. In 2002, PHRI moved to Newark, New Jersey, when it became associated with the University of Medicine and Dentistry of New Jersey.

78. Andrei Slavuckij shared these sentiments with us (Olga Shevchenko and Renée Fox) in 2013 as part of his highly detailed review of a draft of this chapter that we sent to him for his comments, criticisms, and corrections. In turn, he passed the manuscript on to three colleagues closely connected with MSF's TB-related activities (Nicolas Cantau, Myriam Henkens, and Francis Varain), and asked for their input to it. The four of them compiled their feedback to us in the form of extensive, computerized marginal notes throughout the pages of the manuscript. Natalia Vezhnina also read this chapter in manuscript in an earlier version than the one seen by Slavuckij et al. We are grateful to all of them for their invaluable contributions.

CODA: Remembering the Past and Envisioning the Future

1. Saint-Denis was also the site of a vigorous socialist movement; and until the mid-1930s, virtually all of its mayors were members of the French Communist Party. It is still called *la ville rouge* (the red city) or the *banlieue rouge* (red suburb). It has a high crime rate. And according to the *Wikipedia*, in 1999, 35.6 percent of its residents were "born outside of metropolitan France." (This is the definition of an "immigrant" in France. Persons who have become French citizens since moving to France are still defined as immigrants in French statistics.) See "Saint-Denis," http://en.wikipedia.org/wiki/Saint-Denis.

2. See "Basilica of St. Denis," http://en.wikipedia.org/wiki/Basilica_of_St_Denis.

3. See "Menier Chocolate," http://en.wikipedia.org/wiki/Menier_Chocolate.

4. In alphabetical order, these representatives were affiliated with MSF Australia, Austria, Belgium, Canada, Denmark, France, Germany, Greece, Holland, Hong Kong, Italy, Japan, Luxembourg, Norway, Spain, Sweden, Switzerland, the United Kingdom, and the United States.

5. Unni Karunakara, personal communication to Renée Fox, June 6, 2011. I had previously made it known to Karunakara and to several other MSF members that I would welcome an opportunity to attend the meeting. In addition, by prearrangement, they cordially agreed to my request that my colleague Judith P. Swazey accompany me to the meeting. Notwithstanding Karunakara's invitation to me to participate in the discussion that took place at the meeting, I confined my role to that of an observer and to informal interaction with many MSF members who I already knew and some who I met for the first time on this occasion. In his opening remarks on December 16, 2011, Karunakara introduced me as a professor of sociology at the University of Pennsylvania, "a longtime friend of MSF," and "a sort of historian."

6. Rip Hopkins, Jean Lacouture, and Rony Brauman *Sept fois à terre, huit fois debout* [Seven Times on the Ground, Eight Times Standing] (Paris: Chêne, 2011).

7. Ibid., "Mérite, engagement et T-shirts [Merit, Commitment and T-Shirts]," 7.

8. The last photograph in the book is of Hopkins himself in an MSF T-shirt, holding two nude, squirming, crying, auburn-haired babies in his arms, who look like twins and as if they are his children. The photo is subtitled "je le fais pour moi" (I do it for myself), "Rip Hopkins, photographe iconoclaste" (iconoclastic photographer).

9. Hopkins, "Mérite, engagement et T-shirts," 7.

10. Serra and Thiebaut were ultimately freed in Somalia in July 2013 after 644 days

in captivity, the longest kidnapping in MSF history. "During every one of those days," Sophie Delauney, the Executive Director of MSF USA, has written, "an MSF team working on nothing else labored to secure their release as the entire organization held them close in their hearts. And now we are thrilled that we can collectively welcome them home and support them however we can in the days to come. . . . [K]nowing that Mone and Blanca are safe at home allows us to go forward with fuller hearts." "Humanitarian Space," Alert 14, no. 3 (Summer 2013), p. 2.

11. Karunakara did not mention that rather than accepting contributions specifically earmarked for Japan, MSF drew on its unrestricted donations funds. In response to a contribution that I had sent in the aftermath of the earthquake and tsunami, I received a message thanking me, informing me of MSF's policy of not accepting donations specifically designated for this purpose, and offering to return mine unless I earmarked it for the general fund.

12. With the adoption of the new statutes in June 2011 that reformed MSF's international governance structure, the International Council had been replaced by the International General Assembly.

13. Marie-Pierre Allié, introduction titled "Agir à tout prix?" / "Acting at Any Price?" in Claire Magone, Michaël Neuman, and Fabrice Weissman, eds., *Agir à tout prix? Négotiations humanitaires: L'expérience de Médecins Sans Frontières* (Paris: La Découverte, 2011) / *Humanitarian Negotiations Revealed: The MSF Experience* (New York: Columbia University Press, 2011), 1. Many of the contributors to this volume are affiliated with MSF's research center in Paris, the Centre de Réflexions sur l'Action et les Savoirs Humanitaires (CRASH). The English-language edition contains an Afterword by David Rieff that is not included in the French-language edition.

14. Cited in the preceding note.

15. The presentation that preceded this long-awaited session was a keynote address—"What Access to Health Care for the 7 Billion?"—delivered by Hans Rosling, a Swedish physician, trained in public health and statistics, as well as medicine, who is a professor of international health at the Karolinska Institutet, a Stockholm medical school. He spent many years studying outbreaks of konzo, an epidemic paralytic disease, among rural populations in Africa, which opened onto his research on the relationship between economic development, agriculture, poverty, and health in Latin America and Asia, as well as in Africa. He is the developer of so-called Trendanalyzer software that converts statistical data into animated, moving graphs. He was also one of the initiators of MSF in Sweden.

Using Trendanalyzer software to visualize global demographic developments, Rosling delivered a riveting and highly entertaining lecture on the fact that the world's population may reach more than seven billion persons by mid-century, the probable consequences for health, the provision of health care, and access to it in high-, middle-, and low-income countries, and the implications for MSF's actions and aspirations.

16. Jean-Hervé Bradol and Marc Le Pape, "Innovation?" in Bradol and Claudine Vidal, eds., *Medical Innovations in Humanitarian Situations: The Work of Médecins Sans Frontières* (New York: MSF USA, 2011), 3–21, at 5.

17. For a fuller account of this episode in the founding of MSF, see Chapter 2, "Origins, Schisms, Crises."

18. East Pakistan became the nation of Bangladesh at the end of 1971.

19. Evidence that this intrepid spirit still exists in these physician-founders of MSF can be found in the book *Sept fois à terre, huit fois debout* (cited n. 8 above). Wearing an MSF T-shirt, the white-haired Pascal Grellety-Bosviel posed for one of the photos in this book, sitting shoeless on a carpeted floor, holding a large volume with BIAFRA printed in capital letters on its spine. The caption that he chose for his photo was "Même si ça me fait chier, **j'y vais**" ("Even if that makes me crap, **I go there**").

20. See chap. 6 in this book.

21. See chap. 3 in this book.

22. New sections of MSF were created in the United States and Greece in 1990; in Canada and Italy in 1991; in Japan in 1992; in Sweden, Denmark, Germany, and the United Kingdom in 1993; in Australia, Austria, and Hong Kong in 1994; and in Norway in 1995.

23. Out of the approximately 27,000 MSF workers in the field, some 22,000 are national staff.

24. For a more extensive discussion of "expatriates/nationals" issues, see chap. 6.

25. The already-appointed members of the International Board—the presidents of MSF's five operational centers, its international president, and its international treasurer—included five physicians.

26. In addition to the position that Morten Rostrup had held as founding president of the MSF Norway section, Jean-Marie Kindermans had served as president of MSF Belgium (2002–2010), and Darin Portnoy as president of MSF USA (2004–2009). As indicated previously, Rostrup had also been vice president and president of the International Council. Kindermans held the post of secretary-general of the International Office from 1996 to 2001. And after serving as flying coordinator (2006–2007), Fotiadis became the International Association coordinator (2007–2011). Among the elected International Board members, Fotiadis and Rostrup had been the most actively involved in MSF's inner reform. Fotiadis is the husband of Reveka Papadopoulou, general director of MSF Greece.

27. "MSF Shocked and Deeply Saddened by the Killing of Two Staff Members in Mogadishu, Somalia," www.msf.org/article/msf-deeply-shocked-and-saddened-killing-two-staff-members-serious-incident-mogadishu-somalia.

28. www.msf.org/article/msf-closes-its-largest-medical-centres-mogadishu-after-kill ings.

29. See Max Weber, *The Theory of Social and Economic Organization*, trans. A. M. Henderson and Talcott Parsons (New York: Oxford University Press, 1947), 358–373.

Index